Bacterial Protein Toxins

Zentralblatt für Bakteriologie Mikrobiologie und Hygiene I. Abteilung

Supplemente

Supplement 17
Fehrenbach et al. (Eds.), Bacterial Protein Toxins

Gustav Fischer · Stuttgart · New York · 1988

Bacterial Protein Toxins

Third European Workshop
Überlingen, June 28 – July 3, 1987

Editors F. J. Fehrenbach
Robert Koch-Institut, Berlin

J. E. Alouf
Institut Pasteur, Paris, France

P. Falmagne
Université de l'Etat à Mons, Mons, Belgium

W. Goebel
Lehrstuhl für Mikrobiologie, Würzburg

J. Jeljaszewicz
National Institute of Hygiene, Warsaw, Poland

D. Jürgens
Robert Koch-Institut, Berlin

R. Rappuoli
Sclavo Research Center, Siena, Italy

131 Figures and 48 Tables

Gustav Fischer · Stuttgart · New York · 1988

CIP-Titelaufnahme der Deutschen Bibliothek

Bacterial protein toxins : ... europ. workshop / ... Europ.
Workshop on Bacterial Protein Toxins. - Stuttgart ; New York :
Fischer.
NE: European Workshop on Bacterial Protein Toxins

3. Überlingen, June 28 - July 3, 1987. - 1988
   (Zentralblatt für Bakteriologie, Mikrobiologie und Hygiene : Abt. 1 :
   Supplemente ; 17)
   ISBN 3-437-11173-6 (Stuttgart) kart.
   ISBN 0-89574-233-0 (New York) kart.
NE: Zentralblatt für Bakteriologie, Mikrobiologie und Hygiene / 01 /
   Supplemente

All business correspondence should be made with:
Gustav Fischer Verlag GmbH & Co. KG, Wollgrasweg 49, D-7000 Stuttgart 70

For USA and Canada:
VCH Publishers Inc., 303 N.W. 12th Avenue, Deerfield Beach,
Florida 33442-1705, U.S.A.

Printed and bound by F. Pustet, Regensburg
Printed in Germany
ISBN 3-437-11173-6
ISBN 0-89574-260-8
ISSN 0172-5629

Preface

This book contains the contributions presented at the 3rd European Workshop on Bacterial Protein Toxins, in Überlingen/F.R.G., June 29th - July 3rd 1987. The conference was organized and held in the tradition of the two preceeding conferences in Seillac, (France, 1983) and Wepion, (Belgium, 1985). The success of the three conferences completely justified the continuity of the European Workshops on Bacterial Protein Toxins as a series of conferences to be held every two years.

Research in the field of Bacterial Toxinology has necessarily become interdisciplinary and therefore attracts scientists from diverse fields of research. The continuing success of these conferences reflects the consistently high standard of the scientific contributions, their timeliness, relevance and breadth of appeal.

The conferences are always held in late June to early July in a pleasant area of the host european country. The selected locations are always remote from large and busy cities, and provide facilities conducive to a relaxed atmosphere, where accompanying families can also enjoy a holiday. The number of participants is limited to about 120 active scientists and ample time is provided between the lectures to allow the continuation of extended discussions.

It is also an important aim of these conferences to attract young scientists and to encourage their participation by providing them with some financial support. Already this policy has promoted considerable scientific cooperation between numerous laboratories and in particularly has promoted the exchange of visiting junior and senior scientists.

The proceedings of each workshop are published to ensure rapid distribution of the information provided at the conferences. The communications of the 3rd European Workshop on Bacterial Protein Toxins again covers major aspects of Bacterial Toxinology:

Molecular architecture of toxins in relation to function

Toxin/cell surface interactions

Genetic aspects of toxinogenesis

Toxin/secretion and internalization

Toxin-lipid interaction

Toxins as virulence factors

Applied toxinology

It is clear from these conferences that the pace of research in the various aspects of toxinology continues to increase. At the same time, new areas of investigation are unfolding and will become subjects for duscussion at forthcoming European Workshops on Bacterial Protein Toxins.

The organizers would like to express their sincere appreciation and profound thanks to all sponsors who provided financial support. It was largely through the contributions of the DEUTSCHE FORSCHUNGSGEMEINSCHAFT that a sound financial basis for the 3rd European Workshop on Bacterial Protein Toxins was established and the success of the conference assured.

F.J. Fehrenbach, Chairman (Berlin)

J.E. Alouf (Paris)   J. Jeljaszewicz (Warsaw)

P. Falmagne (Mons)   D. Jürgens (Berlin)

W. Goebel (Würzburg)   R. Rappuoli (Siena)

Contents

Toxin cell surface interaction

Toxin secretion and internalization

Genetic aspects of toxinogenesis

Toxin - lipid interaction

Toxins as virulence factors

Applied toxinology

Molecular Architecture of Toxins in Relation to Function

Fehrenbach et al. (Eds.), Bacterial Protein Toxins, Zbl. Bakt. Suppl. 17
© Gustav Fischer, Stuttgart, New York, 1988

Studies on the Synthesis, Assembly and Structure of the Heat-Labile Enterotoxin (LT) of Escherichia coli

B. Witholt, H. Hofstra, J. Kingma, S.E. Pronk, W.G.J. Hol, and J. Drenth

Biomolecular Study Centre (BIOS), University of Groningen, Nijenborgh 16,
9747 AG Groningen, The Netherlands

ABSTRACT

Enteropathogenic strains of Escherichia coli produce a heat-labile enterotoxin (LT), the subunits of which are synthesized on membrane-bound polysomes, exported through the cytoplasmic membrane and processed before being released into the periplasm.

LT-B is released rapidly (within 13-14 sec) following initiation of synthesis, and is immediately integrated into high-molecular weight aggregates. LT-A is released only after one to several minutes and binds to LT-B aggregates rather slowly to form holotoxin. While LT-B and LT-A are synthesized in equimolar amounts and LT-B is assembled into holotoxin quantitatively, part of the LT-A is degraded in the cytoplasm (before export) and in the periplasm (after release from the cytoplasmic membrane).

Isolated holotoxin crystallizes in different crystal forms, depending on the crystallization conditions. Form II contains only B_5, and shows five-fold symmetry. Form III contains holotoxin, also shows five-fold symmetry, and yields high resolution data in the rotating anode generator (2.3 A) and the synchrotron (<2.0 A). At least five heavy-atom derivatives show promising results and a $KAuCl_4$ derivative has been analyzed in the Hamburg synchrotron beam.

INTRODUCTION

The heat-labile enterotoxin (LT) produced by enterotoxigenic Escherichia coli strains is a multimeric protein which is closely related to cholera toxin (CT). LT binds to the membrane of target epithelial cells via its binding component LT-B_5, which consists of five identical subunits LT-B. The active component (LT-A) consists of a single polypeptide which, following binding of LT to target membranes (via binding of B_5 to membrane gangliosides GM_1), is cleaved proteolytically into sequences A_1 (22.5 kD) and A_2 (5.2 kD). A_2 remains bound to B_5, while A_1 penetrates the target membrane to trigger a cascade of events culminating in increased Cl^- and water permeability of the target cells (Middlebrook and Durland, 1984).

Since LT as well as CT act directly on the target membranes, they must be exported by E. coli and Vibrio cholerae, respectively. In fact, CT can be produced extracellularly in large amounts (Mekalanos et al., 1978), while LT has also been reported in culture supernatants. Thus, LT as well as CT are considered to be exotoxins, although there is some doubt that LT is similar to CT in this respect, as we will show below.

Enteropathogenic E. coli strains generally produce very small amounts of LT, typically of the order of 0.01 -0.1 % of the total cell protein. Given a molecular weight of 85.000 for the holotoxin, this amounts to about 100-1000 copies of toxin per cell. Most of these toxin molecules are found not in the culture medium, but in the cell envelope, where they appear to associate closely with the bacterial outer membrane (Wensink et al., 1978; Gankema et al; 1980). Gram-negative bacteria normally shed outer membrane fragments or blebs during growth (Hoekstra et al., 1976; Mug-Opstelten and Witholt, 1978), and in the case of enterotoxigenic E. coli, such fragments are enriched with toxin (Wensink et al., 1978). When the cells are endowed with adhesins, which are also localized in or on the outer membrane, the resulting fragments contain adhesins as well as toxin (Middeldorp and Witholt, 1981, 1983).

While E. coli releases only small amounts of outer membrane material (ca. 5%) under laboratory conditions, considerably more outer membrane may be released under in vivo conditions in the gut. E. coli cells adhering to porcine gut surfaces show characteristic "granules" and "blebs" (Nagy et al. 1976) suggesting that gut enzymes might loosen the interactions between the bacterial outer membrane and peptidoglycan, resulting in massive release of outer membrane material.

Summarizing the above, in contrast to Vibrio cholerae, which produces large amounts of extracellular CT, E. coli generally produces modest amounts of LT, which accumulate in the cell envelope, and may bind to the outer membrane, most likely to its inner surface. Adhesins, when made, are localized on the external surface of the outer membrane. When membrane fragments are released, a normal process for growing E. coli and one which may be accelerated during bacterial adhesion to the porcine, human or other gut, such fragments may function as toxin delivery systems. They bind to epithelial gut surfaces via the adhesins, and thus deliver toxin to its site of action (Middeldorp and Witholt, 1981).

Given the above, LT is really an endotoxin; it is part of the cell envelope, rather than an exported protein. CT, on the other hand, is a classical exotoxin, accumulating as a free protein in the culture supernatant. These differences are not likely to be due to the toxins themselves, which closely resemble one another. Instead, they may be related to quantitative effects: thus, a small amount of toxin - LT - binds to the outer membrane, while larger amounts of toxin – CT – accumulate in the medium or in the periplasm. There may also be differences due to the host strains; that is, easy **toxin export** by V. Cholerae and **toxin accumulation** by E. coli. In addition to the above differences, there are also similarities, since both LT and CT are exported through the cytoplasmic membrane. In this paper we will review results of studies on this export process and the subsequent assembly of holotoxin in the periplasm and we will present preliminary results of studies on the 3-D structure of LT.

TRANSPORT OF ENTEROTOXIN TRHOUGH THE CELL ENVELOPE

The transport of a multimeric protein through the bacterial cell envelope raises several interesting questions. In which form are LT and CT transported through the cytoplasmic membrane? Where is the holotoxin assembled? How are subunits or holotoxin transported through the peptidoglycan layer and the outer membrane, if at all? What are the time scales involved?

To answer these questions it is necessary to examine the kinetics of subunit synthesis, subunit membrane transport, subunit processing, and holotoxin assembly in various cell compartments. These experiments must be done on a time-scale of several seconds to several minutes, during which time 1 to 10 copies of toxin are produced per cell. Since these must be followed quantitatively in a background of 3×10^6 other protein molecules per cell, it is very difficult to carry out such kinetics experiments for proteins expressed at very low levels.

One solution is to work with E. coli strains with much higher toxin levels. We have therefore examined the synthesis and assembly of LT in E. coli C600 (EWD 299), a recombinant strain with a multi-copy LT-encoding plasmid produced by Falkow and co-workers, which contains about 50-80 fold more porcine LT than its natural counterpart. The recombinant strain contains 0.8% LT (w/w) relative to total protein, or about 10.000 copies of LT per cell (Pronk et al., 1985).

Less than 0.2% of this LT finds its way into the medium, so that we can truly speak of an endotoxin. Very little toxin (< 0.4%) is associated with either cytoplasmic or outer membranes. The bulk of the toxin is located in the periplasmic fraction, as determined by cell fractionation and as seen by immuno-electron microscopy of ultra-thin sections (Hofstra et al., 1984). Thus, in E. coli C600 (a K-12 derivative) LT is exported through the cytoplasmic membrane and accumulates in soluble form in the periplasm. Accordingly, this recombinant strain lends itself to studies on the export, processing and assembly of LT. Since large amounts of LT can be produced with this strain, it is also useful in further analysis of the structure of LT.

KINETICS OF TOXIN SYNTHESIS, PROCESSING AND RELEASE FROM THE CYTOPLASMIC MEMBRANE

We have studied the synthesis, processing and release of LT subunits from the cytoplasmic cell membrane into the periplasm (Hofstra and Witholt, 1984). Such experiments were carried out as follows. Exponentially growing cells were pulse-labeled simultaneously with ^{3}H - tyrosine and ^{35}S - methionine for 20 sec., after which the labels were chased with a 1000 - fold excess of unlabeled amino-acids. Samples were taken at different times during a 6 min chase (10 sec intervals during the early part and larger intervals during the later part of the chase), protein synthesis and processing were stopped by cooling in an appropiate inhibitor cocktail, and the cells were subsequently fractionated into spheroplasts and periplasmic fractions. Analysis of LT-A and LT-B was by immuno-precipitation with appropriate antibodies, while precursors and mature form were separated by SDS-PAGE.

The results of these experiments show that LT precursors (pre-A and pre-B) are transported through the cytoplasmic membrane, processed to mature LT-A and LT-B, and released into the periplasmic space with different kinetics. The times involved in these different processes are indicated schematically in Fig. 1.

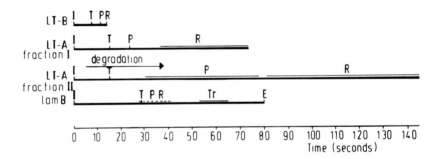

Fig. 1. Synthesis and export of LT subunits through the cytoplasmic membrane. Following initiation of synthesis (I), precursors are transported through the cytoplasmic membrane (T), processed to the mature form (P), and released into the periplasm (R). The kinetics of LT-A processing and membrane release suggest there are two subfractions, one of which is processed and released relatively rapidly (I), while the other fraction is processed and released rather slowly (II).

For comparative purposes, the kinetics of processing of Lam B (an inducible outer membrane protein), its assembly into trimers (Tr), and its exposure at the outer cell surface (E) are also shown (Vos-Scheperkeuter and Witholt, 1984). It is clear that these different cell envelope processes take place om comparable time scales.

Following initiation of synthesis, about 7-8 and 14-16 sec are estimated to be necessary for completion of pre-B and pre-A, respectively. Processing to mature B and A subunits occurs within a few seconds after termination of precursor synthesis, and may occasionally occur co-translationally.

Since immunoprecipitates of the periplasmic fraction showed only mature subunits, processing always preceeded release of LT-A and LT-B from the cytoplasmic membrane. Subunit release followed closely on precursor processing for LT-B, and considerably less tightly for LT-A. Thus, after initiation of LT-B synthesis by intracellular polysomes, only 14 sec elapse before the mature molecule is freely available in the periplasm. For LT-A, the situation is more complex. Most of the LT-A (fraction I, about 70 %) is synthesized, transported, processed and released to the periplasm in a total time of about 40-70 sec. The remaining LT-A (fraction II) is released into the periplasm only very slowly, however.

Interestingly, not only is LT-A processed and released from the cytoplasmic membrane with more difficulty than LT-B, but half of the LT-A originally synthesized is degraded before it is ever transported through the cytoplasmic membrane (Hofstra and Witholt, 1984).

ASSOCIATION OF LT SUBUNITS

The LT subunits oligomerize in the periplasm, following processing and release from the cytoplasmic membrane (Hofstra and Witholt, 1985). This is not an orderly, stoichiometric process. Instead, LT-B monomers oligomerize rapidly into high molecular weight aggregates, subsequently slowly binding LT-A monomers.

Interestingly, no B_5 assemblies are detectable in the periplasmic fraction. Thus, LT-B occurs only as a monomer, or in high molecular weight assemblies. On binding LT-A however, holotoxin (B_5A) is formed.

The kinetics of the process are such that all LT-B has segregated into the periplasm within one minute after termination of synthesis. Within this minute, about 80 % of the LT-B has assembled to a high-molecular weight form, about half of which has been converted to holotoxin by binding LT-A. The remaining 20 % LT-B remains in the monomer form, and disappears into aggregates more slowly with a half-time of 1 min.

LT - A segregates into the periplasm much more slowly than LT-B. Basically, it appears to be solubilized by LT-B oligomeric material. It remains unclear how LT-B aggregates (enterogenoid) are converted to B_5A holotoxin by binding of LT-A; perhaps the A subunit interacts with an LT-B aggregate such that a B_5 unit is broken off the aggregate. It takes at least 2 min and as much as 20 minutes before a newly synthesized LT-A subunit is incorporated into holotoxin. The LT-A which remains free before binding to LT-B oligomers is subject to degradation in the periplasm, with a half-time of about 20 min. These results preclude the possibility that simultaneously synthesized LT-A and LT-B products of the same polycistronic mRNA are found in the same holotoxin molecule.

The above results are summarized in Fig. 2. It appears that LT-A and LT-B are synthesized in approximately equimolar amounts. However, while LT-B is transported, processed, released into the periplasm and assembled into higher oligomers in what appears to be an efficiently linked process, LT-A goes through these same processes more slowly and less efficiently. About half of the LT-A is degraded before being transported through the cytoplasmic membrane. Following processing the remainder is released rather ineffectively, and of the free LT-A in the periplasm, half binds rather slowly to LT-B, while the other half is once again degraded. The net result is that in the holotoxin, one LT-A subunit is bound to five LT-B subunits, while in addition the periplasm contains a considerable pool of free LT-A which awaits either degradation or binding to newly formed LT-B.

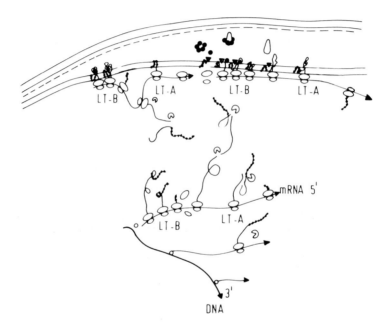

Fig. 2. Model for the synthesis and assembly of LT in the periplasm of E. coli

PREPARATION OF LARGE AMOUNTS OF HIGHLY PURIFIED LT

E. coli C600(EWD299) is routinely grown to a density of about 10 gm (dry mass)/l in a minimal medium in a 10 L Biostat Model E automated fermentor (Braun, West-Germany). Glucose and all of the necessary salts are present in non-limiting quantities or fed into the bioreactor as needed. The pH is maintained at 7.0, and pO_2 is kept above 50% saturation as long as possible.

Under these conditions, about 80-100 gm cells (dry mass) can be harvested at the end of a 15 h fermentation, with a total LT content of about 300-400 mg. Several fermentor batches are usually combined before LT purification is started.

All of the LT is located in the periplasm. Although we initially prepared a periplasmic fraction, it is easier to isolate the LT from total cell lysates. These are prepared by spheroplasting the cells to make the cells more susceptible to sonication, sonicating the spheroplast suspension (to liberate LT still present in the periplasm of these spheroplasts, since our spheroplasting procedure leaves the outer membrane of E.coli largely intact), and collecting the LT by adsorption to Controlled Pore Glass. After desorption with high salt, LT is concentrated and purified by sequential chromatography over agarose (elution with galactose) and Sephacryl S200, as described by Clements and Finkelstein (1979).

The resulting LT preparations are concentrated to about 8 mg/ml in TEAN (50 mM Tris-HCl, 1m M EDTA, 3 mM NaN_3, 200 mM NaCl, pH 7.6), and contain at least 99.5% LT. At most 0.5% of the LT-A occurs in the nicked form. From this LT, highly purified LT-A and LT-B are prepared by chromatography on Sephacryl-S300 under dissociating conditions. They are concentrated to about 2 mg/ml and stored in TEAN.

CRYSTALLIZATION OF LT

To produce LT crystals, it is necessary to start the crystallization from highly concentrated LT samples (Pronk et al., 1985). We found the solubility of LT to decrease dramatically at lower ionic strength. At pH 8.0, solubility decreased from 24 mg/ml at I = 0.2 to less than 4 mg/ml at I < 0.07. LT is essentially insoluble at ionic strength below 0.05. pH effects were examined in less detail. It is clear however that the solubility of LT is lowered at pH < 8.0.

Based on solubility information, a large number of crystallization experiments has been carried out in the past 4 years (Pronk et al., 1985). Although LT forms sizeable crystals quite easily in TEAN (pH 9.7) on standing at 4 $^{\circ}$C, and these diffract beyond 3.0 A, they are useless for structure determination due to twinning.

Three crystal forms have been obtained thus far. Form I is related to the crystals formed spontaneously in TEAN. By slightly modifying the buffers used to dissolve LT (ammonium sulphate instead of sodium chloride, addition of 3 % methanol or 3 % ethanol, removal of EDTA) and using 25 % PEG 6000 in the second solution, crystals which showed reduced twinning could be obtained. However, they were rather small and the resolution decreased from 2.8 to 3.2 A.

Form II, obtained in the presence of 0.3 M $CdCl_2$ diffracted to 3.0 A and showed no disorder. However, it contained only the B_5 component; LT-A was apparently dissociated as a result of the interaction with Cd^{2+}.

Form III is the most promising crystal form obtained thus far. It was obtained under several conditions (dialysis of LT in 1.5 M NaCl against salt free buffer; exposure of LT in glycine-NaOH (pH 10) to the same buffer with 20 % ethanol in the two-layer method; exposure of LT in a dilute TEAK buffer (pH 7.5) containing 0.3 M KF (instead of 0.2 M NaCl) against the same buffer containing 15 % PEG 6000 in the two-layer method).

The crystals formed in 0.3 M KF and polyethylene glycol were the best, showing diffraction beyond 2.0 A and no disorder, and variations of this crystal type have been used during the last two years for structure determination.

X-RAY DIFFRACTION OF LT CRYSTALS

Analysis of type III crystals showed that they belong to the $P2_12_12_1$ space group, with axial dimensions of a = 65.5 A, b = 98.0 A, c = 119.5 A. The unit cell contains four AB_5 molecules, while the asymmetric unit contains a single holotoxin molecule. Excellent diffraction patterns are obtained for type III crystals, and a complete solution of the tertiary LT structure now hinges on the preparation of suitable heavy atom derivatives. Isomorphous replacement by soaking type III crystals in various heavy metal solutions has yielded several derivatives. So far, none of these have yet allowed an unambiguous placement of a limited number of heavy atoms, although one pentagon of Hg sites has almost certainly been located.

LT crystals have also been analysed in the Desy synchrotron in Hamburg. Synchrotron radiation has the advantage of being highly monochromatic and intense, yielding higher resolution in shorter times than that obtained with a rotating anode generator. As an example, an LT crystal soaked in $KAuCl_4$, which was stable for only one day, was examined in the Desy synchrotron, to yield a complete data set (to 4 A resolution) in four hours, using a single crystal. With the rotating anode generator, this would have taken at least one week and therefore many more crystals. The synchrotron data are currently being processed using the supercomputer in Amsterdam.

PRELIMINARY CONCLUSIONS

1. Type II crystals, which contain B_5 only, have been analyzed to 7 A resolution, and show 5-fold symmetry.

2. Type III crystals, which contain AB_5, have been analyzed to 2.3 A and also show 5-fold symmetry. The 5-fold axis is approximately parallel to the a-axis of the unit cell. Although no phase information is yet

available, there are 5 promising heavy atom derivatives. The Hg and Cd derivatives appear to contain many sites; one pentagon of sites has almost certainly been defined.

3.   The various crystals are large and good enough for the generation of high resolution data (beyond 2 A) using synchrotron radiation.

REFERENCES

Clements, J.D., and Finkelstein, R.A. (1979). Isolation and characterization of homogeneous heat-labile enterotoxins with high specific activity from Escherichia coli cultures. Infect. Immun. 24, 760 - 769.

Hoekstra, D., Laan van der, J.W., Leij de, L. and Witholt, B (1976). Release of outer membrane fragments from normally growing Escherichia coli. Biochim. Biophys. Acta 455, 889-899.

Gankema, H., Wensink, J., Guinee, P.A.M., Jansen, W.H. and Witholt, B. (1980). Some characteristics of the outer membrane material released by growing enterotoxigenic Escherichia coli. Infect. Immun. 29, 704-713.

Hofstra, H. and Witholt,B. (1984). Kinetics of synthesis, processing and membrane transport of heat-labile enterotoxin (LT), a periplasmic protein in Escherichia coli. J. Biol. Chem. 259, 15182-15187.

Hofstra, H., Dorner, F., Kingma, J. and Witholt, B. (1984). Escherichia coli LT enterotoxin and its relationship to the cell envelope. in Bacterial Protein Toxins (Alouf, T.E., and Wadström, T.,eds) p.p. 89-97,Academic Press, London

Hofstra, H., and Witholt, B. (1985). Heat-labile enterotoxin of Escherichia coli: Kinetics of association of subunits into periplasmic holotoxin. J. Biol. Chem. 260, 16037-16044.

Mekalanos, J.J., Collier, R.J., and Romig, W.R. (1978). Purification of cholera toxin and its subunits: new methods of preparation and the use of hypertoxinogenic mutants. Infect. Immun. 20, 552-558.

Middeldorp, J.M. and Witholt, B. (1981). K88-mediated binding of Escherichia coli outer membrane fragments to porcine intestinal epithelial cell brush borders. Infect. Immun. 31, 42-51.

Middeldorp, J.M. and Witholt, B. (1983). An in vitro system to study interactions between bacteria and epithelial cells at the molecular level. J. Gen. Microbiol. 129, 179-190.

Middlebrook, J.L., and Dorland, R.B. (1984). Bacterial toxins: mechanisms of action. Microbiol. Rev. 48, 199-221.

Mug-Opstelten, D. and Witholt, B. (1978). Preferential release of outer membrane fragments by exponentially growing Escherichia coli. Biochim. Biophys. Acta 508, 287-295.

Nagy, B., Moon, H.W., and Isaacson, R.E. (1976). Colonization of porcine small intestine by Escherichia coli: ileal colonization and adhesion by pig enteropathogens that lack K88 antigen and by some acapsular mutants. Infect. Immun. 13, 1214-1220.

Pronk, S.E., Hofstra, H., Groendijk, H., Kingma, J., Swarte, M.B.A., Dorner, F., Drenth, J., Hol, W.G.J., and Witholt, B. (1985). Heat-labile enterotoxin of Escherichia coli: characterization of different crystal forms. J. Biol. Chem. 260, 13580-13584.

Vos-Scheperkeuter, G.H., and Witholt, B. (1984). Assembly pathway of newly synthesized LamB protein, an outer membrane protein of Escherichia coli K-12. J. Mol. Biol. 175, 511-528.

Wensink, J., Gankema, H., Jansen, W.H., Guinee, P.A.M. and Witholt, B (1978). Isolation of the membranes of an enterotoxigenic strain of Escherichia coli and distribution of enterotoxin activity in different subcellular fractions. Biochim. Biophys. Acta 514, 128-136.

Fehrenbach et al. (Eds.), Bacterial Protein Toxins, Zbl. Bakt. Suppl. 17
© Gustav Fischer, Stuttgart, New York, 1988

Crystallographic Studies of Pseudomonas Aeruginosa Exotoxin A: Mapping the Enzymatic Active Site

B. J. Brandhuber and D. B. McKay

Department of Chemistry and Biochemistry, University of Colorado, Boulder, Colorado 80309 0215 USA

ABSTRACT

Crystallographic studies of ligand binding and iodination of $\underline{P}$. $\underline{aeruginosa}$ exotoxin A, combined with biochemical data and sequence homology searches, suggest a model for NAD^+ binding that would be similar in both exotoxin A and diphtheria toxin.

KEYWORDS

$\underline{P}$. $\underline{aeruginosa}$ exotoxin A, ADP-ribosyl transferase, x-ray crystallography, sequence homology, NAD^+ binding

INTRODUCTION

Exotoxin A of $\underline{Pseudomonas\ aeruginosa}$ is a secreted bacterial toxin which inhibits protein synthesis in target eukaryotic cells by ADP-ribosylation of a specific modified histidine residue (titled "diphthamide") of protein synthesis elongation factor 2 (EF-2), as the last step of an intoxication process that requires the trans-membrane translocation of, at a minimum, the enzymatic domain of the molecule into the target cell cytoplasm (Iglewski and Kabat, 1975). The proenzyme form of exotoxin A, as it is secreted from $\underline{P}$. $\underline{aeruginosa}$, has been crystallized (Collier and McKay, 1982), and its three-dimensional structure has been solved in our laboratory (Allured and coworkers, 1986). The molecule manifests three distinct structural domains (referred to as I, II and III) which were originally proposed (Allured and coworkers. 1986), and subsequently confirmed by deletion analysis of the exotoxin A gene (Hwang and coworkers, 1987), to have essentially separable functions of receptor binding, facilitation of membrane translocation, and enzymatic activity.

The three-dimensional structure of the enzymatic domain (domain III) of exotoxin A, albeit constrained in a proenzyme conformation within the intact molecule, may provide a useful foundation for elucidating its catalytic mechanism. In the following discussion we summarize some of the recent results of our efforts in this direction.

MATERIALS AND METHODS

The detailed methodology of our crystallographic and biochemical experiments is presented elsewhere. Here we briefly outline a few essential aspects of the experiments.

Iodination of exotoxin A crystals: We have iodinated exotoxin A crystals at pH 5.5, collected 6.0 Å resolution datasets by diffrac-tometer, and located the major sites of iodination in the crystal by difference Fourier methods. We have, further, shown that the protein in the iodinated crystals, after dissolution, is inactive in the ADP-ribosyl transferase reaction. We have also found that iodination of exotoxin A in solution under conditions similar to those used for the crystals, either before and after enzymatic activation, abolishes the ADP-ribosyl transferase activity (Brandhuber, Allured and McKay, 1987).

Ligand binding studies in exotoxin A crystals: Although NAD$^+$ and nonhydrolyzable analogs of NAD$^+$ fail to bind specifically to ex-otoxin A in our crystals, we have been successful in binding, and locating by difference Fouriers, adenosine (8 mM, peak S/N[1] = 3.3 at 6.0 Å resolution and 2.6 at 2.7 Å resolution); AMP (5mM, S/N = 1.9 at 6.0 Å resolution); and ADP (40 mM, S/N = 1.2 at 6.0 Å resolution) (Brandhuber, Falbel and McKay, 1987).

Sequence homology searches: Searches for sequence homology between exotoxin A and diphtheria toxin were effected by computing the number of identical or equivalent amino acids within a sliding "window" ranging in size from 21 to 51 amino acids in length. Since the arginine-to-lysine ratio is substantially higher in the en-zymatic domain of exotoxin A (19 to 3 in residues 401-613) than in fragment A of diphtheria toxin (7 to 16 in residues 1-193), arginine and lysine were considered equivalent.

RESULTS

Iodination Iodination of exotoxin A in the crystals yielded iodine peaks as three major sites: His 118 in domain I, Tyr 289 in domain II, and Tyr 481 in the cleft of domain III. The fact that (i) iodination in the crystal abolished enzymatic activity, (ii) iodina-tion of exotoxin A in solution, both prior to and subsequent to enzymatic activation, also abolished activity, and (iii) Tyr 481 is the only iodinated residue within the enzymatic domain strongly suggest that the modification of Tyr 481 is responsible for the loss

---

[1] The signal-to-noise (S/N) in the difference Fouriers is defined as the magnitude of the largest positive peak divided by the magnitude of the largest (in absolute value) negative peak.

of enzymatic activity. Strictly speaking, the seemingly unlikely
possiblilty that iodination at the sites found in the crystal interfere with the activation of exotoxin A (achieved by incubation in 4
M urea, 1 mM dithiothreitol for 15 minutes at room temperature) has
not been definitively excluded, although the fact that iodination
after activation abolishes enzymatic activity argues against this
possibility.

Ligand binding: An adenosine model could readily be fit to the 2.7
Å resolution difference Fourier map. The adenosine is bound in a
pocket in the cleft of domain III. The difference Fourier showed no
negative peaks that could be interpreted as conformational changes
within the protein. The 6.0 Å AMP and ADP difference Fourier peaks
showed a shape similar to, and extensive overlap with, the 6.0 Å
adenosine peak.

Sequence homology: Sequence homology searches between diphtheria
toxin and exotoxin A showed one stretch of approximately 60 amino
acids of significant homology within the enzymatic domains (Fig. 1
and 2), with one deletion of 3 amino acids in exotoxin A relative to
diphtheria toxin. Within this region, 24 of 60 residues (40% of the
residues) are identical or equivalent (Arg = Lys).

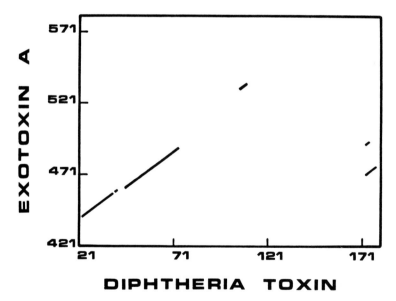

Fig. 1: Contour plot of sequence homology search
between exotoxin A and diphtheria toxin. Window
size: 41 amino acids; Lys and Arg considered equivalent; numbers on axes are sequence numbers of
center amino acid in window. Contours are plotted 4
sigma (4 x 1.8 amino acids) above the mean (3.3
amino acids) homology for the 41 residue window.

```
DT    GLY ALA ASP ASP VAL VAL ASP SER SER LYS
                                               10
ETA   GLU ARG LEU LEU GLN ALA HIS ARG GLN LEU
                                               429

DT    SER PHE VAL MET GLU ASN [PHE] SER SER [TYR]
                                                  20
ETA   GLU GLU ARG GLY TYR VAL [PHE] VAL GLY [TYR]
                                                  439

DT    [HIS GLY THR] LYS PRO GLY TYR VAL ASP [SER]
                                                  30
ETA   [HIS GLY THR] PHE LEU GLU ALA ALA GLN [SER]
                                                  449

DT    [ILE] GLN LYS [GLY] ILE GLN [LYS] PRO [LYS SER]
                                                       40
ETA   [ILE] VAL PHE [GLY] GLY VAL [ARG] ALA [ARG SER]
                                                       459

DT    GLY THR GLN GLY ASN TYR [ASP] ASP ASP [TRP]
                                                  50
ETA   .....(GLN ASP LEU).....[ASP] ALA ILE [TRP]
                                                  466

DT    [LYS GLY PHE TYR] SER THR ASP ASN LYS TYR
                                                  60
ETA   [ARG GLY PHE TYR] ILE ALA GLY ASP PRO ALA
                                                  476

DT    ASP [ALA] ALA [GLY TYR] SER VAL [ASP] ASN [GLU]
                                                       70
ETA   LEU [ALA] TYR [GLY TYR] ALA GLN [ASP] GLN [GLU]
                                                       486

DT    ASN PRO LEU SER [GLY LYS] ALA GLY GLY VAL
                                                  80
ETA   PRO ASP ALA ARG [GLY ARG]
                               492
```

Fig. 2: Sequence alignment showing homology between exotoxin A (ETA) and diphtheria toxin (DT).

DISCUSSION

Although the region of apparent sequence homology between exotoxin A
and diphtheria toxin covers less than a third of the enzymatic
domains, inspection of the molecular model of exotoxin A reveals
that nearly all the residues found homologous between the two
proteins lie within the cleft region of the domain. Presumably, this
strong local sequence homology is manifesting the shared necessity
of the two molecules to bind and act catalytically upon identical
substrates.

The sequence homology around the observed adenosine binding site,
coupled with the observation that adenosine is a competitive (with
respect to NAD^+) inhibitor of the ADP-ribosyl transferase reaction
in both an enzymatically active chymotryptic fragment of exotoxin A
(K_I ~ 0.1 M, Lory and Collier, 1980) and the activated intact
toxin (K_I ~ 0.1 M, Brandhuber, Falbel and McKay, 1987) suggest that
the observed adenosine binding mimics, to a good approximation, the
binding of the adenosine moiety of NAD^+ in the active toxin. The
fact that we are unable to observe specific binding of NAD^+ or
nonhydrolyzable analogs thereof to the proenzyme form of exotoxin A
in our crystals suggests that conformational shifts of an unknown
magnitude are required for productive NAD^+ binding. With this caveat
in mind, we have modeled possible NAD^+ binding sites in exotoxin A.

We have found one model in which the entire NAD^+ molecule can be
accomodated within the cleft region of exotoxin A with only minor

shifts in the conformation of the peptide backbone and side chains. This model provides testable suggestions of specific functions for amino acid residues in both exotoxin A and diphtheria toxin. In our model, the adenosine moiety of NAD^+ is constrained to the binding site observed crystallographically for adenosine alone. Particularly notable in this model is the extensive interactions the conserved pentapeptide Trp 466 – Tyr 470 would have with NAD^+. The nicotinamide ring would stack on the indole ring of Trp 466 (Trp 50 in diphtheria toxin), and could be responsible for the tryptophan fluorescence quenching reported for diphtheria toxin (Kandel, Collier and Chung, 1974). The positively charged side chains of Arg 458 and Arg 467 (Lys 39 and Lys 51 in diphtheria toxin) could form ionic salt bridges with the negatively charged phosphates of NAD^+. Replacement of these residues with uncharged residues, such as methionines, should substantially reduce the affinity of the molecules for NAD^+. The phenolic hydroxyl of Tyr 470 (Tyr 54 in diphtheria toxin) would be positioned near the nicotinamide–ribose bond broken during catalysis; whether Tyr 470 participates directly in catalysis could be tested by examining whether replacing it with phenylalanine abolishes activity. The phenolic ring of Tyr 481 (Tyr 65 in diphtheria toxin) appears to interact with the purine ring of adenosine, but is remote from the proposed catalytic site. It is apparent in this model that abolition of enzymatic activity by iodination of Tyr 481 could result from steric hinderance of NAD^+ binding; if this were the case, replacement of this tyrosine with phenylalanine should not dramatically affect enzymatic activity.

One potentially controversial aspect of this proposed model for NAD^+ binding is that it does not bring the nicotinamide ring into close proximity of Glu 553, a constraint suggested by Carroll and Collier (1987) on the basis of photolabelling studies.

In summary, a crystallographic approach to questions of the enzymology of exotoxin A, when one is constrained to crystals of the proenzyme form of the molecule, yields results which may appear to be dissatisfying for their inability to provide a definitive interpretation of substrate binding and catalytic mechanism, but at the same time may be invaluable for their presentation of explicit testable proposals.

ACKNOWLEDGEMENTS

This work was supported by award AI-19762 and Research Career Development Award AI-00631 from the National Institutes of Health (NIH) to D.B.M. We thank R. J. Collier for toxin supplied for this work under support from awards AI-22021 and CA-39217 from NIH.

REFERENCES

Allured, V.S., R.J.Collier, S.F.Carroll, and D.B.McKay (1986). Structure of exotoxin A of Pseudomonas aeruginosa at 3.0 angstrom resolution. Proc. Natl. Acad. Sci. USA 83, 1320–1324.
Brandhuber, B.J., V.S.Allured, and D.B.McKay (1987). In preparation.
Brandhuber, B.J., T.G.Falbel, and D.B.McKay (1987). In preparation.

Carroll, S.F., and R.J.Collier (1987). Active site of Pseudomonas aeruginosa exotoxin A: glutamic acid-553 is photolabeled by NAD and shows functional homology to glutamic acid-148 of diphtheria toxin. J. Biol. Chem., in press.

Collier, R.J., and D.B.McKay (1982). Crystallization of exotoxin A from Pseudomonas aeruginosa. J. Mol. Biol. 157, 413-415.

Hwang, J., D.J.Fitzgerald, S.Adhya, and I.Pastan (1987). Functional domains of pseudomonas exotoxin identified by deletion analysis of the gene expressed in E. coli. Cell 48, 129-136.

Iglewski, B., and D.Kabat (1975). NAD-Dependent inhibition of protein synthesis by Pseudomonas aeruginosa toxin. Proc. Natl. Acad. Sci. USA 72, 2284-2288.

Kandel, J., R.J.Collier, and D.W.Chung (1974). Interaction of fragment A from diphtheria toxin with nicotinamide adenine dinucleotide. J. Biol. Chem. 249, 2088-2097.

Lory, S., and R.J.Collier (1980). Expression of enzymic activity by exotoxin A from Pseudomonas aeruginosa. Infect. Immun. 28, 494-501.

Fehrenbach et al. (Eds.), Bacterial Protein Toxins, Zbl. Bakt. Suppl. 17
© Gustav Fischer, Stuttgart, New York, 1988

Pertussis Toxin

R. Rappuoli, B. Aricò, A. Bartoloni, R. Gross, M. Perugini and M. G. Pizza

Sclavo Research Center, Via Fiorentina 1,
I-53100 Siena

PROTEIN STRUCTURE

Pertussis toxin (PT) is a protein released into the supernatant by virulent Bordetella pertussis, the etiological agent of whooping cough (Sekura et al., 1985). PT is a complex bacterial protein toxin composed of five different subunits which have been named S1 (m.w. 26,220), S2 (21,920), S3 (21,860), S4 (12,060) and S5 (11,770), according to their electrophoretic mobility (Fig. 1).

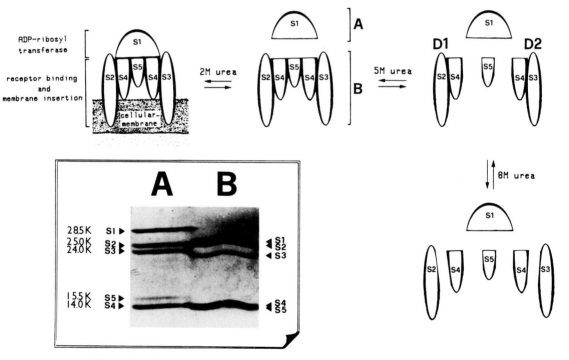

Fig. 1: Structure and properties of pertussis toxin. The insert shows the sodium dodecyl sulphate polyacrylamide gel electrophoresis of purified pertussis toxin under reducing (A) or non-reducing conditions (B).

---

[1] Part of this article is reproduced with the kind permission of Chimica Oggi.

Exposure of PT to 2M urea disassembles the PT into the monomer A (subunit S1) and the oligomer B (which comprises the subunits S2, S3, S4 and S5). Further exposure of the oligomer B to 5M urea disassembles it into two dimers, D1 (comprising S2 and S4), D2 (comprising S3 and S4), and the monomer S5. 8M urea dissociates the two dimers into the single subunits (Fig. 1).

Subunit S1 is an enzyme which, in the presence of NAD, binds the ADP-ribose group to a group of GTP binding proteins which are involved in the translocation of signals across the cellular membrane of eukaryotic cells (Fig. 2). The oligomer B is involved in binding the receptors on the surface of eukaryotic cells, interaction with the cellular membrane and translocation of the enzymatically active subunit S1 into the membrane. A family of glycoproteins containing branched mannose residues are believed to be used as receptors by pertussis toxin which binds them through dimers D1 and D2 and then inserts subunits S2 and S3 into the membrane (Montecucco et al., 1986).

MODE OF ACTION

The proteins, which are covalently modified by the S1 subunit of pertussis toxin, are a family of membrane proteins which bind GTP and regulate enzymes such as adenyl cyclase, phospholipase C, cyclic GMP-phosphodiesterase and others, which release secondary messengers into the cells. Since these enzymes play a key role in cell metabolism, they are regulated by a very fine system. Adenyl cyclase (Adc), for instance, is regulated by two GTP binding proteins: G_s which stimulates the activity of Adc and G_i which inhibits its activity. G_s receives signals from stimulatory receptors (R_s) located on the surface of the eukaryotic cells which in turn receive the messengers from stimulatory hormones (H_s) which are present in the extracellular medium. Similarly, G_i receives signals from inhibitory receptors (R_i) which in turn receive the messengers from inhibitory hormones. The G_s protein is the substrate of cholera toxin which locks it in the active conformation, while the G_i protein is the substrate of pertussis toxin which uncouples it from the receptor R_i. Therefore, cells exposed to pertussis toxin are unable to inhibit the activity of adenyl cyclase.

Other enzymes such as phospholipase C which releases the secondary messengers, inositol-triphosphate and 1,2-diacylglycerol or cyclic GPT-phosphodiesterase are similarly regulated by GTP binding proteins which can be uncoupled from their receptors by pertussis toxin. G proteins with yet unknown function are also modified by pertussis toxin: one of these, G_o, present only in nervous tissues, might explain the neurological lesions which are often associated with pertussis infection or vaccination. The transduction of external signals across the cell membrane mediated by the G proteins is associated with several receptors like beta-adrenergic (R_s), alfa-adrenergic (R_i), colinergic ecc. One of the consequences of pertussis toxin is the blockade of the alfa-adrenergic action. Some of the clinical manifestations of whooping cough may be due to toxin-mediated ADP ribosylation of G_i. Histamine challenge in laboratory animals causes vasodilation and increased vascular permeability, resulting in hypotension. Normal animals respond with a reflex catecholamine release, which causes compensatory vasoconstriction through a predominant alpha-adrenergic mechanism. In animals treated with pertussis toxin, however, the compensatory alpha-

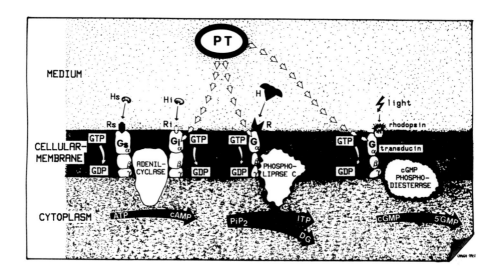

Fig. 2: Signal transduction across eukaryotic cell membranes and action of pertussis toxin. Extracellular signals which can be stimulatory hormones (H_s), inhibitory hormones (H_i), other hormones (H), physical (light) or chemical signals, give their messages to receptors (R_s, R_i, R, Rhodopsin). GTP binding proteins (G proteins) coupled to the receptors transduce the signals to enzymes such as adenyl cyclase, phospholipase C, cGMP phosphodiesterase which release secondary messengers into the cell. The adenylcyclase releases cAMP. Phospholipase C hydrolyzes phosphatidyl-inositol-4,5-phosphate (PIP_2) generating inositol-triphosphate (ITP) and diacylglycerol (DG). ITP mobilizes calcium from non mitochondrial stores, while DG stimulates protein-kinase C. The cyclic GMP phosphodiesterase releases 5' GMP which is the secondary messenger involved in the vision process. Pertussis toxin chemically modifies many of the G proteins and uncouples them from the receptors.

adrenergic effects are blocked, and vasodilation is eventually fatal. This effect of toxin has been termed "histamine sensitization". Alpha-adrenergic blockage may be the cause of hypoglycemia associated with B. pertussis infection; indeed, pertussis toxin was termed "islet-activating protein". Pertussis toxin blocks the alpha-adrenergic response that inhibits insulin release, causing epinephrine to increase insulin production by a normally less efficacious beta-adrenergic mechanism.

By similar mechanisms, pertussis toxin has been shown to interfere with chemotaxis (Backlund et al., 1985), receptor-mediated release of arachidonic acid by neutrophils (Bokoch and Gilman, 1984), excitation-contraction coupling of skeletal muscles (Di Virgilio et al., 1986), calcium mobilization and protein kinase C activation (Lad et al., 1985), lipolysis (Olansky et al., 1983), potassium current in pacemaker atrial cells (Logothetis et al., 1987), transduction of olfactory signals, immune response, lymphokine action and many others.

PT also modifies the growth pattern of CHO or NIH3T3 cells in tissue culture. The cells treated with minute amounts of pertussis toxin (50 picograms/ml) are clustered and overlapping, closely resembling transformed cells (Fig. 3). It is interesting to note that one of the oncogenes (ras) is a G protein which in yeast regulates the adenylcyclase.

In many of the above cases pertussis toxin has allowed identification of the G proteins which are involved in each of the above mechanisms and is a reagent which allows the dissection of the mechanisms of cellular communication.

STRUCTURE OF THE PERTUSSIS TOXIN GENES IN Bordetella pertussis

To clone the genes coding for pertussis toxin, we purified the pertussis toxin, determined the aminoterminal sequence of its subunits and used the aminoacid sequence obtained to identify and clone the genes from the B. pertussis chromosome (Nicosia et al., 1985, 1986; Locht and Keith, 1986). The five genes were found to be contained in a segment of DNA of 3200 base pairs and to have the

Fig. 3: Chinese Hamster Ovary cells (top) and NIH3T3 cells (bottom) grown in tissue culture. A and C: controls. B and D: after 48 hours exposure to 1 ng/ml of pertussis toxin.

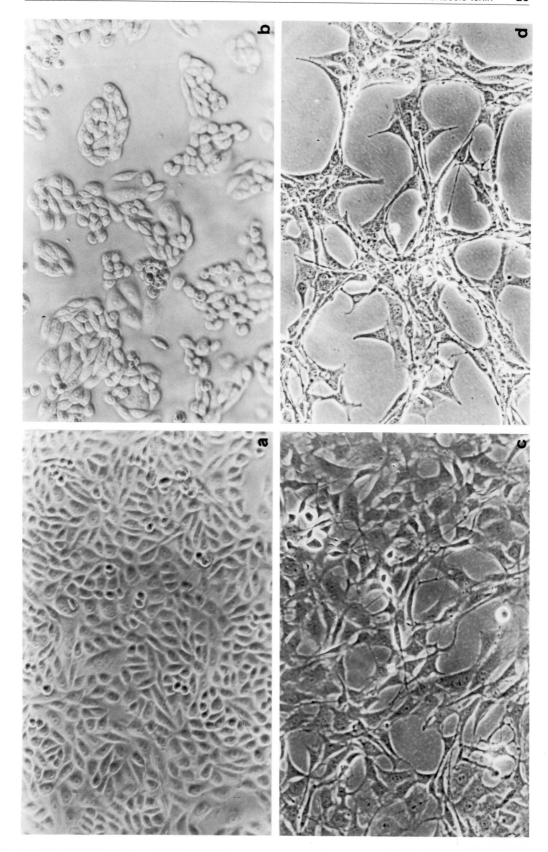

typical features of a bacterial operon: a promoter sequence was found upstream from the first gene and a termination signal was found downstream from the last gene (Fig. 4).

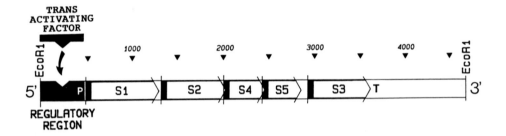

Fig. 4: Structure of the pertussis toxin operon. P: promoter; T: terminator. The black boxes at the 5' end of each gene indicate the sequences encoding the leader peptide.

Each of the five genes is preceded by a sequence encoding for a leader peptide, indicating that the five subunits are secreted separately into the periplasm of the bacteria where the toxin is assembled and subsequently released into the extracellular medium (Nicosia et al., 1986; Nicosia and Rappuoli, 1987). The subunits S2 and S3 were found to be 67% homologous, suggesting a common evolutionary origin of their genes, possibly due to gene duplication. The sequence homology between S2 and S3 subunits is reflected by the functional properties of the two proteins, since both of them form a dimer with the subunit S4 (Fig. 1). The subunit S1 which, like many other bacterial toxins, belongs to the family of the ADP-ribosyl transferases, shares some aminoacid homology with fragment A of cholera toxin.

THE PERTUSSIS TOXIN GENES IN OTHER Bordetella SPECIES

The genus Bordetella comprises the human pathogen B. pertussis, the causal agent of whooping cough, B. parapertussis which causes mild forms of pertussis-like disease in man, and the animal pathogen B. bronchiseptica which causes a variety of serious respiratory diseases in many mammalian species (Pittman, 1984). The classification into these species is based on several minor physiological differences, and this has allowed much speculation. For instance, it has been proposed that B. parapertussis could be simply a non virulent form of B. pertussis and a reservoir for B. pertussis between the epidemic waves of whooping cough (Granstrom and Askelof, 1982).

Among these species, only freshly isolated, virulent (Phase I) B. pertussis produces pertussis toxin. Upon laboratory passage, B. pertussis can lose the ability to produce many virulence factors (including pertussis toxin) and becomes avirulent (phase III). Avirulent (Vir-), B. pertussis have also been obtained by insertion of the transposon TN5 into a single locus of the bacterial chromosome and it has therefore been proposed that a transacting factor (Vir) which is able to activate the virulence-associated genes is responsible for the phase change in Bordetella pertussis (Fig. 4) (Weiss and Falkow, 1984). The availability of the DNA sequence of the pertussis toxin operon has allowed us to tackle the problem at the molecular level and to ask: i) whether B. parapertussis and B. bronchiseptica contain the PT genes, ii) what relationships exist between the various Bordetella species, and iii) why only virulent B. pertussis produces pertussis toxin.

i) Both B. parapertussis and B. bronchispetica were shown to contain mutated PT genes which are not transcriptionally active (Aricò and Rappuoli, 1987). The mutations (72 base pairs in B. parapertussis and 192 base pairs in B. bronchiseptica) are scattered all over the five genes. Some of the mutations were found to be common to B. parapertussis and B. bronchiseptica and remarkably, most of these are clustered in a small segment of DNA upstream from the PT promoter.

ii) The analysis of the nucleotide sequence of the PT genes of B. parapertussis, B. bronchiseptica and other B. pertussis strains such as the type strain BP 18323 and several clinical isolates has allowed us to draw a phylogenetic tree of the genus Bordetella (Fig. 5), which shows that B. parapertussis (BPP) and B. bronchiseptica (BB) derive from a common ancestor which diverged from B. pertussis a long time ago. Furthermore, we have been able to classify the strain BP 18323 as an intermediate in the evolution from B. pertussis to B. parapertussis and B. bronchiseptica. The clinical isolates of B. pertussis are a very homogeneous group and we have found only one base pair difference between the strain BP 165 (isolated in USA in 1950) and the strain BPSA1 (isolated in Italy in 1987). These data allow us not only to draw the phylogenetic tree of the genus Bordetella, but also to conclude that the Bordetella species are of clonal origin and that the proposed conversion from B. parapertussis to B. pertussis is very unlikely (Aricò et al., 1987).

iii) In order to elucidate why only phase I B. pertussis produces pertussis toxin, we cloned the promoter region of the PT genes upstream from the gene coding for the chloramphenicol-acetyl transferase (CAT) and we introduced this plasmid in different Bordetella species. From the analysis of the CAT activity we have been able to establish that the transcription of the PT genes requires 170 base pairs of the 5' untranslated region upstream from the PT promoter and a product which can be furnished in trans by the vir locus of phase I B. pertussis, but not by the same locus of vir- organisms. Phase I B. parapertussis and B. bronchiseptica were also able to trans-activate the promoter of pertussis toxin and therefore their inability to transcribe the PT genes is due to the mutations which are present in the promoter region of the PT genes of B. parapertussis and B. bronchiseptica.

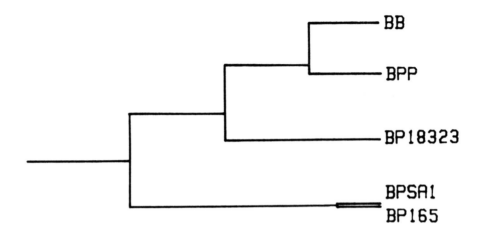

Fig. 5: Phylogenetic tree of the genus Bordetella deduced from the analysis of the nucleotide sequence of the PT genes. BPSA1 and BP165: clinical isolates of B. pertussis isolated in 1987 in Italy and 1950 in USA, respectively. BP18323: type strain of B. pertussis. BPP: B. parapertussis. BB: B. bronchiseptica.

PERTUSSIS TOXIN AND NEW VACCINES AGAINST WHOOPING COUGH

The vaccine which is currently used to prevent whooping cough is composed of entire Bordetella pertussis cells which have been killed and heated to 56°C. This vaccine, although efficacious, can give rise to some undesired side effects such as erythema (70-90% of cases), fever (30-70%), reversible neurological damage (1/100,000) and non reversible neurological damage and death (1/300,000). Chemically detoxified pertussis toxin has been shown to give less side effects and to be as effective as the cellular vaccine in the animal model. It is therefore likely that pertussis toxin will be the main component of a new vaccine against whooping cough. The development of a vaccine containing pertussis toxin involves two major problems: the yield of pertussis toxin is low and the detoxification process is difficult. To overcome these problems, we decided to tackle the problem by the recombinant DNA approach, with the aim of mutating the PT genes in order to make them encode a non-toxic molecule and hyperproduce the new molecule in a suitable host. Since the expression of the PT operon in E. coli is negligible, we expressed each of the five subunits separately as fusion proteins (Fig. 6)(Nicosia et al., 1987).

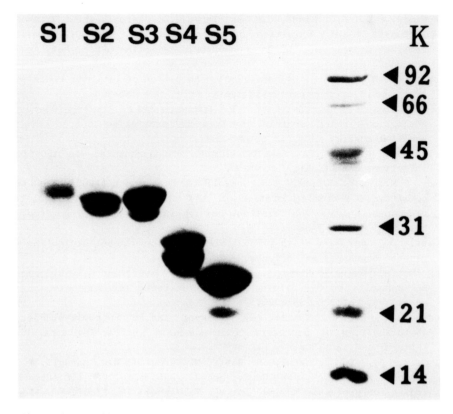

Fig. 6: Sodium dodecyl sulphate gel electrophoresis showing the purified subunits of pertussis toxin produced in E. coli as fusion proteins.

The five subunits expressed in E. coli were then used to immunize rabbits and mice. The antibodies obtained, although able to recognize the native subunits, are not able to neutralize the toxin, indicating that the assembled toxin is required in order to induce protective immunity.

Since the S1 subunit expressed in E. coli maintains the same enzymatic activity as the wild type toxin, we are now able to introduce mutations in this gene by site directed mutagenesis, in order to obtain a gene encoding a non-functional protein. Such a gene will then be introduced into the PT operon which will express a pertussis toxoid which, being immunologically identical to the pertussis toxin but free of toxicity, will form the basis for the construction of a new vaccine against whooping cough.

REFERENCES

Aricò, B., and R. Rappuoli (1987). Bordetella parapertussis and Bordetella bronchiseptica contain transcriptionally silent pertussis toxin genes. J. Bacteriol., 169, 2847-2853.
Aricò, N., R. Gross, J. Smida, and R. Rappuoli (1987). Evolutionary relationships in the genus Bordetella. Molecular Microbiol., in press.

Backlund, P.S., B.D. Meade, C.R. Manclark, G.L. Cantoni, and R.R. Aksamit (1985). Pertussis toxin inhibition of chemotaxis and the ADP–ribosylation of a membrane protein in a human–mouse hybrid cell line. Proc. Nat. Acad. Sci. USA, 82, 2637–2641.

Bokoch, G.M., and A.G. Gilman (1984). Inhibition of receptor mediated release of arachidonic acid by pertussis toxin. Cell, 39, 301–308.

Di Virgilio, F., G. Salviati, T. Pozzan, and P. Volpe (1986). Is a guanine nucleotide-binding protein involved in excitation–contraction coupling in skeletal muscle. EMBO J., 5, 259–262.

Granström, M., and P. Askelöf (1982). Parapertussis: an abortive pertussis infection? Lancet, ii, 1249–1250.

Lad, P.M., C.V. Olson, I.S. Grewal, and S.J. Scott (1985). A pertussis toxin-sensitive GTP-binding protein in the human neutrophil regulates multiple receptors, calcium mobilization, and lectin-induced capping. Proc. Natl. Acad. Sci. USA, 82, 8643–8647.

Locht, C., and J.M. Keith (1986). Pertussis toxin gene: nucleotide sequence and genetic organization. Science, 232, 1258–1264.

Logothetis, D.E., Y. Kurachi, J. Galper, E.J. Neer, and D.E. Clapham (1987). The ß subunits of GTP-binding proteins activate the muscarinic K+ channel in heart. Nature, 325, 321–326.

Montecucco, C., M. Tomasi, G. Schiavo, and R. Rappuoli (1986). Hydrophobic photolabelling of pertussis toxin subunits interacting with lipids. FEBS Letters, 194, 301–304.

Nicosia, A., C. Franzini, G. Ratti, M. Perugini, M.C. Casagli, M.G. Borri, G. Antoni, M. Almoni, P. Neri, and R. Rappuoli (1986). Cloning of the genes coding for pertussis toxin. In: P. Falmagne, J.E. Alouf, F.J. Fehrenbach, J. Jeljaszewicz, and M. Thelestam (Eds.), Bacterial Protein Toxins. Proc. Second European Workshop, Wepion, 1985, Gustav Fischer Verlag, Stuttfart, New York, pp. 289-290.

Nicosia, A., M. Perugini, C. Franzini, M.C. Casagli, M.G. Borri, G. Antoni, M. Almoni, P. Neri, G. Ratti, and R. Rappuoli (1986). Cloning and sequencing of the pertussis toxin genes: operon structure and gene duplication. Proc. Natl. Acad. Sci. USA, 83, 4631–4635.

Nicosia, A., and R. Rappuoli (1987). Analysis of the promoter of the pertussis toxin operon and the production of pertussis toxin. J. Bacteriol., 169, 2843-2846.

Nicosia, A., A. Bartoloni, M. Perugini, and R. Rappuoli (1987). Expression and immunological properties of the five subunits of pertussis toxin. Infect. Immun., 55, 963–967.

Olansky, M., G.A. Myers, S.L. Pohl, and E.L. Hewlett (1983). Promotion of lipolysis in rat adipocytes by pertussis toxin: reversal of endogenous inhibition. Proc. Natl. Acad. Sci. USA, 80, 6547–6551.

Pittman, M. (1984). Genus Bordetella. In: N.R. Krief, and J.G. Holt (Eds.), Bergey's Manual of Systematic Bacteriology, Vol. 1. The Williams and Wilkins Co., Baltimore. pp. 388–393.

Sekura, R.D., J. Moss, and M. Vaughan (Eds.) (1985). Pertussis Toxin. Academic Press.

Weiss, A.A., E.L. Hewlett, G.A. Meyrs, and S. Falkow (1984). Pertussis toxin and extracytoplasmic adenylate cyclase as virulence factors of Bordetella pertussis. J. Inf. Dis., 150 219–222.

Fehrenbach et al. (Eds.), Bacterial Protein Toxins, Zbl. Bakt. Suppl. 17
© Gustav Fischer, Stuttgart, New York, 1988

Tetanus Toxin: Evaluation of the Primary Sequence and Potential Applications

H. Niemann[1], B. Andersen Beckh[2], T. Binz[1], U. Eisel[1], S. Demotz[3], T. Mayer[1] and C. Widman[3]

[1]Institut für Medizinische Virologie, Frankfurter Str. 107, D-6300 Gießen
[2]Rudolf-Buchheim-Institut für Pharmakologie, Frankfurter Str. 107, D-6300 Gießen
[3]Institut de Biochimie, Université de Lausanne, Chemin des Boveresses,
 CH-1066 Epalinges

ABSTRACT

The complete sequence of tetanus toxin has been determined by sequencing the structural gene. The primary sequence is discussed in terms of potential domains involved in the toxicity and the binding process to gangliosides. The promoter of the toxin gene was characterized by primer extension studies as well as by comparative CAT-assays. Expression of nontoxic fragments *in vitro* and in *E. coli* lead to the definition of some of the epitopes of the toxin. Two epitopes of tetanus toxin which could stimulate tetanus toxin specific human T-helper lymphocytes were determined within the heavy chain.

KEYWORDS

Tetanus toxin, Gram-positive promoter, Influenza virus hemagglutinin, Tetanus toxin specific human T-cells.

INTRODUCTION

Tetanus and botulinum toxins are potent neurotoxins produced by anaerobic bacteria of the *Clostridium* genus. The toxins (Fig. 1) are large polypeptides consisting of a heavy chain (mol. wt 100 000) and a light chain (mol. wt 50 000). The subchains are linked by a single disulfide bridge. Tetanus toxin and botulinum toxins cause clinically quite different diseases: While botulinum toxins act on peripheral cholinergic synapses and thus induce flaccid paralyses, tetanus toxin acts in the central nervous system after a retrogradal axonal transport and trans-synaptic migration from the motoneurones to the interneurones by blocking the release of inhibitory transmitters. We have recently elucidated the complete primary sequence of tetanus toxin (Eisel and coworkers, 1986). A comparison with partial amino acid sequences published for botulinum toxins revealed a close relatedness of the clostridial neurotoxins, suggesting that they are derived from a common anchestral gene. In contrast, no homology was found with other toxins nor with 3600 proteins in a protein data bank.

RESULTS AND DISCUSSION

Evaluation of the Primary Sequence of Tetanus Toxin

Studies reported from the group of Boquet have demonstrated convincingly that at low pH tetanus toxin integrates into asolectin vesicles by hydrophobic interaction (Boquet, Duflot, and Hauttecoeur, 1984; Roa and Boquet, 1985). Hydrophilicity analyses of tetanus toxin according to Kyte and Doolittle (1982) indicated several hydrophobic domains predominantly within the L-chain and the N-terminal part of the H-chain. None of these seems to be so pronounced as to suggest an unambigous interaction with membranes. However, one of these domains, extending from amino acids Tyr(223) to Ile(253) (underlined sequence in Fig. 2) contains four of the six histidine residues of the light chain. According to computer predictions (Chou and Fasman 1978) of the tertiary structure, 17 of the amino acids in this stretch are folded into an α-helical structure in which three of the histidine residues (interspaced by three and two amino acids) reside at the same face of the helix as shown in Fig. 3.

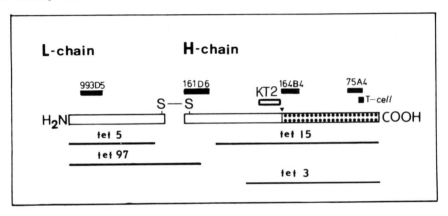

Fig. 1: Structural model of tetanus toxin. The positions of epitopes recognized by monoclonal antibodies are indicated above the model. Two T-cell specific epitopes are indicated by the open box (KT-2) and by a bar above fragment C (dotted part). Peptides tet3, tet5, tet15, and tet97 were expressed in *E. coli* or *in vitro*.

To test whether histidine residues might play a functional role in the establishment of toxicity, we subjected tetanus toxin to treatment with diethylpyrocarbonate and measured the increase in the absorption at 240 nm as detailed by Miles (1977). Under conditions where about 50 % of the histidine residues of the tetanus toxin molecule were carboxyethylated, the preparation was completely nontoxic in mice. Those samples which were treated for a shorter period of time with diethylpyrocarbonate and which therefore contained only about 3 modified histidines per toxin molecule no longer caused tetanus in the test animals but rather caused symptoms generally observed after application of botulinum toxin. We are currently testing whether the modified tetanus toxin is still capable of binding to primary cultures of embryonic rat brain and whether the K^+ stimulated release of acetylcholine is influenced.

Fig. 4 shows an alignment of partial sequences of fragment C from tetanus toxin and of the influenza virus hemagglutinin. The latter glycoprotein plays the key role in binding the virus particle to sialic acid containing host cell receptors and has been crystallized (Wilson, Skehel, and Wiley, 1981). Amino acids Tyr (98), Trp (153), His(183), Glu(190), Leu(194), and Leu(226) of the hemagglutinin

```
         1                    10                      20                        30
NH₂-M P I T I N N F R Y S D P V N N D T I I M M E P P Y C K G L
    D I Y Y K A F K I T D R I W I V P E R Y E F G T K P E D F N
    P P S S L I E G A S E Y Y D P N Y L R T D S D K D R F L Q T
    M V K L F N R I K N N V A G E A L L D K I I N A I P Y L G N
    S Y S L L D K F D T N S N S V S F N L L E Q D P S G A T T K
    S A M L T N L I I F G P G P V L N K N E V R G I V L R V D N
    K N Y F P C R D G F G S I M Q M A F C P E Y V P T F D N V I
    E N I T S L T I G K S K Y F Q D P A L L L M H E L I H V L H
    G L Y G M Q V S S H E I I P S K Q E I Y M Q H T Y P I S A E
    E L F T F G G Q D A N L I S I D I K N D L Y E K T L N D Y K
    A I A N K L S Q V T S C N D P N I D I D S Y K Q I Y Q Q K Y
    Q F D K D S N G Q Y I V N E D K F Q I L Y N S I M Y G F T E
    I E L G K K F N I K T R L S Y F S M N H D P V K I P N L L D
    D T I Y N D T E G F N I E S K D L K S E Y K G Q N M R V N T
    N A F R N V D G S G L V S K L I G L C K K I I P P T N I R E
    N L Y N R T A S L T D L G G E L C I K I K N E D L T F I A E
    K N S F S E E P F Q D E I V S Y N T K N K P L N F N Y S L D
    K I I V D Y N L Q S K I T L P N D R T T P V T K G I P Y A P
    E Y K S N A A S T I E I H N I D D N T I Y Q Y L Y A Q K S P
    T T L Q R I T M T N S V D D A L I N S T K I Y S Y F P S V I
    S K V N Q G A Q G I L F L Q W V R D I I D D F T N E S S Q K
    T T I D K I S D V S T I V P Y I G P A L N I V K Q G Y E G N
    F I G A L E T T G V V L L L E Y I P E I T L P V I A A L S I
    A E S S T Q K E K I I K T I D N F L E K R Y E K T I E V Y K
    L V K A K W L G T V N T Q F Q K R S Y Q M Y R S L E Y Q V D
    A I K K I I D Y E Y K I Y S G P D K E Q I A D E I N N L K N
    K L E E K A N K A M I N I N I F M R E S S R S F L V N Q M I
    N E A K K Q L L E F D T Q S K N I L M Q Y I K A N S K F I G
    I T E L K K L E S K I N K V F S T P I P F S Y S K N L D C W
    V D N E E D I D V I L K K S T I L N L D I N N D I I S D I S
    G F N S S V I T Y P D A Q L V P G I N G K A I H L V N N E S
    S E V I V H K A M D I E Y N D M F N N F T V S F W L R V P K
    V S A S H L E Q Y G T N E Y S I I S S M K K H S L S I G S G
    W S V S L K G N N L I W T L K D S A G E V R Q I T F R D L P
    D K F N A Y L A N K W V F I T I T N D R L S S A N L Y I N G
    V L M G S A E I T G L G A I R E D N N I T L K L D R C N N N
    N Q Y V S I D K F R I F C K A L N P K E I E K L Y T S Y L S
    I T F L R D F W G N P L R Y D T E Y Y L I P V A S S S K D V
    Q L K N I T D Y M Y L T N A P S Y T N G K L N I Y Y R R L Y
    N G L K F I I K R Y T P N N E I D S F V K S G D F I K L Y V
    S Y N N N E H I V G Y P K D G N A F N N L D R I L R V G Y N
    A P G I P L Y K K M E A V K L R D L K T Y S V Q L K L Y D D
    K N A S L G L V G T H N G Q I G N D P N R D I L I A S N W Y
    F N H L K D K I L G C D W Y F V P T D E G W T N D-COOH
```

Fig. 2: Amino acid sequence of tetanus toxin. The first methionine residue used for initiation of translation is not found in the mature protein. The underlined sequence is hydrophobic and contains three of the six histidine residues of the light chain. The double arrow indicates the primary cleavage site between the light and the heavy chain. Cystein(467) participates in the disulfide linkage between the subchains. The papain cleavage site within the heavy chain is indicated by a single arrow.

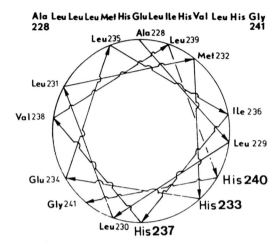

Ala Leu Leu Leu Met His Glu Leu Ile His Val Leu His Gly
228   241

Fig. 3: Prediction of the tertiary structure of a hydrophobic sequence within the light chain. The α-helical structure (3.6 amino acids per winding) positions the histidine residues on top of each other at the same face of the helix.

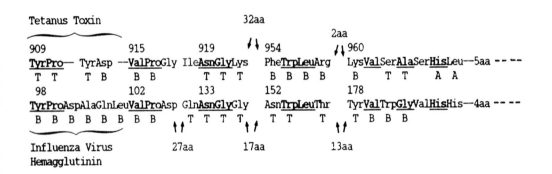

Tetanus Toxin   32aa

| | | | | | 2aa | |
| 909 | 915 | 919 | 954 | 960 | |

TyrPro— TyrAsp --ValProGly IleAsnGlyLys PheTrpLeuArg LysValSerAlaSerHisLeu—5aa -- --
 T T   T B   B B   T T T   B B B B   B   T T   A A
98   102   133   152   178
TyrProAspAlaGlnLeuValProAsp GlnAsnGlyGly AsnTrpLeuThr TyrValTrpGlyValHisHis—4aa -- --
 B B B B B B B B   T T T T   T T   T   T B B B

Influenza Virus   27aa   17aa   13aa
Hemagglutinin

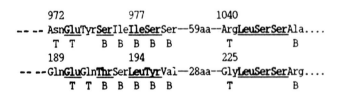

        972   977   1040
-- -- AsnGluTyrSerIleIleSerSer—59aa--ArgLeuSerSerAla....
       T T   B B B B B   T   B
       189   194   225
-- --GlnGluGlnThrSerLeuTyrVal—28aa--GlyLeuSerSerArg....
      T T B B B B B   T   B

Fig. 4: Structural alignment of the primary sequence of tetanus toxin (upper sequence) and the influenza virus hemagglutinin (lower sequence). The letters T (turn), B (β-sheet) and A (α-helix) reflect predictions of the tertiary structure using the computer program according to Chou and Fasman (1978).

are conserved among numerous variant strains of influenza viruses and form a pocket for the neuraminic acid at the distal end of the hemagglutinin molecule (Rogers and coworkers, 1983).
It may be completely accidental that a similar sequential arrangement of amino acids (again containing a histidine residue) can be found within the C-fragment of tetanus toxin. It is well established, however, that this part of the toxin molecule mediates binding to ganglioside receptors (Helting, Zwisler, and Wie-

gandt, 1977). Clearly, the precise localization of the ganglioside binding site requires experimental evidence. Site directed mutation of the individual amino acids of the C-fragment and subsequent expression *in vitro* or *in vivo* will be the approach of choice.

The Promoter of the Tetanus Toxin Gene

Under optimal growth conditions a toxin producing cell contains tetanus toxin up to 15 % of the total mass. This observation reflects the efficient transcription from the toxin promoter. To assess the suitability of this promotor for other genes of Gram-positive cells, we characterized the initiation site for transcription and determined the promoter strength in E.coli. Based on the notion that the toxin gene is flanked by palindromic stem loop structures and supported by expression studies in E. coli, we have postulated that the toxin gene is translated from a monocistronic mRNA. The promoter was functional in E. coli and was postulated to be located immediately upstream from the translation start codon (Eisel and coworkers, 1986).

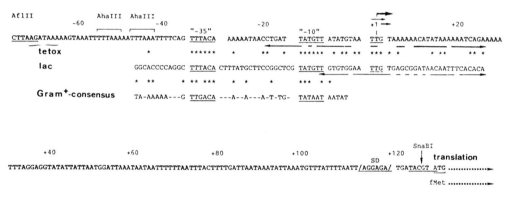

Fig. 5: Characterization of the promoter of the tetanus toxin gene. The initiation of transcription was determined by primer extension. The width of the arrows above the DNA-sequence reflect the intensity of transcription initiated from the particular nucleotide.

To map the site at which transcription begins, we performed primer extension studies using mRNA from *C. tetani* strain E88 as well as *in vitro* synthesized mRNA as templates. A synthetic oligonucleotide the sequence of which was complementary to nucleotides 61 to 77 of the coding region of the toxin gene was used as a primer. Both experimental approaches lead to identical results (data not shown). According to these studies transcription was initiated at the tip of a stem-loop structure 127 nucleotides upstream from the translation start codon (Fig. 5). The "-10"- and "-35"-regions upstream from the transcription initiation site were found identical to the corresponding regions of the lac promoter. In addition, a considerable degree of homology was observed between the toxin promoter and a consensus sequence obtained from 29 different promoters from Gram-positive cells (Graves and Rabinowitz, 1986). The observed homology between the toxin promoter and the lac-promoter are in keeping with the previous finding that the promoter is functional in E. coli.

To correlate the promoter strength with that of the tac-promoter in *E. coli*, we inserted the promoter region or various truncated forms of it upstream from the chloramphenicol-acetyltransferase gene into a promoter test vector (Brosius and Holy, 1984). This particular vector contains translation termination codons in all

three reading frames between the polylinker and the ATG-codon of the CAT gene in
order to prohibit translational read through into the CAT gene. As shown in Fig.
6, the toxin promoter was about 3.5-fold weaker in *E. coli* than the tac promoter.
Deletions of 121 or 151 base pairs from the 5' end of the promoter reduced its
activity to 43% or 28 % of the wild type promoter.

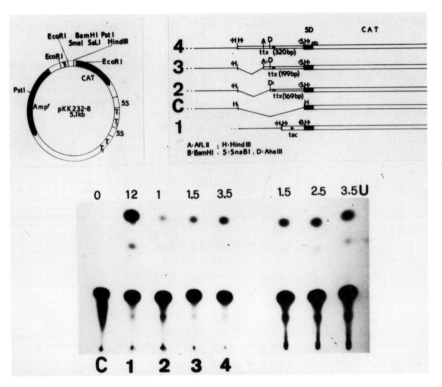

Fig. 6: Characterization of the promoter strength in *E. coli*. The promoter test
vector pKK232-8 was cleaved with HindIII, and the 5'-protruding ends were filled
with Klenow polymerase. Fragments derived from the promoter region were inserted
as indicated. Recombinant 3 x 10⁸ E. coli cells were lyzed and CAT-activity was
assayed according to Gorman and coworkers (1982).

Expression of tetanus toxin specific fragments *in vitro* and *in vivo*

The synthesis of suitable amounts of tetanus toxin specific fragments is a prerequisite for the study of functional domains at a molecular level. We have cloned
individual fragments from the toxin gene into pSP65 to synthesize the corresponding mRNA *in vitro*. The mRNA was capped at the 5'-end with 7m-G(5'PPP5')G and
translated in cell free wheat germ extract or reticulocyte lysate (Fig. 7, lanes 1
and 2). The peptides tet5 and tet97 had the authentic N-terminus of the light
chain. In both cases several peptides of lower molecular weight were formed. The
notion that fragments of identical size were obtained from tet5- and tet97-trans-
lations suggests that these shorter peptides are predominantly formed by premature
termination of translation. Similar observations were made when the products of a
combined transcription/translation in *E. coli*-lysates were analyzed (Fig. 7, lanes
3). For these reasons we have begun to develop a clostridial transcription/trans-
lation system (lanes 4). Although this system is still not as efficient as the *E.
coli*-lysate, it is obvious that this system yields, in contrast to all the other

systems, almost exclusively the homogeneous products of the expected size. The amounts of toxin-specific fragments obtained by *in vitro* synthesis are high enough to establish an epitope map (compare Fig. 1) or to stimulate human T-helper lymphocytes (see below).

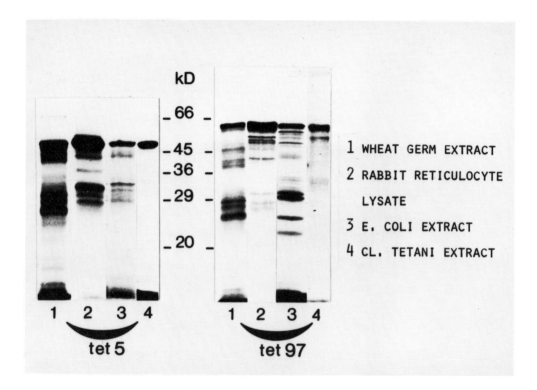

Fig. 7:   Synthesis of radiolabelled tetanus toxin-specific fragments *in vitro*. Lanes 1,2: DNA-fragments encoding tet5 or tet97 were cloned into pSP65-vectors. Capped mRNA was obtained with SP6-polymerase according to standard protocols. The homogeneity of the resulting mRNA was assessed on agarose gels. Translation assays were performed as indicated in the presence of ^{35}S-methionine. Samples were ana-lyzed on 13 % SDS-polyacrylamide gels. Lanes 3,4: Circular pEJ5- or pEJ97-DNA (Eisel and coworkers, 1986) was added to the corresponding transcription transla-tion system. The reactions in E. coli lysates and clostridial extracts werewas performed according to Chen and Zubay (1983) and Andersen and coworkers (1987).

The synthesis of fusion proteins in *E. coli* was another approach to study the immunogenic properties of tetanus-specific fragments. Fig. 8 shows that the syn-thesis of such fragments could be induced in *E. coli* 537-cells transfected with recombinant pEX31-vectors (Strebel and coworkers, 1986). The results from two clones are shown that encode either most of the light chain (tet5) or most of the heavy chain (tet3). Induced cells produced the desired peptide in up to about 5 % of the total cellular mass. By expression of various deletion mutants (including additional clones that are not listed), the epitopes recognized by the monoclonal antibodies were mapped as indicated in Fig. 1. The immunogenic properties of these bacterial clones were tested by immunizing mice and rabbits. From these studies it is quite clear that bacterial lysates containing minute quantities of tet3- or tet15-fragments (about 5 µg per mouse) are highly immunogenic and give rise to antibodies that can actively and passively protect mice (data not shown).

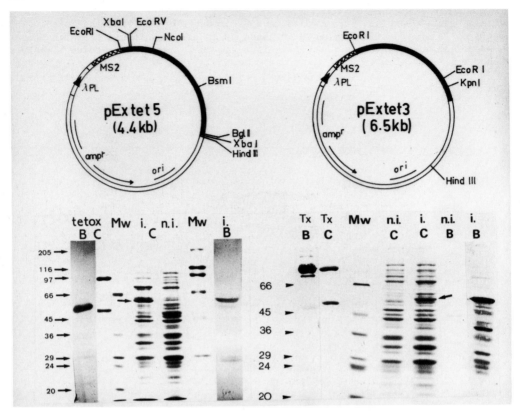

<u>Fig. 8:</u> Expression of fusion proteins in *E. coli*. Tetanus specific fragments were cloned into the pEx31-vectors as illustrated and expression of the corresponding peptides was induced in transformed 537-cells by temperature shifts. Induced (i) and non-induced (n.i.) lysates were analyzed on 13 % SDS-polyacrylamide gels and either stained by Coomassie brilliant blue (C) or blotted onto nitrocellulose. Antibodies 993D5 and 164B4 (for epitopes see Fig. 1) were used in enzyme linked immunosorbent assays.

Epitope mapping of tetanus toxin specific B- and T-helper lymphocytes.

The bacterial expression system was used to further characterize human tetanus-specific B- and T-cells previously established by Lanzavecchia (1985). It is generally accepted that T-cells recognize polypeptide antigens as proteolytic fragments in conjunction with the major histocompatibility complex after processing by antigen presenting cells (Fig. 9). The fact that tetanus toxin is highly immunogenic and that almost all human beings are immunized make this antigen an excellent tool for such studies. In addition, the gene technological construction of fusion antigens between tetanus toxin and foreign antigens might provide a key to induce T-cell specific immunity.

Fig. 9 shows the stimulation of a human T-cell clone (KT-2 cells) by an Eppstein Barr virus transformed human B-cell clone (KK:35) that was preincubated with the lysate of 10^6 induced bacterial cells expressing individual tetanus toxin specific fragments. Each of the lysates contained approximately 10 ng of tetanus toxin specific fragments. After 48 h incubation in RPMI, 1 µCi ^{3}H-thymidine was added and the incorporation of radioactivity was determined after 20 h. While the tet3- and tet15-peptides could stimulate T-cell growth, the light chain specific peptides tet5 and tet97 were completely inactive. Reduction and carboxymethylation of the tet15 preparation abolished its stimulatory properties. Since these T-cells could be stimulated in a parallel experiment by fragment B (i. e. tetanus toxin without fragment C), it may be concluded that the epitope recognized by the T-cell clone KT-2 is present within the 122 C-terminal amino acids of Fragment B. In a similar set of experiments the epitope of a different cell line was assigned to the peptide sequence involving amino acid residues 1273-1284 of tetanus toxin (Demotz and coworkers, 1987)

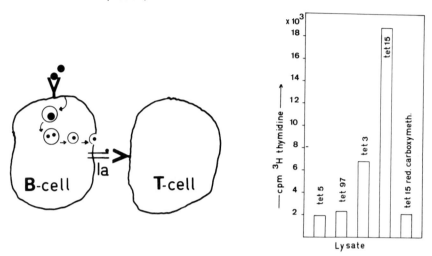

Fig. 9: Epitope mapping of tetanus toxin specific T-cells. 2 x 10⁴ KK35 B cells and 2 x 10⁴ KT-2 cells were incubated with the lysate of 10⁶ induced bacteria expressing individual domains of tetanus toxin (see Fig. 1). After 48 h thymidine incorporation was determined.

Acknowledgements
This work was supported by a grant from the Deutsche Forschungsgemeinschaft (Schwerpunkt Gentechnologie and SFB47).

REFERENCES

Andersen, B., Mayer, T., Eisel, U., and Niemann, H. (1987). Cell-free synthesis of tetanus-toxin specific polypeptides. Manuscript submitted.

Boquet, P., Duflot, E., and Hauttecoeur, B. (1984). Low pH induces a hydrophobic domain in the tetanus toxin molecule. Eur. J. Biochem., 144, 339-344.

Brosius, J. and Holy, A. (1984). Regulation of the ribosomal RNA-promoters with a synthetic lac operon. Proc. Natl. Acad. Sci. USA. 81, 6929-6933.

Chen, H.-Z. and Zubay, G. (1983). Prokaryotic coupled transcription-translation. Methods Enzymol. 101, 674-690.

Chou P.Y. and Fasman G.D. (1978). Prediction of the secondary structure of proteins from their amino acid sequence. Advances in Enzymology 47, 45-148.

Demotz, S., Lanzavecchia, A., Eisel, U., Niemann, H., Widman, C., and Corradin, G. (1987) manuscript submitted.

Eisel, U., Jarausch, W., Goretzki, K., Henschen, A., Engels, J., Weller, U., Hudel, M., Habermann, E., and Niemann, H. (1986). Tetanus toxin: primary structure, expression in E. coli and homology with botulinum toxins. EMBO J., 5, 2495-2502.

Gorman, C.M., Moffat, L.F., and Howard, B.H. (1982). Recombinant genomes which express chloramphenicol acetyltransferase in mammalian cells. Mol. Cell. Biol. 2, 1044-1051.

Graves, M.C. and Rabinowitz, J.C. (1986). In vivo and in vitro transcription of the Clostridium pasteurianum ferredoxin gene. J. Biol. Chem. 261, 11409-11415.

Helting, T.B., Zwisler, O. and Wiegandt, H. (1977). Structure of tetanus toxin. II. Toxin binding to ganglioside. J. Biol. Chem. 252, 194-198.

Kyte, J. and Doolittle, R.F. (1982). A simple method for displaying the hydropathic character of a protein. J. Mol. Biol. 157, 105-182.

Lanzavecchia, A. (1985). Antigen-specific interaction between T and B cells. Nature 314, 537-539.

Miles, E.W. (1977). Modification of histidyl residues in proteins by diethylpyrocarbonate. Methods in Enzymology 47, 431-442.

Roa, M. and Boquet, P. (1985). Interaction of tetanus toxin with lipid vesicles at low pH. J. Biol. Chem. 260, 6827-6835.

Rogers, G.N., Paulson, J.C., Daniels, R.S., Skehel, J.J., Wilson, I.A., and Wiley, D.C. (1983). Single amino acid substitutions in influenza hemagglutinin change receptor binding specificity. Nature 304, 76-78.

Strebel, K., Beck, E., Strohmaier, K., and Schaller, H. (1986) Characterization of foot-and-mouth disease virus gene products with antisera against bacterially synthesized fusion proteins .J. Virol. 57, 983-991.

Wilson, T.A., Skehel, J.J., and Wiley, D.C. (1981). Structure of the hemagglutinin membrane glycoprotein of influenza virus at a 3 A resolution. Nature 289, 366-373.

Fehrenbach et al. (Eds.), Bacterial Protein Toxins, Zbl. Bakt. Suppl. 17
© Gustav Fischer, Stuttgart, New York, 1988

Comparative Properties of Natural and Synthetic Staphylococcal Delta Toxin and Analogues

J. E. Alouf[1], J. Dufourcq[2], O. Siffert[1] and C. Geoffroy[1]

[1]Unité des Antigènes Bactériens, Institut Pasteur, Paris, Rue du Docteur-Roux, 28, F-75724 Paris Cedex 15
[2]CNRS, Centre de Recherche Paul Pascal, F-33405, Talence Cedex

ABSTRACT

A twenty six amino acid peptide (hexacosane peptide) having the linear amino acid sequence of delta toxin produced by human strains of **Staphylococcus aureus** has been synthesized by solid phase peptide synthesis. The synthetic peptide mimicked the natural toxin in its hemolytic and antigenic properties. Several analogues of delta toxin as well as shorter peptides (1-11 and 11-26) were also synthesized to elucidate structure-activity relationship using hemolytic assays on erythrocytes from various species, immunoprecipitation and interaction with lipid vesicles monitored by tryptophan residue fluorescence.

KEYWORDS

Staphylococcal delta toxin, hemolysis, synthetic peptides, tryptophan fluorescence, lipid vesicles.

INTRODUCTION

Clinical isolates of **Staphylococcus aureus** of human origin secrete a number of protein exotoxins including four membrane-damaging agents alpha, beta, gamma and delta toxins (also called cytolysins, hemolysins or lysins) (Freer and Arbuthnott, 1983). The properties of delta toxin which is a surface active polypeptide have been reviewed (Freer and Arbuthnott, 1983; Thelestam, 1983; Freer, Birkbeck and Bhakoo, 1984). The toxin is lytic for erythrocytes and other mammalian cells, intracellular organelles and bacterial protoplasts and spheroplasts (see Stearne and Birkbeck, 1980 for references). The toxin has also many other effects on various cell systems such as activation of membrane phospholipase A2, stimulation of prostaglandin synthesis and inhibition of the binding of epidermal growth factor to cell surface receptors (see Bernheimer and Rudy, 1986 for a review). It also activates lymphocytes, generates chemiluminescence by human polymorphonuclear leukocytes (Tomita, Monroi and Kanegasaki, 1984), inhibits water absorption and activates adenylate cyclase in the ileum and increases vascular permeability in guinea pig skin (see Birkbeck and Whitelaw, 1980).

Delta toxin is relatively stable to boiling and soluble in methanol and other organic solvents. It has been shown to interact with many types of phospholipid monolayers as well as cod and sheep erythrocyte lipid films (Bhakoo, Birkbeck and Freer, 1982) suggesting an amphiphilic structure. The toxin forms an unusually stable monolayer and induces membrane permeability changes of large unilamellar vesicles composed of structurally defined lipids (Bhakoo, Birkbeck and Freer, 1985). The hemolytic activity of the toxin is inhibited by usual phospholipids, cardiolipin and both alpha- and beta-lipoproteins of human serum (Whitelaw and Birkbeck, 1978) indicating a strong affinity for these lipid components.

The primary structure of delta-toxin purified from a human **S. aureus** strain has been determined by Fitton, Dell and Shaw (1980). It is a 2962-dalton polypeptide of 26 amino acid residues (hexacosane peptide) having the following sequence:

```
        1                              11                                                    26
Formyl-Met-Ala-Gln-Asp-Ile-Ile-Ser-Thr-Ile-Gly-Asp-Leu-Val-Lys-Trp-Ile-Ile-Asp-Thr-Val-Asn-Lys-Phe-Thr-Lys-Lys
```

The toxin which has been recently crystallized (Thomas, Rice and Fitton, 1986) contains no cysteine, arginine proline and tyrosine. It has N-terminal formyl-methionine residue, 14 hydrophobic residues, a high percentage of non ionizable side chain amino acids and single tryptophan residue. This is of high interest since this residue may serve as an intrinsic fluorescent probe as shown in this work.

Molecular weight estimates of toxin preparations have ranged from 5600 to 210,000 (Birkbeck and Whitelaw, 1980) suggesting that the toxin exists at a neutral pH as a multimeric assembly of identical monomers. At extremes of pH the aggregate will dissociate into tetramers as determined by Fitton (1981) who suggested by the method of Chou and Fasman that the toxin has a secondary structure consisting of the helical domains (residues 1-6 and 11-18) joined by a hinge flexible region (residues 7-10). Circular dichroism studies support this view. The toxin is predominantly (80%) alpha helical in aqueous ethanol solution and somewhat less helical (40%) in aqueous solution at neutral pH.

The primary sequence reveals a distribution of polar and ionisable residues such that if distributed or an alpha-helix they would result in a laterally amphiphatic rod with hydrophilic and hydrophobic faces distributed on opposite sides of the long axis. The length of the rod would be sufficient to span a biological membrane. According to Freer and Birkbeck (1982) association of six such monomers in a cell membrane may result in the formation of a transmembrane "pore" lined by the hydrophilic faces of the monomer.

An interesting approach for a better evaluation of structure-activity relationship for delta toxin would be the use of synthetic analogues and shorter synthetic peptides for comparative study of their lytic effect and interaction with phospholipids monitored by fluorescence techniques. We report here the successful synthesis of delta toxin and analogues by the solid phase method and the study of some biological antigenic and physicochemical properties of these polypeptides.

MATERIALS AND METHODS

Natural Delta Toxin. Highly purified toxin samples were kindly provided by Dr Harry Birkbeck (University of Glasgow, U.K.). The toxin was also produced (strain NCTC 10345) and purified in our laboratory as described by Bhakoo, Birkbeck and Freer (1982).

Rabbit Antiserum. Antiserum raised in rabbits against delta toxin was generously provided by Dr H. Birkbeck.

Synthetic Peptides. The following peptides named B, C, D, E, F, G, were prepared by one of us (O. Siffert) by the solid phase method. Polypeptide A is the natural toxin.

A. Formyl-Met-Ala-Gln-Asp-Ile-Ile-Ser-Thr-Ile-Gly-Asp-Leu-Val-Lys-Trp-Ile-Ile-Asp-Thr-Val-Asn-Lys-Phe-Thr-Lys-Lys

B. Synthetic δ-toxin

C. Synthetic unformylated δ-toxin

D. Asp-Leu-Val-Lys-Trp-Ile-Ile-Asp-Thr-Val-Asn-Lys-Phe-Thr-Lys-Lys

E. Formyl-Met-Ala-Gln-Asp-Ile-Ile-Ser-Thr-Ile-Gly-Asp

F. Formyl-Met-Leu-Gln-Asp-Leu-Leu-Ser-Ser-Leu-Gly-Asp-Leu-Leu-Lys-Ser-Trp-Leu-Asp-Thr-Leu-Asn-Lys-Phe-Thr-Lys-Lys

G. Unformylated peptide F

The detailed experiments procedure of peptide synthesis will be described elsewhere. All peptides were purified by gel filtration on Biogel P4 followed by ion-exchange chromatography. All peptides were identified by determination of amino acid composition. Their sequence, determined by Edman degradation was kindly performed by Dr Paul Falmagne (University of Mons, Belgium). The synthesized peptides were kept in the lyophilized state. Peptides D and E correspond respectively to 11-26 and 1-11 fragments of natural toxin (A). Peptide F is an analogue in which Trp residue is shifted to position 16 (as compared to Trp 15 in delta toxin) in addition to various substitutions. This peptide was designed so that to obtain an amphipathic profile (Fig. 1) similar to that obtained with delta toxin when analyzed by the helical wheel axial projection as described originally by Schiffer and Edmundson (1967) and applied to delta toxin, mellitin a 26-residue hemolytic and surface active peptide from bee venom (De Grado, Kezdy and Kaiser, 1981) and a 20-residue peptide of human C3a anaphylatoxin (Hoeprich and Hugli, 1986).

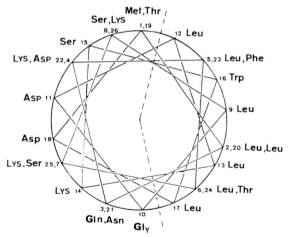

Fig. 1. Helicoidal wheel projection of delta toxin analogue F

Hemolytic Assay. Human, horse, sheep, rabbit and guinea pig blood was centrifuged (5000 g, 5 min) and the erythrocyte pellets were washed three times in 150 mM-sodium PBS, pH 6.8. The blood cells were suspended (about 2.5% v/v) in PBS such that a 30-fold dilution of this suspension in distilled water gave an A_{541} of 0.200. This standard suspension (about 6×10^8 cells/ml for sheep erythrocytes and 3×10^8 cells/ml for the other erythrocytes) were kept at 4°C and used within 2 days. The hemolytic titer was then determined as described for streptolysin S titration (Loridan and Alouf, 1986). In the assay system of Table 1, all peptides dissolved in PBS buffer pH 6.8 were tested at a concentration of 75 μg/ml. One ml of peptide solution was incubated with 0.5 ml of erythrocyte suspension and the percentage of hemolysis was determined.

RESULTS

Hemolytic Activity of the Synthetic Peptides. The peptides (75 μg in assay system) were tested on the erythrocytes of the species mentioned in Table 1.

TABLE 1. Hemolytic Effect of Natural and Synthetic Delta Toxin and Analogues on Erythrocytes from Various Species

Toxin preparation	Man	Horse %	Sheep lysis	Rabbit	Guinea pig
A	100	84	78	100	100
B	51	43	2	22	55
C	60	50	8	25	58
D*	0	0	0	0	0
E	0	0	0	0	0
F	4	12	0	0	36
G	13	31	13	35	34

A and B: natural and synthetic toxin, C: unformylated toxin, D: peptide 11-26, E: peptide 1-11, F: formylated analogue, G: unformylated analogue.
(*) Weakly active (10-20% lysis) at 250 μg in assay system on man and horse erythrocytes.

The formylated and unformylated synthetic peptides B and C were lytic although their hemolytic potency was 2 to 5 fold weaker than that of the natural toxin (A) as regards human, horse, rabbit and guinea pig erythrocytes. Almost no lysis was observed with sheep erythrocytes whereas these cells were lysed by the natural toxin. The interpretation of these differences of activity awaits further investigation. One possibility would be the presence of inhibitors contaminating the peptides due to traces of the organic materials used in solid phase synthesis. Conformational differences between the synthetic peptides and the natural toxin may also explain the differences.
The synthetic C-terminal fragment 11-26 is highly hydrophilic and contains the four lysin groups of the toxin. At a concentration of 75 μg the peptide was not hemolytic. A lytic effect was observed at a concentration of 250 μg on human and

horse erythrocytes. The synthetic N-terminal fragment 1-11 (peptide E) did not show any lytic effect for both concentrations.

The 26-residue analogue F was inactive at the concentration of 75 µg on sheep and rabbit erythrocytes. Human, horse and guinea pig erythrocytes exhibited various degrees of sensitivity as compared to the natural toxin. Analogue G which is the unformylated form of analogue F was more active.

Antigenic Reactivity of the Synthetic Peptides. The synthetic formylated and unformylated toxin (peptides B and C) and analogues F and G gave a pattern of total identity with the natural toxin tested by double immunodiffusion in agar against the homologous immune serum (Fig. 2). The hexadecapeptide D gave a partial cross-reactivity as evidenced by the formation of a spur. Peptide E did not form any precipitation line with the immune serum.

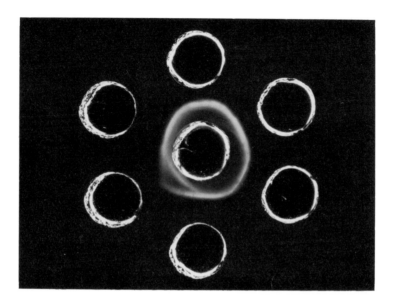

Fig. 2. Double Immunodiffusion pattern of delta toxin and synthetic peptides tested against anti-delta toxin serum (central well). Top well: natural delta toxin:. then in clockwise order peptides B, C, E, D and G.

Tryptophan Fluorescence of the Synthetic Peptides

$Trp_{15}$of natural delta lysine has already been used to monitor autoassociation state of the peptide in solution and its binding to lipid vesicles (Fitton, 1980; Dufourcq and co-workers, 1986; Yianni, Fitton and Morgan, 1986). It is concluded from the emission maximum and anisotropy changes that the peptide is severely autoassociated with a burying and immobilization of Trp_{15} even at a few uM concentration (Dufourcq and co-workers, 1986; Freer, Birkbeck and Bhakoo, 1984). The synthetic peptide with similar sequence but unformylated aminoterminal group (analogue C) has quite a different emission spectrum since its maximum at about 348 nm indicates a Trp residue exposed to solvent at 3 µM. This emission is only slightly shifted towards 345 nm when egg lecithin single unilamellar vesicles are added (EPC-SUV) the quantum yield increasing by about 20%.

The fragment 11-26 (analogue D) again is quite different since in similar conditions its Trp, still equivalent to position 15 of natural delta-toxin, is totally exposed to solvent with an emission centered at 351 nm. As seen in Fig. 3 in the presence of phospholipids very significant blue shifts are observed. This shift depends on the nature of the lipids added with a steep curve plateauing at 338 nm for a lipid to peptide similar ratio: (Ri = PS/pept ≤ 5). At variance with EPC vesicles a very progressive shift occurs and the plateau is not observed even for Ri = 170. Concomitantly net quenching of the fluorescence occurs in the presence of PS (Fig. 3a) while a weak increase is detected with EPC. Such a different behavior of D analogue towards lipids according to their charge was not already found for natural delta-toxin on experiments using monolayers of lipids (4) nor following the escape of small solutes (Freer, Birkbeck and Bhakoo, 1984).

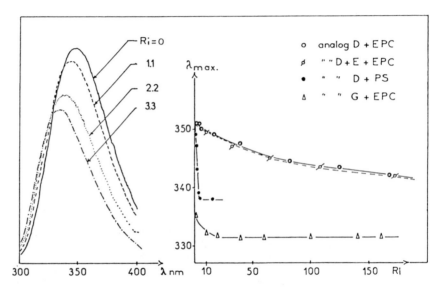

Fig. 3. Interaction of delta toxin and analogues with phospholipid vesicles as followed by Trp fluorescence. Excitation wavelength 275 nm, peptide concentration 2.9 μM. Experiments are done by stepwise addition of small unilamellar vesicles of the desired lipid: EPC egg lecithin, PS natural phosphatidylserine, Tris acetate 20 mM, 1 mM EDTA, pH = 7.5, T = 25°C.

The 1-11 fragment, E analogue, has no chromophore and cannot be detected in fluorescence, but its effect on fluorescence of analogue D has been investigated. The fluorescence changes of analogue D are unsensitive to the presence of E, and its presence even in a ten-fold excess does not change the interaction of D, monitored by its Trp residue, with lipids (Fig. 3). This holds whatever E is added prior or after the lipid vesicles. One then concludes that peptide E is unable to bind significantly lipids, at least in the presence of D. Its affinity for lipid membrane is then probably very weak compared to that of analogue D.

Finally, the fluorescence of G analogue has been analyzed. Its emission maximum corresponding to Trp_{16} at about 335 nm for the peptide alone indicates severe burying. This maximum does not shift in the presence of PS vesicles but is significantly blue shifted to 332 nm in the presence of EPC vesicles. In parallel in both cases very drastic increases of the quantum yield are observed allowing to conveniently monitor the interaction with lipid vesicles. Again a few molecules of negatively charged PS are sufficient to afford the fluorescence changes while several tens of EPC are needed in order to get the spectroscopic characteristics of the peptide totally bound.

Competition of several peptides for the same lipid interface could allow to get at least relative affinities of the different peptides. This has been performed by first allowing interaction of the studied analogues with PS vesicles, the fluorescence of peptides initially totally bound is then followed when adding protamine a strongly basic peptide which has a high affinity for PS but lacks of any aromatic amino-acid residue. For D analogue, addition of protamine results in a rapid recovery of the fluorescence parameters of D alone in solution, which is interpreted by a release of Trp from the bilayer environment. At the opposite when analogue F which has the full 1–26 length of delta-toxin but a modified sequence, the fluorescence of Trp $_{16}$ for the peptide in solution is only progressively recovered and a 10-fold excess of protamine, on a molar basis, is needed. Then we propose that analogue F has a much higher affinity for the lipids when compared to D.

CONCLUSION

The synthetic peptides except the fragment 1–11 were lytic to various degrees towards human, horse, sheep, rabbit and guinea pig erythrocytes. The active peptides cross-reacted with the natural toxin by immunoprecipitation test.

From their emission spectra at concentration in the range of a few μM the different analogues free in solution display a variety of Trp exposures which are probably reflecting different auto-association states.

From fluorescence data it is obvious that all analogues, out of peptide E which is a very acidic one, bind to lipid vesicles but the affinity of peptide D is probably decreased compared to that of analogues with full length. These findings correlate quite well with their activity towards erythrocytes when looked in a rather simplistic manner: peptide E has no activity because it does not bind to lipids, peptide D has a low activity revealing probably its lower affinity for the membrane. Then one can speculate that when similar amounts of peptide D will be bound they should lead to efficient lysis, i.e. the hexadecapeptide is intrinsically able to lyse efficiently and thereby active. In order to try to address the problem of the structure of delta toxin bound to lipid the synthesis of other analogues with Trp on different position and their behavior in the presence of lipid are in progress.

REFERENCES

Bernheimer, A.W. and B. Rudy (1986). Interactions between membranes and cytolytic peptides. Biochim. Biophys. Acta, 864, 123–141.

Bhakoo, M., T.H. Birkbeck and J.H. Freer (1982). Interaction of **Staphylococcus aureus** delta-lysin with phospholipid monolayers. Biochemistry, 21, 6879–6883.

Bhakoo, M., T.H. Birkbeck and J.H. Freer (1985). Phospholipid-dependent changes in membrane permeability induced by staphylococcal delta-lysin and bee venom melittin. Can. J. Biochem. Cell Biol., 63, 1–6.

Birkbeck, T.H. and D.D. Whitelaw (1980). Immunogenicity and molecular characterisation of staphylococcal delta haemolysin. J. Med. Microbiol., 13, 213–221.

DeGrado, W.F., F.J. Kézdy and E.T. Kaiser (1981). Design, synthesis and characterization of a cytotoxic peptide with melittin-like activity. J. Am. Chem. Soc., 103, 679-681.

Dufourcq J., E.J. Dufourc, J.F. Faucon, T.H. Birkbeck and J.H. Freer (1986). Interaction of Staphylococcus aureus delta-lysin with phospholipids: a fluorescence and deuterium NMR study. In P. Falmagne and co-workers (Ed.),Bacterial Protein Toxins, Gustav Fischer, Stuttgart, pp. 109-110.

Fitton J.E., A. Dell and W.V. Shaw (1980). The amino acid sequence of the delta haemolysin of Staphylococcus aureus. FEBS Letters, 115, 209-212.

Fitton, J.E. (1981). Physicochemical studies on delta haemolysin, A staphylococcal cytolytic polypeptide. FEBS Letters, 130, 257-260.

Freer, J.H. and T.H. Birkbeck (1982). Possible conformation of delta-lysin, a membrane-damaging peptide of Staphylococcus aureus. J. Theor. Biol., 94, 535-540.

Freer, J.H. and J.P. Arbuthnott (1983). Toxins of Staphylococcus aureus. Pharmac. Ther., 19, 55-106.

Freer, J.H., T.H. Birkbeck and M. Bhakoo (1984). Interaction of staphylococcal delta-lysin with phospholipid monolayers and bilayers - A short review. In J. E. Alouf and co-workers (Ed.), Bacterial Protein Toxins, Academic Pres, London, pp. 181-189.

Hoeprich, P.D. Jr and Hugli T.E. (1986). Helical conformation at the carboxy-terminal portion of human C3a is required for full activity. Biochemistry, 25, 1945-1950.

Loridan, C. and J.E. Alouf (1986). Purification of RNA-core induced streptolysin S, and isolation and haemolytic characteristics of the carrier-free toxin. J. Gen. Microbiol., 132, 307-315.

Stearn, L.E.T. and T.H. Birkbeck (1980). The action of formaldehyde on staphylococcal delta-haemolysin. J. Med. Microbiol., 13, 223-230.

Schiffer, M. and A.B. Edmundson (1967). Use of heelical wheels to represent the structures of proteins and to identify segments with helical potential. Biophys. J., 7, 121-135.

Thelestam M. (1983). Modes of membrane damaging action of staphylococcal toxins. In C.S.F. Easmon and C. Adlam (Ed.), Staphylococci and Staphylococcal Infections, Academic Press, London, pp. 705-744.

Thomas D.H., D.W.. Rice and J.E. Fitton (1986). Crystallization of the delta toxin of Staphylococcus aureus. J. Mol. Biol., 192, 675-676.

Tomita, T., K. Momoi and Kanegasaki S. (1984). Staphylococcal delta toxin-induced generation of chemiluminescence by human polymorphonuclear leucocytes. Toxicon, 22, 957-965.

Whitelaw, D.D. and T.H. Birkbeck (1978). Inhibition of staphylococcal delta-haemolysin by human serum lipoproteins. FEMS Microbiol. Letters, 3, 335-338.

Yianni, Y.P., J.E. Fitton and Morgan C.G. (1986). Lytic effects of melittin and delta-haemolysin from Staphylococcus aureus on vesicles of dipalmitoyl-phosphatidylcholine. Biochim. Biophys. Acta, 856, 91-100.

Fehrenbach et al. (Eds.), Bacterial Protein Toxins, Zbl. Bakt. Suppl. 17
© Gustav Fischer, Stuttgart, New York, 1988

Botulinum ADP-Ribosyltransferase C3 Modifies A 21 KDA G-Protein

K. Aktories[1], S. Rösener[1], M. Laux[1] and G. S. Chhatwal[2]

[1]Rudolf-Buchheim-Institut für Pharmakologie, [2]Institut für Bakteriologie und Immunologie, Frankfurter Str. 107, D-6300 Gießen

Keywords: Botulinum toxins, ADP-ribosylation, botulinum neurotoxin C1, GTP-binding protein, ADP-ribosyltransferase C3, guanine nucleotides.

Certain strains of Clostridium botulinum type C produce botulinum toxins C1, C2 and D. Whereas C1 and D are typical neurotoxins, whose molecular mechanism is not known at present, the binary botulinum C2 toxin is a peripherally acting cytotoxin. Recently, it has been shown that botulinum C2 toxin possesses ADP-ribosyltransferase activity and modifies non-muscle actin, which thereby loses its ability to polymerize. Besides botulinum C2 toxin culture medium of Clostridium botulinum contains another ADP-ribosyltransferase, which we called botulinum C3 in order to distinguish this novel enzyme from botulinum C2 and C1 toxins (Aktories and others, 1987). Here we report about studies on the novel enzyme and its eukaryotic substrate.

The novel ADP-ribosyltransferase was purified from the culture medium of Clostridium botulinum Type C by ammoniumsulfate precipitation, anionic exchange chromatography and HPLC gel filtration. The purified enzyme migrated as a single band on SDS-polyacrylamide gels with an apparent molecular mass of about 25 kDa. ADP-ribosyltransferase C3 was stable against trypsin treatment (100 ug/ml) and heating (10 min, 95°C). In the presence of ^{32}PNAD the enzyme catalyzes the labelling of a protein with a molecular weight of about 21 kDa. In platelet membranes the labelling of the 21 kDa substrate was prevented by prior heating or trypsin treatment of the platelet membranes indicating the proteinaceous nature of the substrate. Labelling was blocked by addition of NAD (100 uM), nicotinamide (100 mM) but not by ADP-ribose (100 uM). Also pretreatment of ^{32}PNAD with NADase prevented the labelling of the 21 kDa protein.

Recently, it has been reported that botulinum neurotoxins C1 and D also possess ADP-ribosyltransferase activities (Ohashi and Narumiya, 1987). Furthermore, the substrate of C1 was reportedly also a 21 kDa protein. Therefore, we compared the ADP-ribosyltransferase activities of highly purified botulinum neurotoxin C1 with C3. Under the conditions used C3 was about 1000 times more potent than C1 in ADP-ribosylating the 21 kDa protein. Furthermore, antibodies produced against purified C3 recognized only C3 but not C1, indicating that C3 is not an active fragment of botulinum neurotoxin C1.

Studies from recent years have shown that GTP-binding proteins (G-proteins), which are involved in protein synthesis or transmembrane signal transduction, are substrates of microbial ADP-ribosyltransferases. On the other hand, guanine nucleotides modify the properties of G-proteins to serve as substrate of these toxins. In order to examine, whether the substrate of C3 is also a G-protein, we studied the influence of guanine nucleotide on C3-induced ADP-ribosylation. GTPγS but not ATPγS potently inhibited the C3-catalyzed ADP-ribosylation. A maximally inhibitory effect (about 70 - 90 %) was found at 10 uM GTPγS. Also Gpp(NH)p and Gpp(CH$_2$)p were inhibitory. However, GTPγS was much more potent and efficient. In contrast GTP and GDP did not reduce C3-catalyzed ADP-ribosylation. Moreover in the presence of ATP and with creatine phosphate/creatine kinase as a regenerating system, conditions which largely reduce unspecific GTPase activity, GTP was not inhibitory on ADP-ribosylation. In the presence of GTP, however, higher concentrations of GTPγS were necessary to elicit the inhibitory effects. Effects of GTPγS on ADP-ribosylation of the 21 kDa protein were largely affected by Mg^{++}. In the absence of added Mg^{++} and with EDTA (1 mM) GTPγS was not inhibitory but rather stimulatory on C3-catalyzed ADP-ribosylation. With equimolar concentrations of Mg^{++} and EDTA, GTPγS was inhibitory. The inhibitory effect increased with increasing concentrations of Mg^{++} up to 10 mM. In order to clarify, whether ADP-ribosyltransferase C3 itself or the 21 kDa eukaryotic substrate is modified by GTPγS, platelet membranes were pretreated with GTPγS. Thereafter the membranes were extensively washed and then used for the ADP-ribosylation assay. ADP-ribosylation was drastically reduced in GTPγS-pretreated membranes. Further addition of GTPγS to the ADP-ribosylation assay did not enhance inhibition of ADP-ribosylation of the 21 kDa substrate.

The data indicate that C3-catalyzed ADP-ribosylation is potently regulated by guanine nucleotides and suggest that an unknown eukaryotic G-protein is the substrate of the novel ADP-ribosyltransferase C3.

REFERENCES

Aktories, K., U.Weller and G.S.Chhatwal (1987). Clostridium botulinum type C produces a novel ADP-ribosyltransferase distinct from botulinum C2 toxin. FEBS Lett., 212, 109-113.
Ohashi, Y. and S.Narumiya (1987). ADP-ribosylation of a M$_r$ 21,000 membrans protein by type D botulinum toxin. J. Biol. Chem., 262, 1430-1433.

Fehrenbach et al. (Eds.), Bacterial Protein Toxins, Zbl. Bakt. Suppl. 17
© Gustav Fischer, Stuttgart, New York, 1988

Chemical Modification of Clostridium Difficile Toxin B

M. Caspar, I. Florin and M. Thelestam

Karolinska Institute, Department of Bacteriology, Box 60400, S-104 01 Stockholm

ABSTRACT

Clostridium difficile produces two toxins involved in the pathogenesis of the antibiotic-associated diarrhoea and colitis caused by this organism (1). Toxin A is
enterotoxic while toxin B is a potent cytotoxin.

Toxin B is internalized into fibroblasts by endocytosis (2,3). The ensuing actinomorphic change in the target cell involves an irreversible disorganization of the
microfilament system (4,5) but the molecular details are unclear as yet. The MW
of toxin B has not been firmly established. Reports range from 150 to 500 kD
(5,6). Low amounts of histidine, arginine, tryptophan and cysteine have been detected in the toxin while glycine, aspartic acid and glutamic acid are abundant,
making toxin B an acidic protein with at least 1/3 nonpolar residues (5,7).

Studying functional characteristics, we find that the toxin is stable between pH
5 and 9.8. It is inactivated by urea concentrations above 1.5 M if treated for
more than 20 minutes. EDTA at concentrations above 10 mM also inactivates the
toxin.

With the method of chemical modification of specific amino acids (8), we investigated residues essential for cytotoxicity. In these experiments, toxin was incubated with modifying reagent at different concentrations and in the appropriate
buffers. After one hour at 22° C the toxin was separated from reagent by gel
filtration. Modified toxin was applied to fibroblasts and cytotoxicity scored
after 24 hours and compared to controls exposed to native toxin. The minimal
inhibitory concentration (MIC) of each reagent is shown in Table 1 which also indicates the group specificities of the reagents. The MIC is defined as the lowest
concentration of reagent which caused a complete loss of cytotoxic activity.

As seen spectrophotometrically, diethylpyrocarbonate did not modify histidine,
but it did inactivate the toxin (see Table 1) presumably by a side reaction with
lysine. Successful modification of SH-groups required presence of 1 M urea.
Furthermore, the toxin could be reactivated with DTT after slight loss of activity
due to repeated thawing and freezing.

TABLE 1   Minimal Inhibitory Concentrations of Modifying Reagents

Reagent	Specificity	MIC (mM)
trinitrobenzenesulfonate	lys	10
succinic anhydride	lys > SH	10
acetylimidazole	tyr > lys	5
N-bromosuccinimide	trp > tyr	0.5
dinitrophenylsulfonyl chloride	trp	10
N-ethylmaleimide + 1M urea	SH	10
p-chloromercuribenzoate + 1M urea	SH	5
iodoacetamide at pH 8.3	SH > his	13
iodoacetamide at pH 6	his > SH	No inhibition at 100 mM
diethylpyrocarbonate	his > lys	10
N-ethyl-5-phenylisoxazolium-3'-sulfonate	COOH	> 10
1-ethyl-3-(3-dimethylaminopropyl) carbodiimide	COOH	10
1,2-cyclohexanedione	arg	No inhibition at 100 mM
phenylglyoxal	arg	No inhibition at 100 mM

Concluding remarks

Lysine, tyrosine, tryptophan, SH- and carboxyl groups appear essential for main-
taining cytotoxicity, but at which level in the target cell we cannot determine
at present. Modification of these residues may either destroy the active conformation or specific sites involved in binding, membrane passage or enzymatic
action.

References

1) Borriello, S.P. (1984). Antibiotic-associated diarrhoea and colitis. Martinus
   Nijhoff Publishers BV, Haag.
2) Florin, I. and Thelestam, M. (1983). Internalization of C. difficile Cytotoxin
   into Cultured Human Lung Fibroblasts. Biochim. Biophys. Acta, 763: 383.
3) Florin, I. and Thelestam, M. (1986). In: Falmagne et al., (Eds) Bacterial
   Protein Toxins, Suppl. 15, p. 207. Gustav Fischer. Stuttgart.
4) Thelestam, M. and Brönnegård, M. (1980). Interaction of Cytopathogenic Toxin
   from C. difficile with Cells in Tissue Culture. Scand. J. Infect. Dis.,
   Suppl. 22, 16.
5) Pothoulakis, C., Barone, L., Ely, R., Faris, B., Clark, M., Franzblau, C.,
   LaMont, J.T. (1986). Purification and Properties of C. difficile Cytotoxin
   B. J. Biol. Chem. 261(3):1316.
6) Banno, Y., Kobayashi, T., Kono, H., Watanabe, K., Ueno, K., Nozawa, Y.
   (1984). Biochemical Characterization and Biologic Actions of Two Toxins from
   C. difficile. Rev. Inf. Dis. Vol. 6, Suppl. 1, p, S11.
7) Lyerly, D.M., Roberts, M.D., Phelps, C.J., Wilkins, T.D. (1986). Purification
   and Properties of Toxins A and B of C. difficile. FEMS Microbiol. Lett.
   33:31.
8) Cohen, L.A. (1968). Chemical Modification as a Probe of Structure and Function.
   Ann. Rev. Biochem. 37:683.

Fehrenbach et al. (Eds.), Bacterial Protein Toxins, Zbl. Bakt. Suppl. 17
© Gustav Fischer, Stuttgart, New York, 1988

pH Induced Changes in the Conformation of Cholera Toxin and E. coli LT

M. De Wolf[1], B. Witholt[2], G. Van Dessel[3], A. Lagrou[1], H. J. Hilderson[1] and W. Dierick

[1]Ruca, Laboratory for Human Biochemistry, University of Antwerp, Groenenborgerlaan, 171, B-2020 Antwerp
[2]Dept. of Biochemistry, University of Groningen, Nyenborgh 16, 9447 AG Groningen, The Netherlands
[3]UIA, Laboratory for Pathological Biochemistry, University of Antwerp, Groenenborgerlaan, 171, B-2020 Antwerp

ABSTRACT

Quenching of intrinsic fluorescence of cholera toxin (CT), the heat-labile enterotoxin of E.coli (LT) and their respective subunits by brominated Bry 96 indicates that the capacity of detergent binding is as follows : CT A >LT A $\sim$ LT B > CT B $\sim$ CT > LT. In the pH range 7 to 4 a marked salt and time dependent, increase in detergent binding of CT and CT B is observed whereas under similar conditions detergent binding to LT and LT B is not affected. The pH induced detergent binding of CT and CT B is associated with enhanced exposure of the lone Trp 88 of each β-polypeptide chain. The microenvironment of the corresponding Trp 88 in LT B appears to be different as evidenced by its distinct fluorescence properties. Below pH 4.0 CT B and LT B dissociate in their constituent monomers, complexation with GM_1 or oligo-GM_1, however, prevents this dissociation.

KEYWORDS

Cholera toxin, E.coli heat-labile enterotoxin, conformational changes, receptor binding domains.

INTRODUCTION

Cholera toxin (CT; Mr $\sim$84,000) is an oligomeric protein composed of two structural and functional distinct subunits CT A and CT B(Mr $\sim$29,000 and 55,000 respectively). CT B contains five identical polypeptide chains (Mr = 11,600) arranged in a noncovalently associated ring-like pentameric configuration. CT A consists of two polypeptides A_1 or α-chain (Mr= 23,000) and A_2 or γ-chain (Mr= 5,500) linked by a single disulfide bridge. CT action is initiated by rapid binding to the outer cell membrane through interaction between CT B and the monosialoganglioside GM_1 followed by entry of polypeptide A_1 into the cell where it is able to stimulate adenylate cyclase by catalizing the ADP-ribosylation of the $G_{s\alpha}$ subunit of the stimulatory GTP binding regulatory protein. The heat-labile enterotoxin of Escherichia coli (LT) resembles CT not only functionally but structurally and immunologically as well (Clements and co-workers,1980).The B-subunit of LT (LT B) which is responsible for receptor-binding displays significant(79%) amino-acid sequence homology with the B-subunit of CT (CT B) (Dallas and Falkow, 1980). Binding studies and competition experiments, however, indicate that membrane receptors for CT B and LT B are similar but not identical (Holmgren, 1973). The present study is concerned with the effects of environmental factors (pH, ionic strength, reducing agents) on the structure of CT, LT and their respective subunits with the emphasis on the formation or exposure of hydrophobic domains.

RESULTS AND DISCUSSION

Determination of the ratio of intrinsic fluorescence with dibrominated Bry 96(F) relative to that with unbrominated Bry 96(F_0), at neutral pH and in the presence of 0.2 M NaCl reveals that CT A has a somewhat higher affinity for this mild detergent than intact CT and CT B. Receptor (GM_1 or oligo-GM_1) binding has no influence on the very low detergent binding of CT and CT B. Activation of CT A by treatment with dithiothreitol (20 mM) does also not affect detergent binding. Detergent binding of CT A is only slightly pH dependent whereas upon lowering the pH, detergent binding to CT or CT B becomes significant. In the pH range 6.5 to 4.2 a gradual increase in detergent binding to CT and CT B occurs. In the narrow pH range 4.2 - 4.0 a sharp and time dependent enhancement of Br-Bry 96 quenching is observed. These data suggest the presence of a pH induced conformational change unmasking or forming hydrophobic domains on the CT surface.

The increased quenching with Br-Bry 96 might be the result of either the enhanced accessibility (exposure) of Trp 88 of each β-polypeptide chain of CT B or/ and enhanced binding of detergent. Solute quenching experiments with the neutral quencher acrylamide reveal that upon lowering the pH to 5.0 a marked increase in the exposure of the lone Trp 88 residue in each β-polypeptide chain of CT B occurs. The Br-Bry 96 quenching as a function of pH, however, displays a different profile. Maximal quenching is observed below pH 5.0 indicating that the hydrophobicity is increased independently of further exposure of Trp 88.

In contrast to CT, LT is not quenched by Br-Bry 96 (0.1%) even at pH 4.0 . LT B and LT A display a similar rather low affinity for Bry 96 which is not enhanced at pH 4.0. Activation of LT A, however, significantly enhances detergent binding. These data therefore provide no evidence for a pH induced conformational change unmasking or forming hydrophobic domains on LT or LT B. Moreover, no pH induced increase in exposure of the Trp 88 residue of the β-polypeptide chains of LT B is observed. As previously shown for CT (De Wolf and co-workers,1981), this lone Trp 88 appears to be an important determinant in the association of LT with GM_1. The microenvironments of the Trp 88 residues in CT B and LT B are however distinct as reflected by differences in several fluorescence properties (emission maxima, lifetimes, quenching constants, fluorimetric titration profiles).

Below pH 4.0 a progressive dissociation of CT B and LT B is observed as monitored by the decrease in fluorescence anisotropy (r_s) of dansylated CT B and LT B and coincident changes in elution volumes after gelfiltration on a Biogel P60 column. At 25°C and pH 3.2 dissociation of CT B is first order with time displaying a rate constant of 0.150 min^{-1}. Complex formation with GM_1 or oligo-GM_1 prevents the dissociation of CT B and LT B into its constituent monomers. This stabilizing effect of bound GM_1 (oligo-GM_1) is probably the result of shielding from protonation of amino acid residues committed to subunit association and/or crosslinking of the β-polypeptide chains. This further supports the contention that the binding sites of CT as well as LT are clefts formed by two adjacent polypeptide chains.

REFERENCES

Clements, J. D., R. J. Yaucy, and A. Finkelstein (1980). Properties of homogeneous heat-labile enterotoxin from Escherichia coli. Infect. Immun., 29, 91-97

Dallas, W. S., and S. Falkow (1980). Amino acid sequence homology between cholera toxin and Escherichia coli heat-labile toxin. Nature (London), 288, 499-501

De Wolf, M. J. S., M. Fridkin, M. Epstein, and L. D. Kohn (1981). Structure function studies of cholera toxin and its A and B protomers. Modification of tryptophan residues. J. Biol. Chem. , 256, 5481- 5488

Holmgren, J.(1973). Comparison of the tissue receptors for Vibro cholerae and Escherichia coli enterotoxins by means of gangliosides and natural cholera toxoid. Infect. Immun. 8, 851- 859

This work was supported by grant 5RO1AM32136-03 from the NIADDKD, NIH, USA and grant 3.0083.87 from FGWO Belgium

Fehrenbach et al. (Eds.), Bacterial Protein Toxins, Zbl. Bakt. Suppl. 17
© Gustav Fischer, Stuttgart, New York, 1988

An Investigation of Relationships between Structure and Insecticidal Specificity for a Bacillus Thuringiensis Aizawai Delta-Endotoxin

M. Z. Haider and D. J. Ellar

Department of Biochemistry, University of Cambridge, Tennis Court Road, Cambridge, CB 2 1QW, England

ABSTRACT

The mechanism of action and receptor binding of a dual specificity Bacillus thuringiensis aizawai, ICI δ-endotoxin was studied using insect cell culture. The native protoxin was radiolabelled with ^{125}1, proteolytically activated and the affinity of resulting preparations for insect cell membrane proteins was studied by blotting. The activated native B. thuringiensis δ-endotoxin and a cloned toxin from aizawai 1C1 bound to specific membrane receptors in different cells. D-glucose completely inhibited the toxicity of trypsin-activated native aizawai 1C1 preparation to the Mamestra brassicae cells suggesting the role of this carbohydrate in toxin-receptor interaction.

KEY WORDS

Bacillus thuringiensis, Cytolytic, δ-endotoxin, insect cells, Membrane receptor.

INTRODUCTION

There are currently in excess of 1000 B. thuringiensis strains deposited in culture collections. The protein δ-endotoxins they produce show considerable variation in toxicity spectrum in vivo and in vitro and are composed of polypeptides encompassing a broad size range (Calabrese and co-workers, 1980; Huber and co-workers, 1981). Differences in insecticidal specificity have been attributed variously to quantitative differences in δ-endotoxin production, the presence of unique polypeptides and differences in the biochemistry of larval midgut between various insect groups (Yamamoto and McLaughlin, 1981; Haider and co-workers, 1986). We have previously shown that a change in the specificity of var. aizawai 1C1 δ-endotoxin is accompanied by removal of approximately 15 amino acids by host gut proteases (Haider and co-workers, 1986). In the present study ^{125}1 labelled activated var. aizawai 1C1 δ-endotoxin was blotted against insect cell membranes to identify the membrane receptor(s). The lepidopteran-specific preparation (containing 58 and 55 kDa polypeptides) bound to two (120 and 68 kDa) membrane proteins in the lepidopteran cells and none in the

dipteran cells. The dipteran-specific preparation (53 kDa polypeptide) bound to a 90 kDa membrane protein only in the Aedes albopictus cells and to none of the proteins either in the lepidopteran or Drosophila melanogaster cells. This data strongly suggests that the initial action of the activated toxin at the target cell membrane is a specific binding/interaction with a receptor which determines the specifity of the toxin. Another interesting feature of these studies is that although the 53 kDa polypeptide is derived from the 55 kDa polypeptide (Haider and co-workers, 1986), it binds to a different receptor.
This suggests that a change in protein conformation caused by removal of approximately 15 amino acids alters receptor specificity of δ-endotoxin. A cloned aizawai 1C1 crystal protein was purified from Escherichia coli (Haider and co-workers, 1987; Haider and Ellar, 1987), activated and its toxicity and affinity for membrane proteins was studied. The trypsin-activated cloned toxin (55 kDa) bound to 68 kDa membrane protein in the lepidopteran cells.
The identification of these membrane proteins with affinity for the activated toxin prompted further experiments to test the possibility that these putative toxin receptors may be glycoconjugates. This was studied by preincubating susceptible M. brassicae cells with various sugars before addition of toxin. Of a range of sugars tested only D-glucose and raffinose were found to inhibit the toxicity completely. Lactose, sucrose, lactulose and maltose (dissacharides) gave only partial protection whereas monosaccharides (ribose, mannitol, arabinose, D-glucosides and L-glucose) had no protective effect. Protection by D-glucose is possible due to its being part of toxin receptor while the protective effect of di and trisaccharides (which have high viscometric radii than monosaccharides) is a general osmotic effect consistent with the colloid osmotic lysis mechanism proposed for other B. thuringiensis δ-endotoxins (Ellar and co-workers, 1986; Knowles and Ellar, 1987).
The dual specificity of B. thuringiensis var. aizawai 1C1 is determined by two unique toxin conformations generated by the proteolytic activation of the protoxin and interaction of the appropriate conformation with its specific receptor leading to colloid osmotic lysis of the cells.

REFERENCES

Calabrese, D.M., Nickerson, K.W. and Lane, L.C. (1980) Can. J. Microbiol. 26: 1006-1010.
Ellar, D.J., Knowles, B.H., Drobniewski, F.A. and Haider, M.Z. (1986) In: Fundamental and Applied Aspects of Invertebrate Pathology (Samson, R.A. and co-workers, eds.) pp7-11. Foundation of the Fourth International Colloquium of Invertebrate Pathology, Wageningen, The Netherlands.
Haider, M.Z., Knowles, B.H. and Ellar, D.J. (1986) Eur. J. Biochem. 156: 531-540.
Haider, M.Z., Ward, E.S. and Ellar, D.J. (1987) Gene 52: 285-291.
Haider, M.Z. and Ellar, D.J. (1987) Mol. Microbiol. 1: (in press).
Knowles, B.H. and Ellar, D.J. (1987) Biochim. Biophys. Acta. (in press).
Yamamoto, T. and McLaughlin, R.E. (1981) Biochem. Biophys. Res. Commun. 103: 414-421.

Fehrenbach et al. (Eds.), Bacterial Protein Toxins, Zbl. Bakt. Suppl. 17
© Gustav Fischer, Stuttgart, New York, 1988

Comparison of Bacillus Thuringiensis Delta-Endotoxinns Originating from Different Genes

F. Jaquet[1], M. Geiser[2] and P. Lüthy[1]

[1]Institute of Microbiology, Swiss Federal Institute of Technology, CH-8092 Zürich
[2]Biotechnology Department, CIBA-GEIGY Ltd, CH-4002 Basel

KEYWORDS:

B. thuringiensis, delta-endotoxin, toxicity, genes, monoclonal antibodies.

The many existing B. thuringiensis strains differ not only in their activity towards different insect species, but also in the relative potency of their delta-endotoxins (Jaquet and co-workers, 1987). One of the factors contributing to these differences is the composition of the crystal protein. Depending on the strain, one or more genes are coding for delta-endotoxin. Kronstad and Whiteley (1986) reported that three classes of homologous genes can be distinguished in certain strains of B. thuringiensis on the basis of hybridization experiments using a gene-specific probe: the 4.5-, 5.3-, and 6.6-kb classes.
In the work described below, we used different methods for comparing delta-endotoxins expressed by one, two, or three genes.

All the strains used originate from B. thuringiensis subsp. kurstaki (Table 1).

TABLE 1. List of the Strains Used in this Study

Strain	Genes			Supplied by
HD1-4449	4.5	5.3	6.6	H.T. Dulmage, USDA, Brownsville, Texas, USA
HD1-9		5.3		B.C. Carlton and J.M. Gonzalez (1985)
HD73-4443			6.6	our institute's collection
HD1-4432	4.5	5.3	6.6	our institute's collection
HD1-CG1	4.5			CIBA-GEIGY, Ltd, Basel, Switzerland
HD1-CG2	4.5	5.3		CIBA-GEIGY, Ltd, Basel, Switzerland
HD1-CG3	4.5		6.6	CIBA-GEIGY, Ltd, Basel, Switzerland

The cultures were grown as previously described (Jaquet and co-workers, 1987). The crystals were separated from the spores according to the method of Mahillon and Delcour (1984). Solubilization of the crystals, production of toxin, and bioassays were performed as previously described (Jaquet and co-workers, 1987). ELISA was carried out according to Huber-Lukac and co-workers (1986). The method of Laemmli (1970) was used for SDS-PAGE.

Indirect ELISA was used to test the avidity of 10 monoclonal antibodies (MAbs), produced previously against the protoxin from strain HD1-4432 (Huber-Lukac and co-workers, 1986), for protoxin and toxin of the different strains. No difference could be detected between the reference strain HD1-4432 and the strains HD1-4449, HD1-9, HD1-CG1, HD1-CG2, and HD1-CG3. Only strain HD73-4443 showed a different reaction: 5 out of the 10 MAbs showed crossrection with the protoxin, and one with the toxin.

On SDS-PAGE, the molecular weights (MW) of the protoxins were as follows: 135,000 for the strains HD1-CG1, HD1-CG2, HD1-CG3, and HD73-4443; 130,000 for the strain HD1-9; a broad band of 130,000-135,000 was observed for the strains HD1-4449 and HD1-4432. These results are in line with The SDS-PAGE patterns observed by Whiteley and co-workers (1985). On the other hand, a single band of MW about 60,000 was found for the toxins of all the strains.

Bioassays performed by force-feeding of fifth-instar larvae of Pieris brassicae disclosed no significant differences between the strains.

It can be concluded that differences among delta-endotoxins encoded by different genes are difficult to detect by analysis of the molecular weights and immunological reactivity with monoclonal antibodies. Furthermore, these differences have little influence on the insecticidal activity against Pieris brassicae larvae, perhaps because of a competition for the same receptor on the target cell. Moreover, microscopical observations allow the statement that a strain containing three genes does not produce significantly more toxin than a strain harboring only a single gene.

Carlton, B.C., and J.M.Gonzalez (1985). Plasmids and delta-endotoxin production in different subspecies of Bacillus thuringiensis. In: J.A.Hoch and P.Setlow (Ed.), Molecular Biology of Microbial Differentiation. American Society for Microbiology, Washington, D.C., pp. 246-252.

Huber-Lukac, M., F.Jaquet, P.Lüthy, R.Hütter, and D.G.Braun (1986). Characterization of monoclonal antibodies against a crystal protein of Bacillus thuringiensis subsp. kurstaki. Infect. Immun., 54, 228-232.

Jaquet, F., R.Hütter, and P.Lüthy (1987). Specificity of Bacillus thuringiensis delta-endotoxin. Appl. Environ. Microbiology, 53, 500-504.

Laemmli, U.K. (1970). Cleavage of structural proteins during the assembly of the head of Bacteriophage T4. Nature (London), 227, 680-685.

Mahillon, J., and J.Delcour (1984). A convenient procedure for the preparation of highly purified parasporal crystals of Bacillus thuringiensis. J. Microbiol. Methods, 3, 69-76.

Kronstad, J.W., and H.R.Whiteley (1986). Three classes of homologous Bacillus thuringiensis crystal protein genes. Gene, 43, 29-40.

Whiteley, H.R., J.W.Kronstad, and H.E.Schnepf (1985). Structure and expression of cloned Bacillus thuringiensis toxin genes. In: J.A.Hoch and P.Setlow (Ed.), Molecular Biology of Microbial Differentiation. American Society for Microbiology, Washington, D.C., pp. 225-229.

Fehrenbach et al. (Eds.), Bacterial Protein Toxins, Zbl. Bakt. Suppl. 17
© Gustav Fischer, Stuttgart, New York, 1988

Structure-Function Relationships of the S1 Subunit of Pertussis Toxin: Biochemical and Genetic Approaches

J. M. Keith, W. Cieplak, C. Locht and H. Sato[1]

National Institute of Allergy and Infectious Diseases, Laboratory of Pathobiology, Molecular Pathobiology Section, Rocky Mountain Laboratories, Hamilton, MT 59840 USA
[1]National Institute of Health, Tokyo, Japan

The S1 and S2 subunits of pertussis toxin were expressed in Escherichia coli under lac operon transcription and translation control using pUC8 and pUC18 as expression vectors. Various versions of the subunits were detected using anti-S1 or anti-S2 monoclonal antibodies. Recombinant S1, but not S2 subunit, contained the enzymatic NAD-glycohydrolase and NAD:Gi ADP-ribosyltransferase activities. Both activities were also expressed by a truncated version of the S1 subunit in which the 48 carboxy-terminal amino acid residues, including a predicted Rossman structure and one of the two cysteines, had been deleted. The epitope for an anti-S2 monoclonal antibody was localized to the N-terminal 40 amino acid region of the S2 subunit. Both the S1 and S2 subunits expressed in E. coli reacted with human hyperimmune serum. The full length and the truncated recombinant S1 subunit were also found to react in Western blots with a neutralizing and protective monoclonal anti-S1 antibody. The different versions of S1 and S2 subunits expressed in E. coli are useful for mapping active sites, epitopes and regions that interact with receptors or the other subunits in the holotoxin. These recombinant subunits will also facilitate the development of a safer, new-generation vaccine against whooping cough.

Fehrenbach et al. (Eds.), Bacterial Protein Toxins, Zbl. Bakt. Suppl. 17
© Gustav Fischer, Stuttgart, New York, 1988

Two 130 KDa Toxins in the Crystalline Inclusion from a Single Strain of Bacillus Thuringiensis Differ in their Specificity

B. H. Knowles and D. J. Ellar

University of Cambridge, Department of Biochemistry, Tennis Court Road,
Cambridge, CB2 1QW, UK

ABSTRACT

The crystalline protein inclusions synthesised by strains of Bacillus thuringiensis (Bt) during sporulation contain one or more polypeptides in the form of inactive protoxins. These δ-endotoxins are active against insect larvae from orders Lepidoptera, Diptera or Coleoptera. Bt var. aizawai is of particular interest because of its toxicity towards pests from the genus Spodoptera (Kalfon and de Barjac, 1985; Lecadet and Martouret, 1987) which are relatively insensitive to other Bt toxins.
We describe here an indirect method of assessing the relative contribution to toxicity of 2 different but related 130 kDa δ-endotoxins from var. aizawai HD-249. Our results show that when activated one toxin is active against Choristoneura fumiferana CF1 cells in vitro while the other lyses Spodoptera frugiperda cells, suggesting that in this strain there is no synergistic or additive relationship for in vitro toxicity.

KEYWORDS

Bacillus thuringiensis, δ-endotoxin, insecticide, toxin specificity.

INTRODUCTION

Var. aizawai HD-249, like most Bt strains, produces more than one δ-endotoxin of around 130 kDa, which are difficult to separate using standard methods. To date, therefore, it has not been possible to determine the relative contribution of these proteins to toxicity, for example whether they act in an independent or synergistic manner (Whiteley and Schnepf, 1986). Even in the cases where individual toxins have been cloned, bioassays have usually been confined to a single insect species.
The two major 130 kDa crystal proteins from HD-249 were solubilised in 50 mM sodium carbonate/HCl pH 9.5 and 10 mM dithiothreitol, and these protoxins activated with Pieris brassicae gut extract (Knowles and colleagues, 1984). Activation yielded protease-resistant products of 65 and 60 kDa. Antisera against the 60 kDa toxin of var. kurstaki HD-1 (Knowles and colleagues, 1986) reacted predominantly with the 60 kDa toxin of HD-249, and neutralised toxicity against C. fumiferana but not S.frugiperda cells in vitro. Antisera specific to the 65 kDa toxin of HD-249 were purified by affinity chromatography on an HD-229-Sepharose column. These neutralised toxicity against S. frugiperda but not C fumiferana cells in vitro. (HD-229 contains predominantly a 65 kDa active fragment).

These data show that the 130 kDa δ-endotoxins of var. aizawai HD-249 give rise on activation to two distinct toxins, one of 60 kDa active against C. fumiferana cells and one of 65 kDa active against S. frugiperda cells in vitro. Immunoblotting of crystal protoxins suggests that the 60 kDa toxin is derived from a 130 kDa protoxin while the 65 kDa toxin is produced from a 135 kDa protoxin. These results, together with those of Lecadet and Martouret (1987) and Lecadet and colleagues (1986), provide support for the proposal that in vitro toxicity may be related to in vivo activity towards Spodoptera spp. A 130690 Da toxin from var. aizawai that has recently been cloned and sequenced (Oeda and colleagues, 1987) differs from a var kurstaki toxin by only 8 amino acids. It seems likely that this toxin would give rise to a 60 kDa active fragment that cross-reacts with antisera to var. kurstaki 60 kDa toxin.

ACKNOWLEDGEMENTS

We thank Dr. T. Yamamoto for helpful advice on affinity chromatography.

REFERENCES

Kalfon, A.R. and de Barjac, H. (1985) Screening of the insecticidal activity of B. thuringiensis strains against the cotton leafworm Spodoptera littoralis. Entomophaga, 30, 176-185.

Knowles, B.H., Thomas, W.E. and Ellar, D.J. (1984). Lectin-like binding of Bacillus thuringiensis var. kurstaki lepidopteran-specific toxin is an initial step in insecticidal action. FEBS Lett., 168, 197-202.

Knowles, B.H., Francis, P.H. and Ellar, D.J. (1986) Structurally related Bacillus thuringiensis δ-endotoxins display major differences in insecticidal activity in vivo and in vitro. J. Cell Sci., 84, 221-236.

Lecadet, M-M, Martouret, D., Sanchis, V. and Lereclus, D. (1986) What about the δ-endotoxin genes in B. thuringiensis strains active against Spodoptera littoralis? In "Fundamental and Applied Aspects of Invertebrate Pathology" ed. Samson, R.A., Vlak, J.M. and Peters, D. p.397. Foundation IV Int. Coll. Invert. Pathol., Wageningen, NL.

Lecadet, M-M. and Martouret, D. (1987) Host specificity of the Bacillus thuringiensis δ-endotoxin towards Lepidopteran species: Spodoptera littoralis Bdv. and Pieris brassicae L. J. Invertebr. Pathol., 49, 37-48.

Oeda, K., Oshie, K., Shimizu, M., Nakamura, K., Yamamoto, H., Nakayama, I. and Ohkawa, H. (1987) Nucleotide sequence of the insecticidal protein gene of Bacillus thuringiensis strain aizawai IPL7 and its high-level expression in Escherichia coli. Gene, 53, 113-119.

Whiteley, H.R. and Schnepf, H.E. (1986) The molecular biology of parasporal crystal body formation in Bacillus thuringiensis. Ann. Rev. Micribiol., 40, 549-576.

Fehrenbach et al. (Eds.), Bacterial Protein Toxins, Zbl. Bakt. Suppl. 17
© Gustav Fischer, Stuttgart, New York, 1988

Structure and Function of Colicin A: A Model of a Pore from Excitable Membranes

F. Pattus[1], B. Dargent[1], A. Tucker[1], D. Tsernoglou[1], F. Heitz[2], M. Collarini[2], G. Amblard[2], D. Cavard[3], V. Crozel[3], D. Baty[3] and C. Lazdunski[3]

[1]European Molecular Biology Laboratory (EMBL), Meyerhof Str. 1, D-6900 Heidelberg
[2]CNRS, F-34000 Montpellier
[3]Centre de Biochimie et de Biologie Moléculaire du C.N.R.S., 31 Chemin Joseph-Aiguier, BP 71, F-13402 Marseille Cedex 9

ABSTRACT

A large number of mutants introducing point mutations and deletions into the COOH-terminal domain of colicin A have been constructed by using site-directed mutagenesis. The COOH-domain carries the channel activity. The mutated colicin A have been purified and their activity in vivo (on sensitive cells) and in vitro (in planar lipid bilayers) has been assayed. Deletions in the region containing putative helices 4, 5 and 6 (predicted to be involved in pore formation) and the transitions (Ala-Asp492, Phe-Pro493) abolished the activity. Some mutations were found to alter characteristic properties of the single channels. The C-terminal thermolysin fragment of colicin A has been crystallized. The crystals diffract to about 2.6Å. This peptide forms an oligomer upon interaction with dimyristoyl-phosphatidylglycerol, a negatively charged phospholipid.

KEYWORDS

Colicin A, bacteriocin, ionic channel, planar bilayers, site-directed mutagenesis, crystal.

INTRODUCTION

Colicins are bactericidal proteins (60,000 MW) encoded in a plasmid and produced by strains of bacteria harbouring the plasmid. Colicin A kills sensitive E.coli cells by binding to a specific receptor located on the outer membrane of the cell, after which it is translocated across the membrane and depolarization of the inner membrane results. We have shown that colicin A forms voltage dependent channels in planar bilayers, quite similar to those from excitable membranes (Pattus and colleagues, 1983a; Collarini and colleagues, 1987). The pore function is carried by the C-terminal end of the colicin (Martinez, Lazdunski and Pattus, 1983). At neutral and basic pH the N-terminus of colicin A most probably interacts with the C-terminal domain carrying the pore structure influencing its voltage dependence. Upon decreasing the pH this interaction, governed by a pK of 5.5, is disrupted leading to an increase in the affinity of colicin A for membranes and the "acidic" form of the pore (Pattus and colleagues, 1983b; Collarini and colleagues, 1987).

RESULTS

On the basis of CD spectroscopy measurements on colicin A and its C-terminal
fragment and predictions from the amino-acid sequence of secondary structure,
hydrophobicity and hydrophobic moment profiles, we could propose two models of
the structure of the pore formed by colicin A. These models were used to design
site-directed mutagenesis experiments on the structural gene of colicin A. Preliminary characterization of these mutants is reported. They suggest that
helices 4, 5 and 6 built the transmembrane lumen of the channel while helices 2
and 3 may be localised at the mouth of the channel.

A new C-terminal fragment of colicin A was purified after thermolysin digestion.
This fragment, which contains the pore-forming activity, has been crystallised.
The crystals diffract to about 2.6Å. Two heavy atom derivatives have been obtained. This peptide is able to form a complex with dimyristoyl-phosphatidylglycerol (DMPG) at acidic pH. This complex is an oligomer containing 25 DMPG
molecules/monomer. As judged by column chromatography, the complex has a radius
of 6-7 nm and may contain as much as 8-10 monomers. CD spectroscopy and chemical
modification experiments showed that the tryptophan environment within the peptide undergoes drastic changes upon binding to DMPG molecules.

REFERENCES

Collarini, M., G. Amblard, C. Lazdunski and F. Pattus (1987) Gating processes of
    channels induced by colicin A, its C-terminal fragment and colicin E$_1$ in planar
    lipid bilayers. Eur. Biophys. J., 14, 147-153.
Martinez, C., C. Lazdunski and F. Pattus (1983) Isolation, molecular and func-
    tional properties of the C-terminal domain of colicin A. EMBO J., 2, 1501-1507.
Pattus, F., D. Cavard, R. Verger, C. Lazdunski, J.P. Rosenbusch and H. Schindler
    (1983a) Formation of voltage dependent pores in planar bilayers by colicin A.
    In: G. Spach (Ed.), Physical Chemistry of Transmembrane Ion Motions. Elsevier,
    Amsterdam, pp.407-413.
Pattus, F., M.C. Martinez, B. Dargent, D. Cavard, R. Verger and C. Lazdunski
    (1983b) Interaction of colicin A with phospholipid monolayers and liposomes.
    Biochemistry, 22, 5698-5703.

Fehrenbach et al. (Eds.), Bacterial Protein Toxins, Zbl. Bakt. Suppl. 17
© Gustav Fischer, Stuttgart, New York, 1988

Separation of Large Hydrophobic Fragments of Protein B (CAMP-Factor)

J. Rühlmann, D. Jürgens, and F. J. Fehrenbach

Robert Koch-Institut des Bundesgesundheitsamtes, Abteilung für Mikrobiologie, Nordufer 20, D-1000 Berlin 65

KEYWORDS: CAMP-factor, protein B, separation of hydrophobic peptides, reversed phase HPLC, CNBr-fragments

Protein B (CAMP-factor), which has been shown to act as co-cytolysin on sensibilized red blood cells and to bind to the Fc-part of immunoglobulins, was cleaved with CNBr in order to obtain smaller fragments for amino acid sequencing and to enable further studies into structure-function relationship of this biologically active polypeptide.

The separation of the resulting CNBr-fragments with molecular weights of 2-, 10- and 15 kDa was complicated by tenacious aggregation of the large hydrophobic fragments.

Due to this aggregation it was impossible to separate the CNBr-fragments by classical gelfiltration procedures in aqueous solution e.g. on sephadex gels. Poor separation was achieved by gelfiltration on Sephadex LH-60 in ethanol : 88 % formic acid (4 : 1, v/v).

Although the use of reversed phase HPLC (RP-HPLC) for purification of polar peptides is well established, the separation of larger hydrophobic peptides remains still difficult.

We report on the succesfull separation of the large hydrophobic CNBr-fragments of protein B by reversed phase HPLC on Nucleosil 300-5 C18 using 0.1 % heptafluorbutyric acid (HFBA) as ion-pairing reagent (Bennett, H.P.J., C.A.Browne, S.Solomin (1980): The use of perfluorinated carboxylic acids in the reversed-phase HPLC of peptides. J.Liquid Chromatogr., 3, 1353-1365).

The efficiency of this separation was mainly due to the use of HFBA as a hydrophobic counterion, because the substitution of HFBA by trifluoracetic acid (TFA) or triethyl-amin-TFA gave unsatisfactory results.

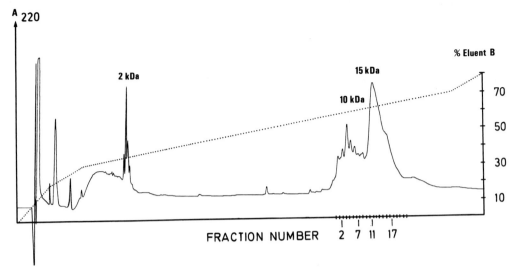

Fig. 1: Separation of the CNBr-fragments of protein B by reversed phase HPLC on Nucleosil 300-5 C18 (column: 250 x 8 mm). Purified protein B was subjected to CNBr-cleavage in 70 % formic acid for 20 h in the dark (CNBr/methionine ratio: 100/1). 0.7 mg protein were applied to the column in 50 µl 6 M guanidine hydrochloride in 0.1 % heptafluorbutyric acid (HFBA). The eluents were: A = 0.1 % HFBA in water, B = 0.08 % HFBA in acetonitrile. Flow rate was 0.5 ml/min. The gradient applied was 0 % B to 20 % B for 10 min, 20 % B to 30 % B for 10 min, 30 % B to 70 % B for 120 min, 70 % B to 80 % B for 10 min. Peptides were detected at 220 nm and 1.0 AUFS. Fractions of 0.5 ml were collected.

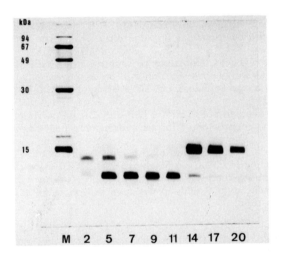

Fig. 2: Analytical SDS-PAGE (T = 15 %, C = 2.7 %) of fractions 2, 5, 7, 9, 11, 14, 17, and 20 (see chrom. fig. 1). 80 µl of each fraction were analysed.
M = marker protein (M_r: 15 - 94 kDa)
In addition to the 10- and 15 kDa-fragments a 13 kDa-fragment is found as a product of partial hydrolysis of an acid labile Asp-Pro peptide bond of protein B cleaved under the acidic conditions used for CNBr-cleavage.

Fehrenbach et al. (Eds.), Bacterial Protein Toxins, Zbl. Bakt. Suppl. 17
© Gustav Fischer, Stuttgart, New York, 1988

Epitope Mapping of Clostridium Perfringens Alpha Toxin

A. D. Shuttleworth, D. A. Percival and R. W. Titball

CDE Porton Down, Salisbury, Wilts, UK, SP4 OJQ

ABSTRACT

A panel of twelve monoclonal antibody-secreting hydrbidomas have been developed
to a formaldehyde-toxoid of the Clostridium perfringens type A alpha toxin. The
monoclonal antibodies were specific for the toxoid, native toxin and genetically
cloned toxin. Competitive binding studies allowed the construction of an
epitope map, illustrating the spatial relationships of the epitopes recognised by
the various antibodies. This indicated that the antibodies were specific for
overlapping epitopes, all lying within a single immunodominant region of the
toxin molecule. Monoclonal antibody 3A4D10 inhibited the toxin's phospholipase
activity in vitro and lethal activity in vivo.

KEYWORDS

Clostridium perfringens alpha toxin, phospholipase C, hybridoma, monoclonal
antibody, epitope mapping.

INTRODUCTION

The alpha toxin of Clostridium perfringens type A is one of the most potent
bacterial phospholipase C's (EC 3.1.4.3) that catalyses the hydrolysis of
lecithin to phosphorylcholine and 1,2-diglyceride (Macfarlane and Knight, 1941).
The alpha toxin has characteristic lethal, haemolytic and dermo-necrotic
properties and these play a central role in the pathophysiology of
Cl. perfringens induced disease (Ispolotovskya, 1971). Despite a detailed
understanding of the biological and biochemical properties of the toxin, it's
structure remains unclear; although an amino acid analysis (Mitsui and co-
workers, 1973) indicates that the structure of the toxin may be quite unusual and
this may explain some of the toxins biochemical properties.

We have investigated the antigenic properties of the toxin using polyclonal and
monoclonal reagents in an attempt to clarify the structure/function relationship
of the toxin and, ultimately, to assess the immunogenicity of cloned toxoids
designed for prophylactic use.

RESULTS AND DISCUSSION

Hyperimmune mouse sera to the alpha toxin were produced by immunising BALB/c mice
with either: sub-lethal doses of low specific activity toxin or with a

formaldehyde toxoid (Ito, 1968., Ito, 1970). Sera raised to both forms of antigen proved specific for native toxin, cloned toxin and toxoid and were used to develop an ELISA assay for the screening of monoclonal antibodies (MAb's).

A panel of twelve hybridoma lines secreting MAb's specific for alpha toxin were produced by fusing hyperimmune splenocytes with X63.Ag8.653 myeloma cells. Antibody secreting clones were selected by growth in hypoxanthine-aminopterin-thymidine (HAT) medium, screened for toxin specificity by ELISA and re-cloned three times to ensure clonality. Suitable hybridomas were expanded _in vitro_ and as ascites. Isotype analysis by ELISA revealed that nine of the twelve MAb's were IgG$_1$, one was IgG$_{2a}$, one IgG$_{2b}$, and one was IgE.

MAb 3A4D10 inhibited the action of the alpha toxin _in vitro_ and increased the time-to-death in mice given a simultaneous 40 LD challenge. This indicates that the epitope recognised by 3A4D10 is the active site of the enzyme, or is at a site sterically linked to the active site.

Competition studies were performed using a two-site immunometric assay and these indicated that the toxin possessed a single immunodominant domain consisting of at least nine overlapping epitopes. This information has been used to produce a "map" of the spatial relationships of these epitopes in relation to the 3-dimensional structure of the toxin.

Comparison of the specificity of the monoclonal antibodies for the native toxin and the cloned toxin demonstrated that the cloned product is immunologically, as well as biochemically similar to the native _Cl. perfringens_ alpha toxin.

Work is in progress to produce further panels of MAb's to the cloned toxin, in order to clarify the degree of similarity between the native toxin, cloned toxin and cloned toxoids.

REFERENCES

Ispoltovskya, M.V. (1971). Type A Clostridium perfringens Toxin. In: Kadis, S., T.C. Montie and S.J. Ajl (Eds.) _Microbial Toxins_, Vol. IIA, 1st ed. Academic Press, New York. pp. 109–149.

Ito, A. (1968). Alpha toxoid of Clostridium perfringens. I. Purification and Toxoiding of the Alpha toxin of Clostridium perfringens. _Jap. J. Med. Sci. Biol._, 21, 379–391.

Ito, A. (1970). Alpha Toxoid of Clostridium perfringens. II. Immunogenicity of the Toxoid. _Jap. J. Med. Sci. Biol._, 23, 21–30.

Macfarlane, M.G., and B.C.J.G. Knight (1941). The Biochemistry of Bacterial Toxins. I. The Lecithinase Activity of Clostridium welchii toxins. _Biochem. J._, 35, 884–902.

Mitsui, K., N. Mitsui, and J. Hase (1973). Clostridium perfringens Exotoxins. I. Purification and properties of alpha toxin. _Jap. J. Exp. Med._, 43, 65–80.

Fehrenbach et al. (Eds.), Bacterial Protein Toxins, Zbl. Bakt. Suppl. 17
© Gustav Fischer, Stuttgart, New York, 1988

Diversity of Structure and Specificity of Mosquitocidal δ-Endotoxins

E. S. Ward, D. J. Earp, B. H. Knowles, S. M. Pinnavaia, C. N. Nicholls, T. J. Sawyer, P. E. Granum and D. J. Ellar

Department of Biochemistry, University of Cambridge, Tennis Court Road, Cambridge, CB2 IQW, England

ABSTRACT

B.thuringiensis produces parasporal crystalline protein inclusions (δ-endotoxins), which have been shown to be toxic to a wide range of lepidopteran, some dipteran and coleopteran larvae (Huber and Luthy, 1981; Krieg et al., 1983). Several of the genes encoding mosquitocidal δ-endotoxins have been cloned (Ward, Ellar and Todd, 1984; Waalwijk et al, 1985; Sekar and Carlton, 1985; Bourgouin, Klier and Rapoport, 1986; Thorne et al., 1986; Haider, Ward and Ellar, 1987) and in some cases the nucleotide sequences of the genes reported. In this report we compare and contrast mosquitocidal δ-endotoxins and present data which, on the basis of molecular weights, immunological studies, toxicity assays and DNA sequences, illustrates the diversity of these proteins.

KEYWORDS

B. thuringiensis, δ-endotoxin, mosquitocidal activity, immunological cross-reactivities, gene sequence.

INTRODUCTION

The δ-endotoxins of B.thuringiensis subsp. israelensis, morrisoni PG14 and PG14/11, darmstadiensis 73E-10-2, kyushuensis, morrisoni HD-12, aizawai HD-249 and aizawai IC1 were analysed by polyacrylamide gel electrophoresis and their molecular weights range from 23 to 140 kDa. The number of polypeptides comprising the crystal of a particular subspecies differs from strain to strain, and the toxicity ranges from 1ng/ml to 100 µg/ml. Immunoblotting reveals several antigenically distinct classes of mosquitocidal δ-endotoxin, both within and between strains. Recent data suggests that unrelated crystal proteins may interact synergistically to enhance toxicity (Wu and Chang, 1985; Chilcott and Ellar, 1987).

For several strains (morrisoni HD-12, aizawai IC1 and HD-249) both lepidopteran and dipteran activity is associated with one or more proteins of Mr 130-140 kDa. Interestingly, these cross-react with antisera raised against the lepidopteran specific P1 protein of subsp. kurstaki. Aizawai HD-249 also has a 63 kDa protein which cross reacts with antisera raised against the mosquitocidal P2 polypeptide of subsp. kurstaki (Yamamoto and McLaughlin, 1981). The in vitro toxicity of the high molecular weight proteins of aizawai IC1, HD-249 and morrisoni HD-12 is confined to certain lepidopteran and dipteran cell lines, and in some cases, reflects the in vivo specificity. Of particular interest in this respect is the differential activation of the aizawai IC1 δ-endotoxin to produce either a dipteran or lepidopteran specific δ-endotoxin from the same polypeptide precursor (Haider, Knowles and Ellar, 1986).

By contrast, the δ-endotoxins produced by israelensis, darmstadiensis and PG14 show broad cytolytic and haemolytic activity in vitro. For israelensis this activity can be attributed to a 25/27 kDa polypeptide (Thomas, 1984; Armstrong, Rohrmann and Beaudreau, 1985), which shows strong immunological cross reactivity with a 27 kDa protein of PG14, but no relatedness to darmstadiensis nor kyushuensis. Thus the determinants of the cytolytic activity of darmstadiensis appear to differ from those of israelensis/PG14. In addition, the PG14 27 kDa gene has recently been cloned and sequenced (Earp and Ellar, 1987) and shown to have an identical sequence to that of israelensis with the exception of a pro >ala change at residue 81. The israelensis and PG14 130 kDa doublet proteins also show strong immunological cross-reactivity. The two genes encoding the subsp. israelensis 130 kDa doublet proteins have been cloned (this communication; Sekar and Carlton, 1985; Bourgouin, Klier and Rapoport, 1986), shown to be mosquitocidal, and sequenced (this communication; Yamamoto et al., 1986). The two proteins share considerable homologies in the C-terminal regions. In addition short stretches of homology shared with the kurstaki P1 sequence (Schnepf, Wong and Whiteley, 1985) have been identified which may account for the weak immunological cross-reaction with P1 antisera. These three proteins (israelensis 130 kDa doublet, kurstaki P1) have N-terminal regions of high hydrophobicity. Interestingly, PG14 has a third high molecular weight crystal protein of Mr 140 kDa which appears to be antigenically related to the israelensis/PG14 130 kDa toxins. Data obtained using a derivative of PG14 which harbours only the 140 kDa polypeptide indicates that this protein has mosquitocidal activity.

Despite the structural diversity of the different mosquitocidal δ-endotoxins, results to date indicate that they share a common cytolytic mechanism involving colloid osmotic lysis. Current work is directed towards cloning and sequencing 130-140 kDa mosquitocidal proteins of B. thuringiensis strains in an attempt to learn more of the structural features which determine their insect specificity and potency.

References cited in the text are obtainable from the corresponding author (*) upon request.

Toxin Cell Surface Interaction

Fehrenbach et al. (Eds.), Bacterial Protein Toxins, Zbl. Bakt. Suppl. 17
© Gustav Fischer, Stuttgart, New York, 1988

Pore-Forming Bacterial Cytolysins

S. Bhakdi, G. Menestrina, F. Hugo, W. Seeger and J. Tranum-Jensen

Institute of Medical Microbiology, University of Gießen, Frankfurter Str. 107, D-6300 Gießen

ABSTRACT

Many bacterial cytolysins damage target cells by forming hydrophilic pores in the plasma membrane. Membrane-bound pores may exhibit characteristic ultrastructures, or they may be invisible by present-day electron microscopic techniques. Structured pores are found when native protein molecules self-associate on and in the target lipid bilayer to form oligomeric aggregates. Examples include S.aureus α -toxin and the oxygen-labile cytolysins (e.g.streptolysin-O). Pores devoid of characteristic ultrastructure may arise through insertion of protein monomers into the membrane. E.coli hemolysin is the best-studied cytolysin in this category. Pore-formers can invoke profound secondary pathophysiological reactions. Triggering of the arachidonic acid cascade through passive influx of Ca^{2+} through toxin pores probably generally occurs in nucleated cells to elicit a wide spectrum of tisue reactions. Insertion of streptolysin-O into host cell membranes creates nuclei for secondary self-attack reactions by host antibody and complement.Extracellularly located toxins can form soluble, complement-activating immune complexes that may cause local decomplementation, thus diverting the protective action of host complement away from the bacteria. These diverse, direct and indirect effects of bacterial cytolysins can together account for many pathophysiological phenomena that are encountered in the pathogenesis of bacterial infections.

KEYWORDS

Pore-forming toxins, S.aureus   α-toxin, streptolysin-O, E.coli hemolysin, arachidonate metabolism, complement activation.

INTRODUCTION

The concept of pore-forming proteins has been reviewed recently (Bhakdi and Tranum-Jensen, 1987), and we will therefore confine the present discussion to most recent findings on S.aureus α-toxin, streptolysin-O (SLO), and E.coli hemolysin.
Common features. All pore-forming cytolysins are primarily water-soluble proteins that are secreted by viable bacteria. Upon gaining contact with a target lipid bilayer, they undergo conformational changes that lead to a hydrophilic-amphiphilic transition, enabling their spontaneous penetration into the membrane. We envisage one surface of the membrane-embedded protein to interact via hydrophobic forces

with membrane lipids, whilst the other repels lipids due to its hydrophilic character. As a result, stable transmembrane pores are generated that allow passive flux of ions and small molecules across the bilayer. Such lesions will cause cytolysis of cells that are devoid of membrane turn-over and repair mechanisms such as erythrocytes. In general, nucleated cells can probably repair a limited number of lesions, but ion fluxes across the transiently formed pores may nevertheless trigger secondary reactions which are of pathophysiological relevance in the organism.

One category of pore-formers presents structures that are visible in the electron microscope as arc or rings. These pores arise through non-covalent aggregation of toxin protomers in the bilayer to form supramolecular oligomers (e.g. S.aureus α-toxin and SLO). Other pore-formers such as E.coli hemolysin probably represent monomeric channels and they are not detectable by present-day electron microscopic techniques.

S.AUREUS α-TOXIN

This cytolysin is produced as a single-chained polypeptide of M 34 000 by most strains of S.aureus and is an important factor of bacterial pathogenicity (Bernheimer, 1974; McCartney and Arbuthnott, 1978; Rogolsky, 1979). The toxin probably initially interacts with the choline head group of phosphatidylcholine in the target membrane (Watanabe et al, 1987). The nature of this interaction is under study; it does not display characteristics of a receptor-ligand interaction and appears to be influenced by local membrane factors including surface charge and membrane composition. For example, the presence of cholesterol at molar ratios $\geqslant 0.1:1$ greatly enhances the efficiency of toxin-binding and pore-formation in phosphatidylcholine liposomes.

The process of membrane-binding of α-toxin is temperature-independent. When offered to target rabbit erythrocytes at 0°C in low concentrations ($\sim 10^{-8}$M), the toxin initially absorbs in its monomeric form to the cells. Net binding is ineffective, in the order of 4-8% of toxin offered. When cells are washed in the cold and then re-incubated at 37°C, cell-bound toxin oligomerizes to form predominantly hexamers, and this process coincides with functional pore formation and hemolysis (Reichwein et al, 1987). The use of a very sensitive ELISA has led to an estimate that the formation of less than 10 hexamers per cell induces one functional "hit" (hemolytic lesion)/erythrocyte (Reichwein et al, 1987; Hugo et al, 1987). In essence, this fulfills a one-hit-one-hole prediction derived from the pore concept of toxin action (Füssle et al, 1981; Bhakdi et al,1984a ; Bhakdi and Tranum-Jensen, 1987).

Other cell species, e.g. human erythrocytes, are much less susceptible to lysis by α-toxin. This appears to be due to the inability of the toxin to gain access and absorb to the phosphatidylcholine molecules unless a critical threshold concentration is reached. When the required threshold is exceeded, however, the toxin will bind to human erythrocytes in similar amounts as to rabbit erythrocytes. Hence, α-toxin will never bind in small numbers to human erythrocytes or to other relatively unsusceptible cells : either no binding takes place at all, or a large number of toxin molecules abruptly bind to and lyse the cells.

In accord with the concept of absorptive binding to phosphatidylcholine, α-toxin has also been found to bind to plasma low density lipoprotein (Bhakdi et al, 1983). Hexamerisation on the lipoprotein molecules cause toxin inactivation because the amphiphilic oligomers are unable to dissociate from lipid and cross the water-phase to gain access to target cells. S.aureus α-toxin will also bind to and perturb lipid monolayers (Buckelew and Colacicco, 1971), liposomes (Freer et al, 1968; Arbuthnott et al, 1973), and planar lipid bilayers (Menestrina, 1986).

Many model experiments on the action of α-toxin on nucleated cells have shown thatprofound secondary reactions are elicited, for example, because of Ca^{2+}-influx and triggering of Ca^{2+}-dependent cellular processes. These include the stimulation of arachidonate metabolism (Seeger et al, 1984; Suttorp et al, 1985, 1987), as well as triggering of exocytotic processes in secretory cells (Ahnert-Hilger et al, 1985; Bader et al, 1986). Indeed, experiments with chromaffin cells indicate that α-toxin can become a useful tool to study the minimal requirements for exocytosis (Ahnert-Hilger et al, 1985; Bader et al, 1986).

STREPTOLYSIN-O

This toxin represents the prototype of sulfhydryl-activated, oxygen-labile cytolysins, and we expect that many of the properties found for SLO will also be extendable to other toxins in this category (Bernheimer, 1974; Smyth and Duncan, 1978; Alouf, 1980). SLO is secreted as a single polypeptide chain. The molecular weight is 69 000, the pI 6.4 (Bhakdi et al,1984b). Toxin monomers bind firmly to cholesterol molecules in the target cell membrane (Smyth and Duncan, 1978; Alouf, 1980). Pore formation occurs when the toxin-cholesterol complexes collide in the membrane through lateral aggregation (Hugo et al, 1986). Presumably, toxin-toxin contact triggers a conformational change that cause unfolding of the molecule and membrane insertion. This process is probably analogous to pore-formation by staphylococcal α-toxin. The pores generated by SLO are very large, and may approach 35 nm diameter (see Duncan, 1974; Duncan and Schlegel, 1975; Buckingham and Duncan, 1982; Bhakdi et al,1985a). They are also very heterogeneous depending on the number of toxin protomers present in an individual lesion (Bhakdi et al, 1985a) We have estimated that between 25-80 toxin molecules may aggregate to form ultrastructurally visible arc- or ring-shaped lesions, whereby aggregates of smaller size may also be present but are then invisible in the electron microscope (Bhakdi et al, 1985a).

One aspect of particular interest is the fact that toxin aggregates which are not fully circularized (i.e. arc structures) may nevertheless form true transmembrane pores due to lateral repellment of lipid from the hydrophilic surface. This contention, if corroborated, would imply that transmembrane pores may in other cases also be lined to a certain extent by an edge of free membrane lipid. It is conceivable that such a principle will be encountered, for example, in cases of pore formation by protein monomers; an obvious candidate is presently the hemolysin of E.coli (see below).

Secondary processes triggered by SLO include the stimulation of arachidonate metabolism (Bremm et al, 1985), and induction of auto-attack by autologous antibody and complement on the target cells (Bhakdi et al, 1985b).Both may be expected to enhance inflammatory reactions and necrosis of infected tissues.

E.COLI HEMOLYSIN

This cytolysin has aroused the interest of bacteriologists for several reasons. First, the high incidence of hemolysin producers amongst human pathogenic E.coli strains indicated that hemolysin production enhances bacterial pathogenicity (for review, see Cavalieri et al, 1984). This contention is supported by many experiments in animal models (e.g. Hacker et al, 1983). Second, the hemolysin is the only protein that is genuinely secreted by E coli. Studies on the mechanism of its secretion would be expected to shed light on the poorly understood mechanism of protein transport across the envelope of Gram-negative organisms. Finally, it has been of interest to elucidate the mechanism of toxin action and to place this in context with its pathogenic potential. Recent reviews have covered the molecular genetics of toxin production and secretion (Cavalieri et al, 1984; Mackman et al, 1986), and we will here focus on new evidence concerning the mechanism of toxin action.

Only recently did it become possible to obtain substantial amounts of toxin in active form. Whereas earlier studies reported a molecular weight of 60 000 for native toxin, it became evident that the 60 K polypeptide represents a degradation product; the molecular weight of active hemolysin established by SDS-PAGE and nucleotide sequence analysis is 107-110 000 (Mackman and Holland, 1984; Gonzalez-Carrero et al, 1985; Felmlee et al, 1985). The toxin molecule contains three hydrophobic domains between residues 200 and 400, and has an overall negative charge. The N-terminus does not contain a typical secretion signal sequence and the molecule is not proteolytically processed at either the N- or the C-terminus during secretion to the medium (Felmlee et al, 1985). All the information for secretion of the toxin appears to reside within the terminal 30-50 amino acids (Nicaud et al, 1986; Gray et al, 1986; Mackman et al, 1987).

In a recent study regarding the mechanism of toxin action, Jorgensen et al (1983) detected a rapid influx of extracellular Ca^{2+} into toxin-treated erythrocytes, and accordingly suggested that the toxin acted in a manner akin to a calcium ionophore. Cell-lysis was thought to ensue through secondary effects triggered by influx of Ca^{2+} into the erythrocytes. Studies from our laboratory indicate, however, that E.coli hemolysin produces genuine transmembrane pores of a more non-specific nature. Hemolysis could be inhibited by the addition of Dextran (M_r 4000) to the medium, and ensued after removal of the osmotic protectant (Bhakdi et al, 1986). This demonstrated that hemolysis was due to osmotic swelling and rupture of the cells. Measurements of K^+-efflux and marker influx into the cells under osmotic protection were undertaken, and it was found that rapid K^+-efflux occurred which was essentially complete within 1 min at 25-37°C. Concomitantly, influx of small marker molecules including Ca^{2+} and sucrose was noted. From these data, we concluded that E.coli hemolysin formed pores of approximately 2 nm effective diameter in erythrocyte membranes (Bhakdi et al, 1986).

When erythrocyte membranes lysed with E.coli hemolysin were solubilized with non-denaturing detergent (deoxycholate) and the solubilisates centrifuged through sucrose density gradients, all toxin was recovered as a monomer in the upper gradient fractions. Hence, the cytolysin did not form detergent-stable oligomeric aggregates similar to those previously described for complement, S aureus α-toxin, sulfhydryl-activated cytolysins, and lymphocytolysins (for review, see Bhakdi and Tranum-Jensen, 1987). These results suggested that E coli hemolysin might represent a novel type of pore-forming bacterial cytolysin that inserted as a monomer into mammalian cell membranes (Bhakdi et al, 1986)

Recent studies in planar lipid membranes have provided conclusive support of the pore concept (Menestrina et al, submitted for publication) E coli hemolysin was applied to voltage-clamped lipid bilayers consisting of phosphatidylcholine and phosphatidylethanolamine. Within a few minutes, current steps of homogeneous size were observed that indicated the formation of ion channels in the membrane. The conductivity measurements led to an estimate of effective pore diameter of approximately 1.5 nm, assuming a pore length of 5-7 nm. In contrast to pores formed by S.aureus α-toxin (Menestrina, 1986), the E.coli hemolysin channel displayed a selectivity of cations over anions. Furthermore, channel-opening was dependent on the presence of a correct transmembrane potential : channels opened when the trans-side was negative relative to the cis (application) side, and closed when the trans-voltage became positive ($\geq$ 5 mV) relative to the cis-side. In this respect, E.coli hemolysin displayed similarities to pore-forming colicins. Clear one-hit dose-response curves were obtained in this experimental system, indicating that individual pores are indeed formed by insertion of single toxin molecules into the bilayer.

Since E.coli hemolysin can attack bilayers of pure phosphatidylcholine, it is apparent that surface membrane protein or glycoprotein receptors are not essential for its action. In this respect, E.coli hemolysin resembles the S aureus α-toxin, and we currently place both in the category of "receptorless" cytolysins.

When applied to isolated, ventilated and perfused, blood-free rabbit lungs, E.coli hemolysin causes a dose-dependent release of potassium into the recirculating medium within a few minutes, accompanied by an acute rise in pulmonary artery pressure. Experiments in calcium-free buffer fluid in the presence of cyclooxygenase inhibitors, thromboxane-synthetase inhibitors, and thromboxane-receptor antagonist, together with measurements of toxin-induced lung prostanoid generation indicate a sequelae of events similar to those following application of S.aureus α-toxin in rabbit lungs (Seeger et al, 1984). Transmembrane shift, probably occurring via toxin-created pores, induces stimulation of arachidonate metabolism in lung target cells, and vasoconstriction ensues due to pulmonary generation of thromboxane A2, which surpasses the vasodilatory effect of simultaneously generated prostaglandin I2. In addition to pulmonary hypertension, E.coli hemolysin causes a second pathophysiological event in the rabbit lung which occurs 20 to 60 min after its application and is independent of the cytolysin-induced pressor response. There is a delayed increase in lung weight gain due to edema formation, and measurements of the capillary filtration coefficient and the vascular compliance of the lungs reveal a severalfold increase in the hydraulic conductivity of the pulmonary vasculature. This induction of lung vascular leakage is not reversed by the exchange of lung perfusate with toxin-free buffer, and its underlying mechanisms have not yet been established (Seeger et al, submitted for publication). The capacity of E.coli hemolysin to cause pulmonary edema may well be pathophysiologically relevant to the pathogenesis of pulmonary complications arising during severe infections with toxin-producing organisms.

CONCLUDING REMARKS

The concept of damage to mammalian cell membranes by pore-forming proteins is well documented. New pore-formers are being increasingly recognized, and the spectrum of producers is already known to range from prokaryonts to plants and lower parasitic, as well as mammalian cells. Of these, pore-forming bacterial cytolysins represent some of the best-studied prototypes. Although the first pore-formers to be discovered were those exhibiting typical ultrastructures, it should be stressed that many, and perhaps even the majority of other proteinaceous pores may not present characteristic structures that are detectable by present-day electron-microscopic techniques. Irrespective of whether a pore-former belongs to the oligomerizing category or not, it must be endowed with the unique property of undergoing a hydrophilic-amphiphilic transition upon gaining contact with the target membrane, and be able to subsequently to insert into the bilayer. Despite the rapid progress that is being made at a molecular genetic level, with the amino acid sequences of several pore-formers already available (Gray and Kehoe, 1984; Felmlee et al, 1985), a molecular model for the insertion process has not yet been constructed for any pore-former. With regard to their biological relevance, it is apparent that pore-forming bacterial cytolysins may elicit a wide spectrum of potentially detrimental cellular reactions due to their entry into host cell membranes and perturbation of the membrane permeability barrier. Further study of such secondary reactions will undoubtedly deepen our understanding of the pathogenesis of bacterial infections.

ACKNOWLEDGEMENTS

Work referred to in this review was supported by the Deutsche Forschungsgemeinschaft (Bh 2/2) and the Verband der Chemischen Industrie.

REFERENCES

Ahnert-Hilger, G., S.Bhakdi, and M.Gratzl (1985). Minimal requirements for exocytosis: a study using PC 12 cells permeabilized with staphylococcal α-toxin.
J.Biol.Chem., 260, 12730-12734.

Alouf, J.E. (1980).Streptococcal toxins. Pharmacol.Ther.,11, 661-717.

Arbuthnott, J.P., J.H.Freer, and B.Bilcliffe (1973). Lipid-induced polymerization
of staphylococcal α-toxin. J.Gen.Microbiol.,75, 309-319.

Bader,M.F., D.Thierse, D.Aunis, G.Ahnert-Hilger, and M.Gratzl (1986). Characterization of hormone and protein release from α-toxin permeabilized chromaffin
cells in primary culture. J.Biol.Chem., 261, 5777-5783.

Bernheimer, A.W. (1974). Interactions between membranes and cytolytic bacterial
toxins. Biochim.Biophys.Acta,344, 27-50.

Bhakdi,S., R.Füssle, G.Utermann, and J.Tranum-Jensen (1983). Binding and partial
inactivation of S.aureus α-toxin by human plasma low density lipoprotein.
J.Biol.Chem., 258, 5899-5904.

Bhakdi,S., M.Muhly, and R.Füssle (1984a).Correlation between toxin-binding and
hemolytic activity in membrane damage by staphylococcal α-toxin. Infect.Immun.,
46, 318-323.

Bhakdi,S., M.Roth, A.Sziegoleit, and J.Tranum-Jensen (1984b). Isolation and
identification of two hemolytic forms of streptolysin-O. Infect.Immun., 46,
394-400

Bhakdi,S., J.Tranum-Jensen, and A.Sziegoleit (1985a).Mechanism of membrane damage
by streptolysin-O. Infect.Immun., 47, 52-60.

Bhakdi,S. and J.Tranum-Jensen (1985b). Complement activation and attack on autologous cells induced by streptolysin-O. Infect.Immun., 48, 713-719.

Bhakdi,S., N.Mackman, J.M.Nicaud, and I.B.Holland (1986). E.coli hemolysin may
damage target cell membranes by generating transmembrane pores. Infect.Immun.,
52, 63-69.

Bhakdi,S. and J.Tranum-Jensen (1987). Damage to mammalian cells by proteins that
form transmembrane pores. Rev.Physiol.Biochem.Pharmacol.,107, 147-223.

Buckelew,A.R. and G.Colaccico (1971). Lipid monolayers. Interaction with staphylococcal α-toxin. Biochim.Biophys.Acta, 233, 7-16.

Buckingham, L. and J.L.Duncan (1983). Approximate dimensions of membrane lesions
produced by streptolysin-S and streptolysin-O. Biochim.Biophys.Acta, 729,115-122.

Cavalieri, S.J., G.A.Bohach, and I.S.Snyder (1984). Escherichia coli α-hemolysin:
characteristics and probable role in pathogenicity. Microbiol.Rev., 48,326-343.

Duncan,J.L. (1974). Characteristics of streptolysin-O hemolysis: kinetics of
hemoglobin and 86-rubidium release. Infect.Immun., 9, 1022-1027.

Duncan, J.L. and R.Schlegel (1975). Effect of streptolysin-O on erythrocyte membranes, liposomes, and lipid dispersions. J.Cell Biol., 67, 160-173.

Felmlee, T., S.Pellet, and R.Welch (1985). Nucleotide sequence of an Escherichia
coli chromosomal hemolysin. J.Bacteriol., 163, 94-105.

Freer, J.H., J.P.Arbuthnott, and A.W.Bernheimer (1968). Interaction of staphylococcal α-toxin with artificial and natural membranes. J.Bacteriol., 95,
1153-1168.

Füssle, R., S.Bhakdi, A.Sziegoleit, J.Tranum-Jensen, T.Kranz, and H.J.Wellensiek
(1981). On the mechanism of membrane damage by S.aureus α-toxin. J.Cell Biol.,
91, 83-94

Gonzalez-Carrero, M.I., J.C.Zabala, F. de la Cruz, and J.M.Oritz (1985). Purification of α-haemolysin from an overproducing E.coli strain. Mol.Gen.Genet.,
199, 106-110.

Gray, G.S. and M.Kehoe (1984). Primary sequence of the α-toxin gene from staphylococcus aureus Wood 46. Infect.Immun., 46, 615-618.

Gray, L., N.Mackman, J.M.Nicaud, and I.B.Holland (1986). The carboxy-terminal
region of haemolysin 2001 is required for secretion of the toxin from Escherichia coli. Mol.Gen.Genet., 205, 127-133.

Hacker, J., C.Hughes, H.Hof, and W.Goebel (1983). Cloned hemolysin genes from Escherichia coli that cause urinary tract infection determine different levels of toxicity in mice. Infect.Immun., 42, 57-63.

Hugo, F., J.Reichwein, M.Arvand, S.Krämer, and S.Bhakdi (1986). Mode of trans-membrane pore formation by streptolysin-O analysed with a monoclonal antibody. Infect.Immun., 54, 641-645.

Hugo, F., A.Sinner, J.Reichwein, and S.Bhakdi (1987). Quantitation of monomeric and oligomeric forms of membrane-bound staphylococcal α-toxin by ELISA using a neutralizing monoclonal antibody. Infect.Immun., in press

Mackman, N. and I.B.Holland (1984). Functional characterization of a cloned haemo-lysin determinant from E.coli of human origin, encoding information for the se-cretion of a 107K polypeptide. Mol.Gen.Genet., 196, 123-134.

Mackman, N., J.M.Nicaud, L.Gray, and I.B.Holland (1986). Secretion of haemolysin by Escherichia coli. Curr.Top.Microbiol.Immunol., 125, 159-181.

Mackman, N., K.Baker, L.Gray, R.Haigh, J.M.Nicaud, and I.B.Holland (1987). Release of a chimeric protein into the medium from E.coli using the C-terminal secretion signal of haemolysin. Embo J., in press

Menestrina, G. (1986). Ionic channels formed by S.aureus α-toxin. J.Memb.Biol., 90, 177-190.

Nicaud, J.M., N.Mackman, L.Gray, and I.B Holland (1986). The C-terminal, 23kDa peptide of E.coli haemolysin 2001 contains all the information necessary for its secretion by the haemolysin export machinery. FEBS-Lett., 204, 331-335.

Reichwein, J., F. Hugo, M.Roth, A.Sinner, and S.Bhakdi (1987). Quantitative analys-is of the binding and oligomerisation of staphylococcal α-toxin in target ery-throcyte membranes. Infect.Immun.,in press

Seeger, W., M.Bauer, and S.Bhakdi (1984). Staphylococcal α-toxin elicits hyper-tension in isolated rabbit lungs due to stimulation of the arachidonic acid cascade. J.Clin.Invest., 74, 849-858.

Suttorp, N., W.Seeger, D.Dewein, S.Bhakdi, and L.Roka (1985). Staphylococcal α-toxin stimulates synthesis of prostacyclin by cultured endothelial cells from pig pulmonary arteries. Am.J.Physiol., 248, C127-C135.

Suttorp, N., W.Seeger, J.Zucker-Reimann, L.Roka, and S.Bhakdi (1987). Mechanism of leukotriene generation in polymorphonuclear leukocytes by staphylococcal α-toxin. Infect.Immun., 55, 104-110.

Watanabe, M., T.Tomita, and T.Yasuda (1987). Membrane-damaging action of staphylo-coccal alpha-toxin on phospholipid-cholesterol liposomes. Biochim.Biophys.Acta, 898, 257-265.

Addendum

Bremm, K.D., W.König, P.Pfeiffer, I.Rauschen, K.Theobald, M.Thelestam, and J.E.Alouf (1985). Effect of thiol-activated toxins on the generation of leuko-trienes and leukotriene-inducing and -metabolizing enzymes from human poly-morphonuclear granulocytes. Infect.Immun., 50, 844-851.

Rogolsky, M. (1979). Non-enteric toxins of Staphylococcus aureus. Microbiol.Rev., 43, 320-360.

Fehrenbach et al. (Eds.), Bacterial Protein Toxins, Zbl. Bakt. Suppl. 17
© Gustav Fischer, Stuttgart, New York, 1988

Staphylococcal Gamma-Lysin: A One- or Two-Component Toxin?

T. H. Birkbeck and I. P. Niven

Department of Microbiology, University of Glasgow, Alexander Stone Building, Garscube Estate, Bearsden, Glasgow G61 IQH, Scotland

ABSTRACT

The γ-lysin from S. aureus strain Smith 5R was purified by heparin-agarose affinity chromatography followed by chromatography on hydroxylapatite to yield a a single component toxin of Mr = 33400 and pI = 9.0. A second component which was not haemolytic (termed component A and probably similar to the γ1 component of Taylor and Bernheimer, 1974) was also obtained during hydroxylapatite chromatography. Gamma-lysin was most active against rabbit erythrocytes and although component A did not affect the titre of γ-lysin on rabbit erythrocytes it potentiated the lytic activity on human (4 fold) and sheep erythrocytes (62.5 fold). Gamma-lysin was toxic to mice (LD50 = 10µg by intravenous injection) and this was not enhanced by the presence of component A.

KEYWORDS

Staphylococcus aureus, staphylococcal gamma-lysin, gamma-toxin

INTRODUCTION

Of the four cytolytic toxins of Staphylococcus aureus the α, β, and δ-lysins are well characterised in terms of physicochemical properties and interactions with cells (Freer and Arbuthnott, 1986) but less attention has been paid to the γ-lysin. First recognised by Smith and Price (1938), γ-lysin of strain Smith 5R was produced in aerated fermenter cultures (Bezard and Plommet, 1973) and purified by ion exchange chromatography (Guyonnet and Plommet, 1970) to yield two components, both of which were required for haemolytic and toxic activities. Further characterisation by Taylor and Bernheimer (1974) of material prepared in Plommet's laboratory confirmed the two-component nature of the toxin. Component 1 was a protein of Mr = 29000 and pI = 9.8 and component 2 was of Mr = 26000 and pI = 9.9. The toxin was most active against rabbit erythrocytes and was inhibited by sulphonated polymers such as heparin and agar, trypan blue, and by a range of phospholipids. Gamma-lysin was also purified by Wadstrom and Mollby (1972) and by Fackrell and Wiseman (1976a), neither of whom found evidence for a second component. The lysin of Fackrell and Wiseman (1976a,b) was of Mr = 45000 and pI = 6.0 but others properties were essentially as reported by Taylor and Bernheimer (1974).

METHODS

Growth of S. aureus and Production of Crude Culture Supernates

Staphylococcus aureus strain Smith 5R was obtained from Dr. M. Plommet and rough haemolytic colonies were selected after passage three times in plate culture (Brain Heart Infusion Broth containing 1% agarose and 10% v/v washed human erythrocytes). Sterile cellophane dialysis membranes (24cm x 24cm, Medicell International, London) were overlaid onto Tryptic Soy agarose (TSAg; 250ml tryptic soy broth solidified with 1% w/v agarose) in square petri dishes (24cm x 24cm). Each plate was inoculated with 10ml of a suspension in tryptic soy broth of S. aureus (A600nm = 2) grown overnight on 9cm diameter TSAg plates. Plates were incubated for 24h at 37°C in an atmosphere of 80% O_2 / 20% CO_2 prior to harvesting in 50ml 0.01M potassium phosphate buffer, pH 6.8. Bacterial cells were removed by centrifugation for 20 min at 10000 x g at 4°C.

Purification of Gamma-Lysin

Crude gamma-lysin solution was stirred overnight at 4°C with heparin-agarose (BRL-Gibco Laboratories, Paisley; 1ml packed heparin-agarose per 10000 HU) previously equilibrated in 0.01M potassium phosphate buffer. The heparin-agarose was poured into a 10cm x 1cm diameter column and washed with 0.01M potassium phosphate buffer to remove unbound material. A gradient of 0 to 1.5M NaCl in 0.01M phosphate buffer, pH 6.8, was applied and 3ml fractions collected. The A280nm and haemolytic activity of each fraction were recorded and peak haemo-lytic fractions were pooled, diluted to 50 ml with 0.1M potassium phosphate buffer, pH 6.8, concentrated to 10ml by ultrafiltration over an Amicon PM30 membrane, diluted to 50ml with buffer and reconcentrated to 15ml.

For hydroxylapatite chromatography the above concentrate was stirred overnight at 4°C with hydroxylapatite (Tiselius, Hjerten and Levin, 1956; approximately 1ml per 3000 HU gamma-lysin) equilibrated in 0.1M potassium phosphate buffer, pH 6.8. The hydroxylapatite suspension was packed into a column (10cm x 1.5cm diameter) and unbound material was removed by washing with buffer. Bound mat-erial was eluted by application of a 0.1 to 0.75M gradient of potassium phos-phate buffer, pH 6.8, and collection of fractions of 1.5ml.

Assays for staphylococcal products

The haemolytic activity of gamma-lysin was assayed at 37°C against washed 1% v/v suspensions of rabbit or human erythrocytes in Dulbecco's phosphate-buffered saline. Delta-lysin was similarly assayed at 20°C with suspensions of washed cod erythrocytes in citrate/dextrose/saline buffer (Chao and Birkbeck, 1978) and beta-lysin by its "hot-cold" haemolytic action against sheep erythrocytes (Low and Freer, 1977). In all cases, one haemolytic unit (HU) was the amount of lysin required to produce 50% lysis of 1 ml of a 0.5% (v/v) erythrocyte suspension.

Tests for coagulase, fibrinolysin and deoxyribonuclease were done on a 400ug ml solution of purified γ-lysin and on 1mg ml solutions of heparin-agarose partially-purified lysin. Methods and detection thresholds for such tests has been discussed by Low and Freer (1977).

Properties of Gamma-lysin

Methods for sodium dodecyl sulphate polyacrylamide gel electrophoresis (SDS-PAGE), isoelectric focusing in a Valmet trough apparatus, spectral analysis, preparation of hydroxylapatite, amino acid analysis and immunodiffusion have been published elsewhere (Birkbeck and Whitelaw, 1980; Stearne and Birkbeck, 1980). For N-chlorosuccimimide cleavage of γ-lysin, heparin-agarose partially-purified lysin was subjected to SDS-PAGE in a 12.5% polyacrylamide gel and protein bands were visualised following treatment with 4M sodium acetate. Appropriate bands were excised, digested with N-chlorosuccinimide as described by Lischwe and Ochs (1982) and the resulting peptides from the two bands were compared in 15% polyacrylamide gels and visualised by silver staining (Morrisey, 1981).

RESULTS

Production and Purification of Gamma-lysin

With a wide range of liquid media and gaseous atmospheres only poor yields of haemolysin (titres 0-16 HU ml^{-1}) were obtained. Much superior yields were obtained when bacteria were cultured on cellophane overlayered on agarose containing Tryptic Soy medium in an atmosphere of 80% O_2 / 20% CO_2 as described by Fackrell and Wiseman (1976a); approximately 6400 HU were obtained per 24cm x 24cm plate.
As most of the haemolytic activity in crude culture supernates from S. aureus strain Smith 5R was inhibited by heparin, heparin-agarose was used for affinity chromatography. From 350ml crude culture supernate containg 44800 HU, 18400 HU were recovered on elution with a gradient of NaCl (Fig. 1a).
On SDS-PAGE a characteristic pair of protein bands was found in fractions containing haemolytic activity, together with some material of higher and lower molecular weights (Figure 1b). Chromatography on hydroxylapatite separated the two components, with haemolytic activity associated entirely with the lower molecular weight component (Fig. 2). Because the elution profiles for haemolytic

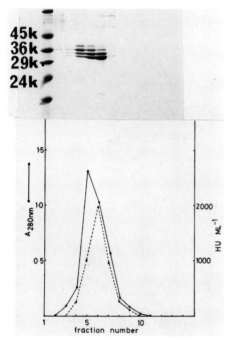

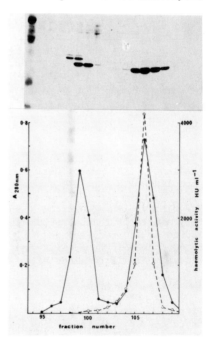

Figs. 1 and 2. Elution profiles and SDS-PAGE of fractions from Heparin-Agarose and from hydroxylapatite chromatography. Molecular weight markers are shown.

activity and for the second component (Mr = 33400) were so similar and because haemolytic activity did not depend on the presence of the higher molecular weight component (Mr = 35000), γ-lysin was considered to be a single component lysin, the action of which did not require the second component. Henceforth, the haemolytic factor will be referred to as γ-lysin and the factor of Mr = 35000 in the first peak eluted from hydroxylapatite as Component A.

Assays for other Staphylococcal Products

Highly purified γ-lysin (400 ug ml^{-1}) and heparin-agarose partially-purified lysin (1 mg ml^{-1}) were not haemolytic towards suspensions of cod erythrocytes (Chao and Birkbeck, 1978) and there was no "hot-cold" haemolytic effect when titrated against suspensions of sheep erythrocytes (Low and Freer, 1977) indicating the absence of detectable levels of β- and δ-lysins. Alpha-, β , and δ-lysins and leucocidin were not detected by immunodiffusion against appropriate monospecific antisera; coagulase, fibrinolysin, deoxyribonuclease and egg yolk factor were also not detected in the above semi-purified (heparin-agarose) or purified γ-lysin preparations.

Physicochemical Properties of Gamma-Lysin

By SDS-PAGE a single protein-staining band was found which migrated with a mobility corresponding to a molecular weight of 33400. Component A had an apparent molecular weight of 35000 by SDS-PAGE. On isoelectric focusing in a Valmet trough apparatus, the pI of γ-lysin was 9.0 (Fig. 3).

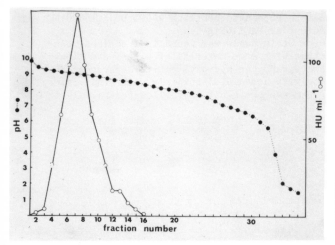
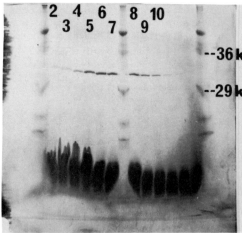

FIGURE 3 Isoelectric focusing of 2.5mg purified gamma-lysin in a pH 9 to 11 gradient (LKB Ampholines, final concentration 0.5%). Anode solution - 1% Ampholines (pH 6 to 8); cathode solution - 1% tetramethylenediamine.

The ultraviolet absorption spectra of both purified γ-lysin and component A were very similar with absorption maxima at 280nm and minima at 251nm. For γ-lysin an A280nm of 1.0 corresponded to a protein concentration of 410 ug ml. On heating to 60°C haemolytic activity was lost rapidly; < 20% of activity remained after 1 min and only 1% remained after 4 min.

Haemolytic Spectrum

Titration of purified gamma-lysin against standardised suspensions of various erythrocytes confirmed the preferential activity against rabbit erythrocytes (Table 1), with mouse and human erythrocytes also being sensitive to the lysin. Horse and cod erythrocytes, which are both sensitive to delta-lysin, were not lysed at the highest concentrations tested.

TABLE 1 Haemolytic Spectrum of Gamma-Lysin

Species	Sensitivity to Gamma-Lysin [*]
Man	100
Rabbit	1600
Mouse	200
Guinea Pig	25
Sheep	6
Horse	<1
Cod	<1

* relative to the sensitivity of human erythrocytes expressed as 100

Inactivation by Phospholipids

All phospholipids tested inhibited the action of gamma-lysin with phosphatidyl-glycerol being the most inhibitory and phosphatidylethanolamine being inactive at the highest concentration tested (Table 2).

TABLE 2. Inhibition of Gamma-Lysin by Phospholipids and Cardiopilin

Lipid	Inhibitory Titre HI per mg
phosphatidylethanolamine	<1
phosphatidyl choline	8
phosphatidyl serine	8
phosphatidic acid	11
phosphatidyl inositol	16
phosphatidyl glycerol	33
cardiolipin	64

* One haemolysin inhibitory unit (HI) was the amount of inhibitor which completely inhibited lysis after 30 min at 37°C (Whitelaw and Birkbeck,1978).

Potentiation of the Activity of Gamma-lysin

Partially-purified gamma-lysin, obtained by heparin-agarose chromatography contained both gamma-lysin and component A and the relative haemolytic activities against rabbit, human and sheep erythrocytes differed considerably from that of purified gamma-lysin (Table 1). Therefore, the combined effect of purified gamma-lysin and component A was tested on suspensions of thes erythrocytes. Component A had no stimulatory (or inhibitory) effect on the activity of gamma-lysin on rabbit erythrocytes , it potentiated haemolytic activity on human and sheep erythrocytes by 4x and 62.5x respectively, to levels similar to those obtained for the partially-purified lysin, and to levels approaching the activity against rabbit erythrocytes (Table 3). In separate studies on the interaction of γ-lysin with the complement system (Niven and Birkbeck, to be published) 32 fold stimulation of the haemolytic titre of complement occurred in the presence of γ-lysin suggesting that the potentiation of the action of γ-lysin by Component A is not a specific function. Purified α- and δ-lysins did not potentiate the lytic activity of γ-lysin.

TABLE 3. Potentiation of the Activity of Gamma-Lysin by Component A

Erythrocyte Species	Specific Activities (HU per mg)				
	Semi-purified lysin	Component A	γ-Lysin	Component A + γ-lysin	Potentiation by Component A
Rabbit	4200	32	4000	4000	0
Human	1050	8	250	1000	4 x
Sheep	2100	4	16	1000	62.5 x

* The low haemolytic activity of Component A was considered to be due to traces of γ-lysin (Figure 2) and not an inherent property of the protein.

Toxicity of Gamma-Lysin to Mice

The LD_{50} of partially-purified lysin (from heparin-agarose and containing both gamma-lysin and component A was 10HU (10µg) by intravenous injection and 100HU (100µg) by intraperitoneal injection. Insufficient purified lysin was available for complete titration of toxicity of purified lysin but 4 of 10 mice injected with 10HU purified lysin died indicating that purified lysin was of similar toxicity to mixtures of lysin and component A.

Relationship between Gamma-Lysin and Component A

Because of the similar molecular weights (33400 and 35000) of γ-lysin and Component A and the similar isoelectric points reported by Taylor and Bernheimer (1973) a relationship between the two proteins could not be discounted (e.g. that component A was a "precursor" of γ-lysin and this was investigated in several ways. The amino acid compositions of γ-lysin and component A were very similar (Table 4), with methionine being absent from both proteins and Asx, Lys, Ser, Glx, Leu, Thr and Gly being the predominant amino acids in both cases. The molecular weights calculated from amino acid analyses were 32500 and 37500 for γ-lysin and component A respectively.

TABLE 4. Amino acid Composition of γ-Lysin and Component A

Amino Acid	Predicted Number of Residues	
	Gamma-Lysin	Component A
Lys	30	29
His	8	6
NH	57	21
Arg	8	12
Asp	41	46
Thr	17	24
Ser	27	30
Glu	27	33
Pro	8	9
Gly	22	28
Ala	11	18
Val	17	17
Met	0	0
Ile	16	17
Leu	24	21
Tyr	13	18
Phe	14	18
Trp	4	6

* The number of amino acid residues predicted for each protein is based on the assumed molecular weights of 33400 and 35000 respectively.

Cleavage of gamma-lysin and component A with N-chlorosuccinimide and comparison of the resulting peptides by SDS-PAGE yielded 7 peptides from component A (molecular weight range 34000 to approximately 12000) and 8 peptides from gamma-lysin (molecular weight range from 32000 to 13000) with 5 peptides from each protein having similar apparent molecular weights.
An antiserum was raised against gamma-lysin containing traces of component A and this reacted on immunodiffusion to give non-identity between gamma-lysin and component A, indicating that although the two proteins are very similar they are serologically distinct.

DISCUSSION

The γ-lysin purified by chromatography on heparin-agarose and hydroxylapatite was clearly a single component toxin which did not require Component A for lytic activity against rabbit erythrocytes or for toxicity. The physicochemical properties of the lysin, in terms of molecular weight and pI, are similar to those reported by Taylor and Bernheimer (1974) for their component 2 and by Mollby and Wadstrom (1972) but apparently different from the molecular weight of 45000 daltons and pI of 6.0 reported by Fackrell and Wiseman (1976b). The higher molecular weight value reported by Fackrell and Wiseman (1976b) is undoubtedly due to the use of gel filtration for molecular weight measurement as they report an identical value for α-lysin, for which the generally accepted molecular weight is approximately 30000 (Freer and Arbuthnott, 1986)

The amino acid compositions of both γ-lysin and Component A are similar to those of staphylococcal α- and β-lysins (Freer and Arbuthnott, 1986) and, given the broadly similar molecular weights (30000 to 35000) and isoelectric points of these and other staphylococcal exoproteins, several may represent a "family" of proteins which have evolved from a common ancestral gene. Thus far, only the sequence coding for the α-lysin gene has been reported (Gray and Kehoe, 1984) and further sequence studies are required to test this hypothesis.

One of the most interesting findings of the present study was that although γ-lysin is haemolytic per se its action on certain cells can be potentiated by Component A or by complement. Although α- and δ-lysins did not act synergistically with γ-lysin one may speculate that many other factors could potentiate lysis by γ-lysin. Inhibitors of γ-lysin have acidic functional groups (Table 2; Wadstrom and Mollby, 1972; Taylor and Bernheimer, 1974) and potentiators may prevent binding of γ-lysin to surface molecules from which membrane penetration does not subsequently occur. Among staphylococcal proteins synergism occurs between β- and δ-lysins in their action on sheep erythrocytes (Marks and Vaughan, 1950) and on human erythrocytes Heatley, 1971), between α- and δ-lysins reacting with rabbit erythrocytes and platelets (Berheimer and others, 1972) and between the F and S components of leucocidin (Noda and others, 1982). Beta-lysin is a sphingomyelinase and δ-lysin is lytic by virtue of its high surface activity .(Freer and Arbuthnott, 1986). Similar synergism occurs commonly between phospholipases and surface active peptides and polypeptides such as melittin ("direct lytic factors") (Mollay and Kreil, 1974) and CAMP factor (Sterzik, Jurgens and Fehrenbach, 1986). Component A did not itself appear to be haemolytic and seems to bear little, if any, relationship to "direct lytic factors" or CAMP factor.
The mode of action of γ-lysin is unknown, but Thelestam and Mollby (1979) classified γ-lysin along with α-lysin in forming small "functional pores" in membranes of fibroblast cells; by analogy with α-lysin, which forms voltage-gated channels in lipid membranes (Menestrina, 1986), γ-lysin may act in this way.

We thank Dr. W. Manson, Hannah Research Institute, Ayr, for amino acid analyses. IPN was in receipt of an SERC studentship.

REFERENCES

Bernheimer, A.W., K.S.Kim, C.C.Remsen, J.Antanavage, S.W.Watson (1972). Factors affecting interaction of staphylococcal alpha toxin with membranes. Infect. Immun., 6, 636-642.

Bezard, G. and M.Plommet (1973). Production de la toxine staphylococcique gamma brute. Ann. Rech. veter.,4, 355-358.

Birkbeck, T.H. and D.D.Whitelaw (1980) Immunogenicity and molecular characterisation of staphylococcal δ-haemolysin. J. Med. Microbiol., 13, 213-221

Chao, L.-P., and T.H. Birkbeck (1978) Assay of staphylococcal δ-haemolysin with
   fish erythrocytes. J. Med. Microbiol., 11, 303-313.

Fackrell, H.B., and G.M.Wiseman (1976). Production and purification of the
   gamma-haemolysin of Staphylococcus aureus "Smith 5R". J. Gen. Microbiol,
   92, 1-10.

Fackrell, H.B., and G.M.Wiseman (1976). Properties of the gamma-haemolysin of
   Staphylococcus aureus "Smith 5R". J. Gen. Microbiol, 92, 11-24.

Freer, J.H., and J.P.Arbuthnott (1986). Toxins of Staphylococcus aureus. In: F.
   Dorner and J.Drews (Eds.), Pharmacology of Bacterial Toxins, Pergammon
   Press, Oxford, pp. 581-634.

Gladstone, G.P., and W.E. van Heyningen (1957). Staphylococcal leucocidins.
   Brit. J. Exp. Pathol., 38, 123-137.

Gray, G.S., and M.Kehoe (1984). Primary sequence of the α-toxin gene from
   Staphylococcus aureus Wood 46. Infect. Immun., 46, 615-618.

Guyonnet, F., and M. Plommet (1970). Hemolysine gamma de Staphylococcus aureus:
   purification et proprietes. Ann. Inst. Pasteur, 118, 19-33.

Heatley, N.G. (1971). A new method for the preparation and some properties of
   staphylococcal delta-haemolysin. J. Gen. Microbiol., 69, 269-278.

Lischwe, M.A., and D.Ochs (1982) A new method for partial peptide-mapping using
   N-chlorosuccinimide urea and peptide silver staining in sodium dodecyl
   sulfate polyacrylamide gels. Analyt. Biochem., 127, 453-457.

Low, D.K.R., and J.H.Freer (1977) The purification of β-lysin (sphingomyelinase
   C) from Staphylococcus aureus. FEMS Letts., 2, 139-143.

Marks, J., and A.C.T.Vaughan (1950). Staphylococcal γ-haemolysin. J. Pathol.
   Bacteriol., 62, 597-615.

Menestrina, G. (1986) Ionic channels formed by Staphylococcus aureus alpha-
   toxin: voltage-dependent inhibition by di- and trivalent cations. J. Membr.
   Biol., 90, 177-190.

Mollay, C., and G.Kreil (1974) Enhancement of bee venom phospholipase A
   activity by melittin, direct lytic factor from cobra venom and polymyxin B.
   FEBS Letts., 46, 141-144.

Morrissey, J.H. (1981) Silver stain for proteins in polyacrylamide gels: a
   modified procedure with enhanced uniform sensitivity. Analyt. Biochem.,
   117, 307-310.

Noda, M., I.Kato, T.Hirayama, and F.Matsuda ((1982). Mode of action of
   staphylococcal leucocidin: effects of the S and F components on the
   activities of membrane-associated enzymes of rabbit polymorphonuclear
   leukocytes. Infect. Immun., 35, 38-45.

Smith, M.L., and S.A.Price (1938). Staphylococcus gamma-haemolysin. J. Path.
   Bact., 47, 379-393.

Stearne, L.E.T., and T.H.Birkbeck (1980) The action of formaldehyde on
   staphylococcal δ-haemolysin. J. Med. Microbiol., 13, 223-230.

Sturzik, B., D.Jurgens, and F.J.Fehrenbach (1986) Structure and function of CAMP
   factor of Streptococcus agalactiae. In P.Falmagne, J.E.Alouf,
   F.J.Fehrenbach, J.Jeljaszewicz and M.Thelestam (Eds.), Bacterial Protein
   Toxins, Gustav Fischer Verlag, Stuttgart, pp. 101-108.

Taylor, A.G., and A.W. Bernheimer (1974). Further characterization of
   staphylococcal gamma-haemolysin. Infect. Immun., 10, 54-59.

Thelestam, M., and R.Mollby (1979) Classification of microbial, plant and animal
   cytolysins based on their membrane-damaging effects on human fibroblasts.
   Biochim. Biophys. Acta, 557, 156-169.

Wadstrom, T., and R. Mollby (1972). Some biological properties of purified
   staphylococcal haemolysins. Toxicon, 10, 511-519.

Whitelaw, D.D., and T.H.Birkbeck (1978) Inhibition of staphylococcal delta-
   haemolysin by serum lipoproteins. FEMS Letts., 3, 335-338.

Fehrenbach et al. (Eds.), Bacterial Protein Toxins, Zbl. Bakt. Suppl. 17
© Gustav Fischer, Stuttgart, New York, 1988

Low pH-Induced Release of Diphtheria Toxin Fragment A to the Cytosol

J. Ø. Moskaug, K. Sandvig and S. Olsnes

Institute for Cancer Research at the Norwegian Radium Hospital, Montebello, Oslo 3, Norway

ABSTRACT

When nicked diphtheria toxin was bound to Vero cells and entry from the surface was induced by exposure to pH < 5.3, the disulfide linking the A- and the B-fragment was reduced in 5-10% of the toxin molecules. Treatment of the cells with pronase showed that the free A-fragment and a 25 kD part of the B-fragment were protected against proteolysis, indicating that they were shielded by the plasma membrane. Fractionation of the cells showed that the A-fragment was in the soluble fraction while most of the B-fragment-derived 25kD polypeptide was associated with the membrane. A number of drugs and conditions that protect cells against intoxication also inhibited the cell-mediated reduction of the interfragment disulfide and the protection of the A-fragment against pronase, indicating that the procedure visualizes A-fragment entry that is relevant for intoxication.

KEYWORDS

Diphtheria toxin, transmembrane transport, anion transport, proton gradient, endosome.

INTRODUCTION

Although diphtheria toxin is synthesized as a single polypeptide chain, only "nicked" toxin (nDT), i.e. toxin that is proteolytically cleaved to yield a molecule consisting of two disulfide linked fragments, is able to enter the cytosol and intoxicate cells (Sandvig and Olsnes, 1981). Under normal conditions the transfer of the enzymatically active A-fragment to the cytosol occurs through the membrane of endosomes. A conformational change in the toxin molecule induced by the low pH of the endosome is required for the entry (Pappenheimer, 1977; Sandvig, Sundan and Olsnes, 1984). The low pH induces exposure of hydrophobic domains in the B-fragment which insert themselves into the membrane and somehow facilitate the transfer of the A-fragment (Kagan, Finkelstein and Colombini, 1981; Montecucco, Schiavo and Tomasi, 1985).

When the endosomal pH is increased by treatment with agents like monensin, the normal entry of diphtheria toxin is prevented and the cells are therefore protected against intoxication. However, when the cells are exposed to low pH, toxin entry is rapidly induced (Sandvig and Olsnes, 1980; Draper and Simon, 1980). A number of control experiments have indicated that this entry occurs directly through the plasma membrane (see Fig. 1). After entry is induced, there is a progressive reduction in the ability of the cells to synthesize protein, as expected, since the A-fragment inactivates its target molecules, elongation factor 2, in a time-dependent manner (Moynihan and Pappenheimer, 1981). The important features of this model system of intoxication is that the process of toxin entry can be synchronized, it occurs rapidly, and it takes place across a membrane where the ionic conditions on both sides can be manipulated in a controlled manner. Finally, it allows proteolytic removal of toxin that has not entered.

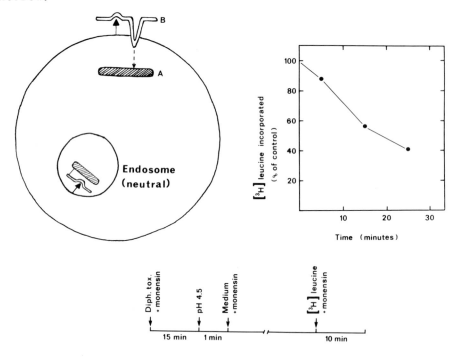

Fig. 1: Rate of protein synthesis inhibition in Vero cells after low pH induced toxin entry. Cells were incubated with hepes medium, pH 7.4, containing 10 uM monensin and 10^{-10} M nDT for 15 min at 37°C. Then the medium was removed, and hepes medium, pH 4.5, was added. After 1 min, the medium was replaced by hepes medium, pH 7.4, containing 10 uM monensin and the incubation was continued. After increasing periods of time, the ability of the cells to incorporate [³H] leucine during 10 min was measured.

CELL-MEDIATED REDUCTION OF THE INTER-FRAGMENT
DISULFIDE

When ^{125}I-labelled nDT is bound to cells and the cells are
subsequently dissolved and analyzed by polyacrylamide gel
electrophoresis (SDS-PAGE) under non-reducing conditions,
essentially all the radioactivity migrated at a rate
corresponding to whole toxin (Fig. 2, lane 1). However, when
the cells were briefly exposed to pH 4.5 before lysis, part of
the toxin migrated corresponding to the A- and B-fragments
(lane 2). Treatment of toxin at low pH in the absence of cells
did not induce disulfide reduction (lane 3). The reason that
only 5-10% of the toxin was reduced in the experiment in lane 2
was not due to incomplete nicking of the toxin molecules. Thus,
after treatment with 2-mercaptoethanol, most of the
radioactivity migrated at rates corresponding to the free A-
and B-fragments (lane 4).

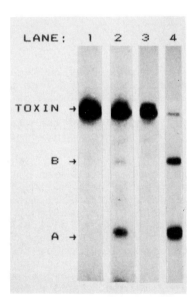

Fig. 2: Cell-mediated reduction of diphtheria toxin.
^{125}I-nDT was bound to Vero cells for 15 min at 37°C in
the presence of 10 uM monensin. The cells were then
exposed for 2 min at 37°C to Hepes medium, pH 7.2
(lane 1) or 4.5 (lane 2). The medium was removed and
Hepes medium, pH 7.2, containing 1 mM N-ethyl
maleimide was added and, after 5 min, the cells were
lysed. The TCA-precipitated proteins were dissolved in
sample buffer without reducing agents and analyzed by
SDS-PAGE and autoradiography. In a control experiment,
labeled toxin was incubated at pH 4.5 in the absence
of cells (lane 3). Lane 4: toxin treated with 1%
2-mercaptoethanol before the electrophoresis.

In order to induce intoxication in monensin-treated cells with
surface bound nDT, it is necessary to treat the cells with
medium adjusted to pH < 5.3. The data in Fig. 3 show a similar
pH-dependence of the cell-mediated reduction of ^{125}I-nDT.

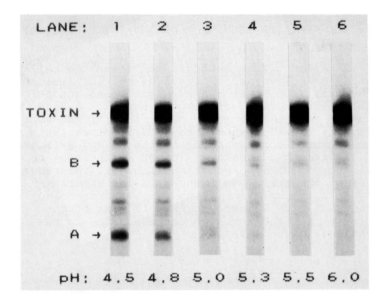

Fig. 3: Effect of pH on the cell-mediated reduction of the interfragment disulfide. Vero cells with bound ^{125}I-nDT were exposed for 2 min at 37°C to hepes medium with pH as indicated. The cells were subsequently dissolved, and the proteins were analyzed by SDS-PAGE under non-reducing conditions and subsequent autoradiography.

A number of conditions have earlier been found to prevent intoxication of cells by diphtheria toxin. These conditions comprize treatment with anion transport inhibitors, such as 4,4'-diisothiocyanostilbene 2,2'-disulfonic acid, acidification of the cytosol and treatment of cells with bound toxin with anti-diphtheria toxin antibodies. The same conditions also inhibited the cell-mediated reduction of the inter-fragment disulfide in ^{125}I-nDT (Moskaug, Sandvig and Olsnes, 1987). Pretreatment of cells with membrane permeant sulfhydryl reagents, such as N-ethylmaleimide and p-chloromercuribenzoic acid prevented the cell-mediated disulfide reduction, whereas non-permeant reagents, such as dithiobis-p-nitrobenzoic acid (Ellman's reagents) did not. This indicates that the reduction takes place at the cytosolic side of the membrane.

PROTECTION OF FRAGMENTS AGAINST PRONASE DIGESTION

To test in more detail to which extent fragments of diphtheria toxin are transferred to the cytosol at low pH, we used pronase E to remove extracellular toxin. Such treatment has been used in a variety of studies to remove proteins facing the exterior of vesicles and cells, whereas proteins in the membrane and in the cytosol are shielded (Schleyer and Neupert, 1985).

The data in Fig. 4 (lane 1), show that such treatment almost completely removed ^{125}I-nDT that had been bound to the cells at neutral pH. However, when the cells were briefly exposed to pH

4.5, two fragments with MW of 25 kD and 20 kD were protected (lane 2). In experiments where the cells were subsequently disrupted and fractionated, the 20 kD protein, which represents the A-fragment, was exclusively found in the soluble fraction (lane 3) while most of the 25 kD protein, which is derived from the B-fragment, was associated with the membrane fraction (lane 4).

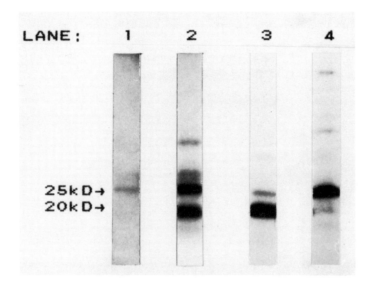

Fig. 4: Ability of low pH to induce protection of diphtheria toxin fragments against extracellular pronase. Vero cells with bound ^{125}I-nDT were exposed for 2 min at 25°C to hepes medium, pH 7.2 or 4.5. The cells were then incubated for 5 min at 37°C with hepes medium containing 3 mg/ml pronase E. Subsequently, the cells were either dissolved (lane 1 and 2) or permeabilized with saponin and separated into a soluble and a particulate fraction (lane 3 and 4). Proteins from dissolved cells and in supernatant and particulate fraction were precipitated with TCA and analyzed by SDS-PAGE under non-reducing conditions and autoradiography. Lane 1, pH 7,2; lane 2, pH 4,5; lane 3, pH 4.5, supernatant; lane 4, pH 4.5, particulate fraction.

EFFECT OF pH ON THE AMPHOPHILIC PROPERTIES OF DIPHTHERIA TOXIN AND THE ISOLATED A-FRAGMENT

It is well established that hydrophobic domains in diphtheria toxin become exposed when the toxin is treated at low pH. Furthermore, it has been reported that the A-fragment associates with liposomes in a reversible manner at low pH (Montecucco et al. 1985). Previous experiments from this laboratory have shown that at low pH diphtheria toxin binds both Triton X-100 and Triton X-114 (Sandvig and Olsnes, 1981; Sandvig and Brown, 1987). To test if diphtheria toxin

A-fragment also acquires hydrophobic properties at low pH, we measured the ability of pure A-fragment to bind Triton X-114 at different pH values.

Triton X-114 is miscible with water at $0^{\circ}C$, whereas at $37^{\circ}C$ a detergent-rich and a detergent-poor phase are formed. For simplicity, the two phases are in the following referred to as the Triton-phase and the water-phase, respectively. A number of proteins with exposed hydrophobic domains have been shown to enter the Triton-phase under these conditions.

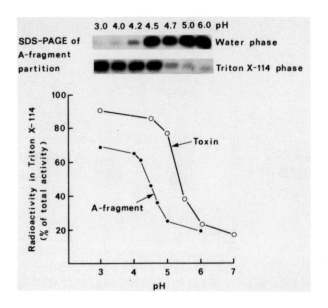

Fig. 5: Effect of pH on the ability of diphtheria toxin and A-fragment to bind Triton X-114. Diphtheria toxin A-fragment and ^{125}I-nDT was added to 400 ul Triton X-114/hepes-medium mixture with the pH indicated at the abscissa and kept at $0^{\circ}C$ for 15 min. The mixture was then transferred to $37^{\circ}C$, incubated for 1 h to separate the two phases and centrifuged for 1 min at 12,000 rpm in an Eppendorf centrifuge. The water phase was removed, the radioactivity in the Triton-phase was measured, and percent radioactivity in the Triton-phase was calculated from the total activity added. In the experiment with A-fragment, the material in the water- and Triton-phases was submitted to SDS-PAGE and autoradiography (top).

When the pH was lowered from 5 to 4, an increasing fraction of the A-fragment entered the Triton-phase (Fig. 5). Whole diphtheria toxin entered the Triton-phase at approximately 1 pH unit higher due to exposure of hydrophobic domains in the B-fragment. The transition of the A-fragment from one phase to the other with varying pH was not complete. Thus, part of the A-fragment molecules (~20%) was in the Triton-phase even at pH 6.0, while ~ 30% of the A-fragments remained in the water-phase at pH 3.0. The data indicate that the A-fragment partitions between the water and the Triton-phase and that low pH favours the partition into the Triton-phase. If this is the case, the A-fragment, which is largely in the Triton-phase at pH 4.0 should return to the water-phase when the pH is increased. This was indeed found to be the case. The results therefore indicate that when the pH is lowered from 5 to 4, a reversible change in the A-fragment takes place that strongly increases its ability to enter the Triton-phase. This change could consist in protonation of carboxyl groups in aspartic and glutamic acid side chains at the low pH.

CURRENT MODEL OF DIPHTHERIA TOXIN ENTRY

The intoxication is initiated by binding of the toxin to receptors present at the surface of susceptible cells (Middlebrook, Dorland and Leppla, 1978). Although the receptor is still not identified with certainty, our experiments with monoclonal antibodies against Vero cell surface proteins indicate that it is a transmembrane glycoprotein with MW   120 kD. Two requirements must be fulfilled for efficient toxin entry: 1) an inward directed proton gradient of > 1 pH unit and 2) permeant anions in the medium and free anion passage (Sandvig and coworkers, 1986; Sandvig and Olsnes, 1986).

It is likely that the conformational change in the toxin molecule that takes place at low pH results in insertion of amphophilic domains into the membrane. These domains, possibly in conjunction with the receptor molecule, may form a transmembrane channel. The A-fragment could interact with this complex on its way through the membrane in such a way that it forms part of the wall of the channel. In this way the A-fragment could present its polar and charged groups to the hydrophilic environment in the channel without the requirement for the bulk of the protein of passing through the channel (Singer, Maher and Yaffe, 1987).

It is likely that the inward directed proton gradient energizes the transport. The requirement for permeant anions is more difficult to explain. One possibility is that anion transport is required to maintain a necessary conformation of the receptor. Another possibility is that an inward directed flux of anions is required to neutralize the cationic parts of the A-fragment on its transfer across the membrane.

ACKNOWLEDGEMENTS

This work was supported by The Norwegian Council for Science and Humanities and by The Norwegian Cancer Society.

REFERENCES

Draper, R.K., and Simon, M.I. (1980). The entry of diphtheria toxin into the mammalian cell cytoplasm: evidence of lysosomal involvement. J.Cell.Biol., 87, 849-854.

Kagan, B.L., Finkelstein, A., and Colombini, M. (1981).
Diphtheria toxin fragment forms large pores in phospholipid
bilayer membranes. Proc.Natl.Acad.Sci.USA., 78, 4950-4954.

Middlebrook, J.L., Dorland, R.B., and Leppla, S.H. (1978).
Association of diphtheria toxin with Vero cells. Demonstration
of a receptor. J.Biol.Chem., 253, 7325-7330.

Montecucco, C., Schiavo, G., and Tomasi, M. (1985).
pH-dependence of the phospholipid interaction of
diphtheria-toxin fragments. Biochem.J., 231, 123-128.

Moskaug, J.Ø., Sandvig, K., and Olsnes, S. (1987).
Cell-mediated reduction of the interfragment disulfide in
nicked diphtheria toxin. A new system to study toxin entry at
low pH. J.Biol.Chem., 262, In press.

Moynihan, M.R., and Pappenheimer, A.M., Jr. (1981). Kinetics of
adenosinediphosphoribosylation of elongation factor 2 in cells
exposed to diphtheria toxin. Infect.Immun., 32, 575-582.

Pappenheimer, A.M., Jr. (1977). Diphtheria toxin.
Annu.Rev.Biochem., 46, 69-94.

Sandvig, K. and Brown, E. (1987). Ionic requirements for entry
of Shiga toxin from Shigella dysenteriae 1 into cells.
Infect.Immun., 55, 298-303.

Sandvig, K., and Olsnes, S. (1980). Diphtheria toxin entry into
cells is facilitated by low pH. J.Cell.Biol., 87, 828-832.

Sandvig, K., and Olsnes, S. (1981). Rapid entry of nicked
diphtheria toxin into cells at low pH. Characterization of the
entry process and effects of low pH on the toxin molecule.
J.Biol.Chem., 256, 9068-9076.

Sandvig, K., and Olsnes, S. (1986). Interaction between
diphtheria toxin entry and anion transport in Vero cells. IV.
Evidence that entry of diphtheria toxin is dependent on
efficient anion transport. J.Biol.Chem., 261, 1570-1575.

Sandvig, K., Sundan, A., and Olsnes, S. (1984). Evidence that
diphtheria toxin and modeccin enter the cytosol from different
vesicular compartments. J.Cell.Biol., 98, 963-970.

Sandvig, K., Tønnessen, T.I., Sand, O., and Olsnes, S. (1986).
Diphtheria toxin entry into cells is inhibited by acidification
of the cytosol. J.Biol.Chem., 261, 11639-11644.

Schleyer, M. and Neupert, W. (1985). Transport of proteins into
mitochondria: Translocation intermediates spanning contact
sites between outer and inner membranes. Cell, 43, 339-350.

Singer, S.J., Maher, P.A., and Yaffe, M.P. (1987). On the
transfer of integral proteins into membranes.
Proc.Natl.Acad.Sci.USA, 84, 1960-1964.

Fehrenbach et al. (Eds.), Bacterial Protein Toxins, Zbl. Bakt. Suppl. 17
© Gustav Fischer, Stuttgart, New York, 1988

The Role of Lipids in the Action of Pseudomonas aeruginosa Cytotoxin on Mammalian Cells

F. Lutz, K. Crowell, N. Lewicki and R. Conrath

Institut für Pharmalogie und Toxikologie im Fachbereich Veterinärmedizin, Justus-Liebig-Universität Gießen, Frankfurter Straße 107, D-6300 Gießen

ABSTRACT

The amount of Pseudomonas aeruginosa cytotoxin bound specifically to erythrocytes of various species correlates with their toxin-response and is found to be inversely related to the sphingomyelin content of the membrane. Treatment of erythrocytes with sphingomyelinase C from B. cereus increases binding capacity and toxin-response, whereas the toxin-membrane dissociation constant remains unchanged. The temperature shift between 21^0 and 30^0 C in the cytotoxin-induced permeability increase was not influenced by alteration of fatty acid composition of Ehrlich ascites tumor cells by fat diet to the tumor-bearing mice. We suppose that sphingomyelin molecules, located close to toxin acceptors, interfere with cytotoxin binding.

KEYWORDS

Pseudomonas aeruginosa, cytotoxin, erythrocytes, Ehrlich ascites, sphingomyelin.

INTRODUCTION

The cytotoxin is one of numerous toxins produced by Pseudomonas aeruginosa. It is an acidic protein with a molecular mass of 25 kDa (Lutz, 1979). Our search for enzymatic activities, including ADP-ribosyl-transferase in the presence of S49 lymphoma cell membranes, platelet cytosol or pig liver actin (Bärmann and Aktories, unpublished results), was negative. The cytotoxin attacks many eucaryotic cells primarily at the plasma membrane. As shown on Ehrlich ascites cells, the interaction starts with the toxin binding to a proteinaceous acceptor (Lutz, 1986). For endothelial cells, rat erythrocytes and Ehrlich ascites cells the creation of pores with a diameter of 2 nm was functionally characterized (Suttorp and others, 1985; Weiner and others, 1985, Lutz and others, 1987). Earlier studies indicated that the lipid phase of the membrane is involved in the intoxication process. Pretreatment of isolated Ehrlich ascites cell plasma membranes with phospholipase A_2 decreased the 125-I-cytotoxin binding (Lutz, 1986). Furthermore, with Ehrlich ascites cells a sharp increase of toxin-induced membrane permeability enhancement was shown in the temperature range of lipid transition, i.e. between 17^0 and 27^0 C (Lutz and others, 1982). In the present study, the role of lipid components in the membrane-toxin interaction is investigated by testing intoxication steps (I) after nutritional change of fatty acid composition of membrane lipids and (II) after enzymatic changes of phospholipid headgroups.

METHODS

Pseudomonas aeruginosa cytotoxin was prepared from autolysates of P. aeruginosa strain 158 according to the method described by Lutz (1979). Its iodination with 125-I was performed enzymatically as described by Lutz and others (1981).

Ehrlich ascites tumor cells were grown in Han-NMRI mice of either sex fed on a normal laboratory diet or a semisynthetic diet containing 16 % unhardened or hydrogenated soya oil according to the pattern of Awad and Spector (1976) with (26 mg D-α-tocopherol equivalents/100 g) or without vitamin E. Weanling mice were nourished on these diets for 5 weeks prior to intraperitoneal transplantation of 5×10^7 cells. The cells were harvested 9 - 14 days after transplantation and, if >98 % of the cells were not stainable with trypan blue, used for experiments. The Ehrlich cells were characterized by the following K^+ and Na^+ concentration: 138+/-8 mM and 41+/-5 mM (fed on a normal laboratory diet; N = 10), 144+/-11 mM and 39+/-9 mM (semisynthetic diet; N = 52). The tumor was intoxicated at cytotoxin concentrations of 12 nM $\times 2^i$ (for i = 0 to 9) for 60 min at 37° as described by Lutz and others (1982).

Fresh citrated blood (1 % sodium citrate) was washed three times at 1000 xg in phosphate buffered saline, pH 7.4, delivered from buffy coat, adjusted to 3.5 % cellular content (cattle: 7×10^8 cells/ml; rabbit, dog, pig, sheep and rat: 4.2×10^8 cells/ml; man: 3.85×10^8 cells/ml) and used for experiments within 3 hr. The erythrocytes of various species were characterized by the following K^+ and Na^+ concentration (N = 3 - 6): 105+/-18 mM and 6+/-3 mM (rat), 95+/-10 mM and 6+/-2 mM (human), 88+/-14 mM and 9+/-3 mM (rabbit), 16+/-3 mM and 51+/-12 mM (cattle), 10+/-3 mM (sheep), and 3+/-0 mM and 116+/-7 mM (dog). In each case the cation with the higher cellular concentration was used for permeability studies. Intoxication was performed with 3.5 % suspension in 0.15 M phosphate buffered K^+ or Na^+ salt, pH 7.4, at cytotoxin concentrations of 30 mM $\times 2^i$ (for i = 0 to 7) at 37° C for 60 min and terminated by centrifugation for 4 min at 10,000 xg. Binding assay was performed as described by Lutz (1986) with the exception that Schleicher and Schüll OE66 0.2 μm filters were used (nonspecific adsorption was about 0.8 % of the total radioactivity). At 4° C 1.2 nM of 125-I-cytotoxin were incubated with 1 % erythrocyte suspension for 2 hr, at 37° C 2.2 nM of 125-I-cytotoxin with 5 % erythrocyte suspension for 30 min, respectively. Unlabelled cytotoxin was present up to 8.9 μM.

Incubation of Ehrlich cells (2.7×10^7 cells/ml) or erythrocytes (3.5 % suspension) with phospholipases was carried out at 37° with sphingomyelinase C from B. cereus (EC 3.1.4.12; purchased from Boehringer, Mannheim), at a concentration between 0.016 - 2 U/ml under conditions described by Ikezawa and others (1978), with phospholipase C from C. perfringens (EC 3.1.4.3; Calbiochem; 0.08 - 1 U/ml; Bangham and Dawson, 1962) with phospholipase C from B. cereus (EC 3.1.4.3; Boehringer, Mannheim; 40 U/ml; Little and Otnäss, 1975) and phospholipase D from S. chromofuscus (EC 3.1.4.4; Boehringer, Mannheim; 0.1 - 10 U/ml in the presence of 10 mM Ca^{++} at pH 8 as described by Imamura and Horiuti, 1979). The cells were subsequently washed at 1000 xg for 2 min (Ehrlich cells: three times; erythrocytes: one time). With the exception of high concentrations of phospholipase C from C. perfringens, no change in the cellular cationic gradient by the treatment with phospholipases was obtained. The suspension of Ehrlich ascites tumor cells or erythrocytes, unchanged in the cationic gradient, were used for intoxication or binding studies.

Liposomes were prepared according to the method of Linder and others (1977) at a concentration of 5 mg/ml sphingomyelin (Serva, Heidelberg) and 2.5 mg/ml ceramide (Sigma, München).

Determination of the cellular K^+ and Na^+ concentration by flame photometry was carried out as described by Lutz and others (1982). Choline and phosphorylcholine were estimated enzymatically in the incubation medium according to the method of Imamura and Horiuti (1978). Lipids were extracted with 10 parts of chloroform: methanol = 2 : 1, washed four times, hydrolized in alkaline methanol and methylated in borotrifluoride, analyzed for fatty acids on a Chromosorb WAW-DMCS column coated with 10 % EGSS in a Hewlett-Packard chromatograph 575G.

The values are given as arithmetical means +/- S.D. Differences were considered significant at $P < 0.05$. N is the number of experiments. The cytotoxin concentration sufficient for a 50 % loss in cellular cationic gradient was calculated from a dose-response curve derived from 4 different cytotoxin concentrations each. 100 % corresponds to the ionic equalization between cells and medium.

RESULTS

Fatty Acid Composition of Ehrlich Cells and Cytotoxin Attack

The fatty acid composition of Ehrlich ascites cells varied corresponding to the diet if host mice were fed for six weeks with a semisynthetic diet containing 16 % fat. The content of the polyenoic fatty acids in the chloroform-methanol extract of the cells animals fed unhardened soya oil (about 62 % polyenoic fatty acids) was 44 %, that of animals fed with hydrogenated soya oil (about 2.5 % polyenoic fatty acids) was 16 - 19 % of the total fatty acids. Sufficient vitamin E supply in the diet of the host animals or omission of vitamin E had no influence on the fatty acid composition of the cell-lipid extracts.

The temperature shift of the cytotoxin effect, tested between 21° and 30° C, was only in part influenced by the fatty acid composition of the cells. If host animals were fed with sufficient vitamin E, Ehrlich cells from animals fed with unhardened soya oil showed a slightly steeper slope of the temperature dependence curve (Fig. 1). Less cytotoxin was required to achieve a 50 % loss of the cellular Na^+ gradient at 21 and 22° C and more cytotoxin was required at 30° C if compared to those cells from animals fed hydrogenated soya oil. Such an effect could not be ascertained for the change of the cellular K^+ gradient. No differences in temperature dependence of the cytotoxin effect on cells were detected for the K^+ and Na^+ gradient from hosts fed with unhardened or hydrogenated soya oil without vitamin E supply.

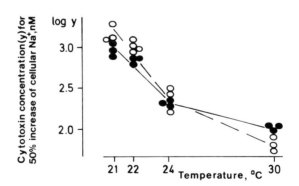

Fig.1: Content of polenoic fatty acids in Ehrlich ascites cells and the temperature slope of the cytotoxin-induced increase of cellular Na^+. Host mice were fed a semisynthetic diet containing 16 % hydrogenated (●——●) or unhardened (o-----o) soya oil at sufficient vitamin E supply. Each point represents one experiment.

Fig. 2: Relation between the release of phosphorylcholine from Ehrlich ascites tumor cells by sphingomyelinase C and their sensitivity to Pseudomonas aeruginosa cytotoxin. 4.1×10^8 cells were preincubated with sphingomyelinase C from B. cereus at concentrations of 16 mU x 2^i/ml (for i = 0 - 5) in 15 ml Krebs-Ringer phosphate buffer, pH 7.4, at 37 ° C. After 30 min the cells were washed three times and aliquots of the supernatant used for phosphorylcholine determination. The cells were resuspended and 5.4×10^7 cells each intoxicated with pseudomonal cytotoxin at concentrations of 6 nM x 2^i (for i = 0 - 5) in a volume of 2 ml. After 60 min the cells were centrifugated at 3000 xg for 3 min and their K^+ and Na^+ concentration determined. Each point represents one experiment. The correlation coefficient was for K^+ (o;————) 0.95 and for Na^+ (▲;------) 0.87.

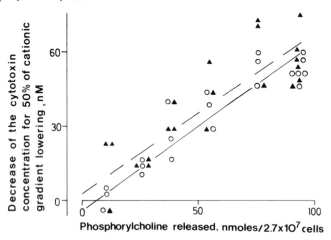

Cytotoxin Toxicity to Ehrlich Cells and Phospholipase Pretreatment

The cytotoxin concentration for a 50 % decrease of cellular cationic gradient of 2.7×10^7 cells/ml was 94+/-20 nM for K^+ and 89+/-23 nM for Na^+ at 37° C within 60 min (N = 36).

A correlation was found between release of phosphorylcholine by sphingomyelinase-active phospholipases and the enhancement of cytotoxin-induced increase in permeability. Sphingomyelinase C from B. cereus cleaved membrane sphingomyelin in a concentration dependent manner to maximally 40 % (94+/-6 nmoles/ 2.7×10^7 cells; Fig. 2) and decreased cytotoxin concentration required for a 50 % loss of cellular K^+ up to 38+/-4 nM (N = 6). Phospholipase C from C. perfringens released up to 10 % of the membrane phosphorylcholine (44+/-8 nmoles/ 2.7×10^7 cells) without cytolysis and decreased the cytotoxin concentration for a 50 % loss of cellular K^+ up to 59+/-10 nM (N = 3). Similar results were obtained for increase of cellular Na^+. Sphingomyelin-inactive phospholipase C from B. cereus cleaved up to 10 % of the membrane phosphatidylcholine (22+/-2 nmoles/ 2.7×10^7 cells) without effect on cytotoxin toxicity.

Presence of liposomes containing sphingomyelin (500 µg/ml) or ceramide (200 µg/ml) in the incubation medium did not influence the cytotoxin toxicity.

Cytotoxin Toxicity and Sphingomyelin Content of Erythrocytes

As shown in Table 1, the sensitivity of erythrocytes to the cytotoxin was found to be directly related to their phosphatidylcholine : sphingomyelin ratio. Red blood cells with low sphingomyelin content (11 - 19 %) of the phospholipids were damaged by 10^{-8} - 10^{-7} M cytotoxin. 1000-fold higher concentrations of the cytotoxin did not increase the permeability of erythrocytes from species containing more sphingomyelin than man (26 %). Up to 83 % of sphingomyelin was cleaved by treatment of erythrocytes from various species with sphingomyelinase C from B. cereus (Table 1), and up to 50 - 55 % of choline released by treatment with phospholipase D from S. chromofuscus (data not shown). Whereas preincubation of erythrocytes with phospholipase D did not influence their cytotoxin sensitivity, sphingomyelinase treatment enhanced the cytotoxin effect in a dose-dependent manner, particularly in erythrocytes with high sphingomyelin content (Table 1).

Cytotoxin Binding to Erythrocytes Depending on Their Sphingomyelin Content

Binding of cytotoxin to erythrocytes was studied using suspensions from rabbits, humans and cattle. Whenever significant binding of 125-I-cytotoxin was achieved, binding was rapid, tight, saturable and temperature dependent. At 37° C steady-state was reached within 25 min ($t_{1/2}$ <1 min) and lasted for several hr. Specific binding was up to 95 % reversible in the presence of 1000-fold excess of cold cytotoxin. At 4° C more 125-I-cytotoxin (rabbit: seven fold) was bound than at 37° C, reaching steady-state within 2 hr.

The amount of 125-I-cytotoxin bound to erythrocytes from rabbits, humans and cattle was found to be directly related to their phosphatidylcholine : sphingomyelin ratio at 37° C (Table 1) and at 4° C (rabbit: 4.7 x 10^{4} molecules/cell; man: 1.4 x 10^{4} molecules/cell; cattle: 10 molecules/cells). The binding capacity was triggered independent of species, but dependend on the phospholipase used. Pretreatment with sphingomyelinase C from B. cereus increased the binding capacity of 125-I-cytotoxin at 37° C (Table 1). At 4° C an increase of the binding capacity was also obtained on human erythrocytes. Erythrocytes from cattle hemolyzed after pretreatment with sphingomyelinase when cooled to 4° C. In contrast, the dissociation constant (5 - 8 x 10^{-8} M for all species) was not changed at different temperatures and after pretreatment.

The influence of liposomes containing sphingomyelin or ceramide on the binding properties of the cytotoxin was tested on rabbit erythrocytes at 4° C. Using up to 250 µg sphingomyelin or 125 µg ceramide per 3 x 10^{7} cells, no changes of binding properties could be observed.

DISCUSSION

The interaction of lipids with other components within plasma membranes occurs at low polarity zones located in the inner part of the membrane at both the hydrocarbon chains (I), and at the polar head groups on the membrane surface (II).

I. Thermal analyses of lipid crystals have shown that saturated and unsaturated fatty acids affect the lipid phase transition considerably (Phillips and others, 1969). Because Ehrlich ascites cells change their sensitivity to the cytotoxin within a small temperature interval from rather insensitive to fully sensitive, we tested the cytotoxin toxicity shift in these temperatures only.

After alteration of fatty acid composition with diet, the temperature sensitivity was found to be almost independent of the fatty acid composition of the cells. This suggests that during the intoxication process the hydrocarbon portion of membran lipids may play a minor role only.

Table 1 Sphingomyelin Content in the Outer Layer of Erythrocyte Membrane and Pseudomonas Cytotoxin Intoxication

Data derived from three independent experiments are given as means +/- S.D. The experiments were performed at 37° C. Cells were pre-incubated for 15 min with sphingomyelinase C from B. cereus in 0.15 M phosphate buffered K^+ or Na^+ salt, pH 7.4. In binding experiments up to 8.9 µM unlabelled cytotoxin was present.

Species	Sphingo-myelin content§	Sphingomyelinase C pretreatment		Toxin concentr. for 50 % loss of cellular catio-nic gradient	Toxin mole-cules bound per erythrocyte
		Sphingomyelin degraded	Enzyme activity		
	Mole % of Phospho-lipids	%	U/ml	µM	x 10^4
Dog	10.8	1+/-1	0	0.20+/-0.02	ND
		83+/-2	0.1	0.18+/-0.03	ND
Rat	12.8	ND		0.23+/-0.02	ND
Rabbit	19.0	1+/-1	0	0.69+/-0.05	0.68+/-0.12
		82+/-2	0.1	0.39+/-0.01‡	0.84+/-0.10‡
Man	26	2+/-0	0	10.4 +/-0.4	NM
		78+/-5	0.2	2.9 +/-0.9‡	0.05+/-0.015
Pig	26.5	7+/-2	0	*	ND
		79+/-6	0.4	20.0 +/-0.4	ND
Cattle	46.2	6+/-2	0	*	NM
		81+/-4	2.0	4.30+/-0.4	0.15+/-0.05
Sheep	51.0	ND		*	ND

§ Data from review of Rouser and others (1968).
ND, not determined.
NM, bound radioactivity was no more than the two fold of the background (about 300 cpm) corresponding to maximal 10 molecules bound per cell.
* No change of cellular cationic gradient emerged with cytotoxin concentrations up to 40 µM.
‡ Significant different from experiments without sphingomyelinase C pretreatment using Student's t-test for paired samples.

II. In the outer plasma membrane layer of mammalian cells cholesterin, sphingomyelin and phosphatidylcholine are the predominant lipid components. Besides about 25 % cholesterin, erythrocyte outer leaflets contain sphingomyelin and phosphatidylcholine in different properties depending on the species.
Any variation of phosphatidylcholine content is generally counterbalanced by an
opposite alteration in sphingomyelin (Rouser and others, 1968).

Erythrocytes from mammals with low sphingomyelin content were sensitive
to the pseudomonal cytotoxin, while others with high sphingomyelin content were
insensitive. Sphingomyelin differs from phosphatidylcholine in a greater hydro-
gen-binding capability (sphingosine moiety). Moreover, experiments on sphingomyelin films indicated strong intermolecular interactions (Long and others,
1972) and Kramer and others (1972) obtained preferential binding of sphingomyelin by a pooled protein fraction from sheep erythrocytes. The isolation of
5'-nucleotidase from rat liver by Widnell and Unkeless (1968) gave evidence
associating sphingomyelin to membrane-bound enzymes in a high lipid:protein
ratio. Sphingomyelin may interact with the cytotoxin intoxication process forming
structures which inhibit this process. When it is ascertained that such preferential interaction does affect the cytotoxin intoxication process, splitting
off the sphingosin head groups may also change these steps, i.e. binding process
and permeability change. Experiments on Ehrlich ascites tumor cells show that
digestion of sphingomyelin results in a remarkable enhancement of the cytotoxin-
induced permeability increase, and digestion of phosphatidylcholine has no
effect. The binding study on erythrocytes from different species with and without sphingomyelinase pretreatment shows that the treatment of erythrocytes
with sphingomyelinase C does not change the dissociation constant of the toxin-
membrane binding. This suggests that at least the binding function of the cytotoxin-binding site may not depend on membrane lipids. The increase of the amount
of cytotoxin molecules bound per cells (supported by the species dependence
of cytotoxin sensitivity of erythrocytes) indicates, however, that the binding sites are probably shielded partially from cytotoxin attack, particularly
in the loosening of lipid-protein interaction induced by sphingomyelinase treatment the osmotic fragility increases as reported by Colley and others (1973),
Ikezawa and others (1978) and Taguchi and others (1983) for erythrocytes from
various species (in response to osmotic, hot-cold and hot hemolysis). Accordingly, we found hemolysis of cattle erythrocytes treated with sphingomyelinase from B. cereus after cooling to 0° C. Also synergistic hemolysis was reported
for other bacterial products (CAMP phenomenon; Linder, 1983). The isolation of
the proteinaceous cytotoxin-binding site (Lutz, 1986) is in progress in order
to allow further studies by performing reconstitution experiments.

Acknowledgements - We thank Miss R. Leidolf for her excellent technical
assistance. The study was supported by the Deutsche Forschungsgemeinschaft.

REFERENCES

Awad, A.B., and A.A.Spector (1976). Modification of the fatty acid composition
of Ehrlich ascites tumor cell plasma membranes. Biochim.Biophys.Acta, 426,
723-731.
Bangham, A.D., and R.M.C.Dawson (1962). Electrokinetic requirements for the
reaction between Cl. perfringens α-toxin (phospholipase C) and phospholipid
substrates. Biochim.Biophys.Acta, 59, 103-115.
Colley, C.M., R.F.A.Zwaal, B.Roelofsen, and L.L.M.van Deenen (1973). Lytic and
non-lytic degradation of phospholipids in mammalian erythrocytes by pure
phospholipases. Biochim.Biophys.Acta, 307, 74-82.

Ikezawa, H., M.Mori, T.Ohyabu, and R.Taguchi (1978). Studies on sphingomyelinase of Bacillus cereus I. Purification and properties. Biochim.Biophys.
Acta, 528, 247-256.
Imamura, S., and Y.Horiuti (1978). Enzymatic determination of phospholipase D
activity with choline oxidase. J. Biochem., 83, 677-680.
Imamura, S., and Y.Horiuti (1979). Purification of Streptomyces chromofuscus
phospholipase D by hydrophobic affinity chromatography on palmitoyl cellu-
lose. J. Biochem., 85, 79-95.
Kramer, R., C.Schlatter, and P.Zahler (1972). Preferential binding of sphingomyelin by membrane proteins of the sheep red cell. Biochim.Biophys.Acta,
282, 146-156.
Linder, R. (1983). Alteration of mammalian membranes by the cooperative and antagonistic actions of bacterial toxins. Biochim.Biophys.Acta, 779, 423-435.
Linder, R., A.W.Bernheimer, and K.-S.Kim (1977). Interaction between sphingomyelin and a cytolysin from sea anemone Stochiactis helianthus. Biochim.Bio-
phys.Acta, 467, 290-300.
Little, C., and A.B.Otnäss (1975). The metal ion dependence of phospholipase C
from Bacillus cereus. Biochim.Biophys.Acta, 391, 326-333.
Long, R.A., F.E.Hruska, H.D.Gesser, and J.C.Hsia (1971). Phase transitions in
sphingomyelin thin films. A spin label study. Biochem.Biophys.Res.Commun.,
45, 167-173.
Lutz, F. (1979). Purification of a cytotoxic protein from Pseudomonas aeruginosa. Toxicon, 17, 467-475.
Lutz, F. (1986). Interaction of Pseudomonas aeruginosa cytotoxin with plasma
membranes from Ehrlich ascites tumor cells. Naunyn-Schmied.Arch.Pharmacol.,
332, 103-110.
Lutz, F., S.Grieshaber, and I. Käufer (1981). Cytotoxin from Pseudomonas aeruginosa in mice: Distribution related to pathology. Toxicon, 19, 763-771.
Lutz, F., S.Grieshaber, and K.Schmidt (1982). Permeability changes of Ehrlich
mouse ascites tumor cells induced by a cytotoxin from Pseudomonas aeruginosa.
Naunyn-Schmied.Arch.Pharmacol., 320, 78-80.
Lutz, F., M.Maurer, and K.Failing (1987). Cytotoxic protein from Pseudomonas
aeruginosa: Formation of hydrophilic pores in Ehrlich ascites tumor cells
and effect on cell viability. Toxicon, 25, 293-305.
Phillips, M.C., R.M.Williams, and D.Chapman (1969). On the nature of hydrocarbon chain motions in lipid liquid crystals. Chem.Phys.Lipids, 3, 234-244.
Rouser, G., G.J.Nelson, S.Fleischer, and G.Simon (1968). Lipid composition of
animal cell membranes, organelles and organs. In: D.Chapman (Ed.), Biological membranes.Physical fact and function. Academic Press, London and New
York, pp. 5-69.
Suttorp, N., W.Seeger, J.Uhl, F.Lutz, and L.Roka (1985). Pseudomonas aeruginosa cytotoxin stimulates prostacyclin production in cultured pulmonary artery
endothelial cells: Membrane attack and calcium influx. J.Cell.Physiol.,
123, 64-72.
Taguchi, R., M.Mizuno, M.Inoue, and H.Ikezawa (1983). Increase in osomotic
fragility of bovine erythrocytes induced by bacterial phospholipase C.
J.Biochem., 93, 403-412.
Weiner, R.N., E.Schneider, C.W.M.Haest, B.Deuticke, R.Benz, and M.Frimmer
(1985). Properties of the leak permeability induced by a cytotoxic protein from Pseudomonas aeruginosa (PACT) in erythrocytes and black lipid
membranes. Biochim.Biophys.Acta, 820, 173-182.
Widnell, C.C., and J.C.Unkeless (1968). Partial purification of a lipoprotein with 5'-nucleotidase activity from membranes of rat liver cells.
Proc.Natn.Acad.Sci. U.S.A., 61, 1050-1057.

Fehrenbach et al. (Eds.), Bacterial Protein Toxins, Zbl. Bakt. Suppl. 17
© Gustav Fischer, Stuttgart, New York, 1988

Release of Lipidmediators (Leukotrienes, PAF) by Bacterial Toxins from Human Polymorphonuclear Granulocytes

K.-D. Bremm[1], W. König[1], J. Brom[1], M. Thelestam[2], F. J. Fehrenbach[3] and J. E. Alouf[4]

Medizinische Mikrobiologie und Immunologie, AG Infektabwehr, Ruhr-Universität Bochum, Universitätsstr. 150, 4630 Bochum
[2]Karolinska Institut, Stockholm, Sweden
[3]Robert-Koch-Institut, D-1000 Berlin
[4]Unité des Antigènes Bactériens, Institut Pasteur Paris, Rue du Docteur Roux, 28, F-75724 Paris Cedex 15

ABSTRACT

Human neutrophil granulocytes (PMN) release leukotrienes when they are stimulated with bacterial toxins. In comparison to other stimuli the toxin-induced generation is quiet low (1). Theta-Toxin (1 HU) activates $1x10^7$ granulocytes to release 9.9 ng LTC_4 and 9.4 ng LTB_4. When PMN are prestimulated with antagonists of calmodulin (W-7) or protein kinase C (dibucaine) the leukotriene release is inhibited between 10% and 80%. In addition to leukotriene release bacterial toxins activate the metabolism of platelet activating factor (PAF).

KEYWORDS

bacterial toxins, leukotrienes, platelet-activating factor (PAF), calmodulin, protein kinase C

RESULTS

Bacterial toxins represent good tools for studying membrane biochemical events in cell activation. It was the purpose of the present investigation to investigate (1)the role of calmodulin and protein kinase C in toxin induced leukotriene release and (2)influence of bacterial toxins on PAF-metabolism. In order to study the participation of the calmodulin and protein kinase C in toxin induced leukotriene release, PMN ($1x10^7$) were prestimulated for ten minutes with specific antagonists. Dibucaine was used to inhibit protein kinase C in a range from $1.6x10^{-4}$ to $1.6x10^{-6}$M and W-7 an inhibitor of calmodulin was used from $3.3x10^{-7}$ to $3.3x10^{-9}$M. After preincubation PMN were stimulated for further 30 minutes with various bacterial toxins. Cell free supernatants were then deproteinized and analysis was performed by reversed-phase HPLC and specific radioimmunoassays for LTC_4 and LTB_4. The results of these experiments are summarized in table 1:

PMN +	dibucaine (M)	W-7 (M)	LTC_4	LTB_4
			(ng/10^7 PMN)	
SLO (10 HU/ml)			9.3±1.9	18.2±3.6
	1.6×10^{-4}		3.3±1.0	4.3±0.5
	1.6×10^{-5}		4.9±1.2	19.8±1.8
		3.3×10^{-7}	2.3±0.6	3.5±0.4
		3.3×10^{-8}	4.5±0.9	7.3±1.2
theta-Toxin (10 HU/ml)			9.9±1.6	9.4±1.6
	1.6×10^{-4}		3.4±0.8	6.9±1.0
	1.6×10^{-5}		6.7±1.4	8.6±1.2
		3.3×10^{-7}	4.6±0.6	2.0±0.6
		3.3×10^{-8}	6.5±1.2	7.1±1.4

As is apparent, a dose-dependent inhibition of toxin induced leukotriene release is observed with both antagonists. It is therefore evident that calmodulin as well as protein kinase C are involved in toxin stimulated activation of lipoxygenase metabolism in PMN. Further studies with more specific antagonist should help to clarify the steps of membrane activation more precisely.

With each molecule of arachidonic acid released from membrane phospholipids a precursor for the platelet-activating factor (PAF) is theoretically available for PAF-metabolism (2). Since PAF is also a very potent mediator of inflammation it is of interest to know whether bacterial toxins also interfere with this metabolic pathway. PMN (1×10^7) were preincubated with 0.37 kBq ^{3}H-lyso-PAF for two minutes and subsequently stimulated with various bacterial toxins for 20 minutes. Incubation was stopped with methanol-chloroform (1:2) and extraction of PAF was performed twice with chloroform. Analysis of lyso-PAF metabolism was performed by TLC. Results are summarized in table 2:

PMN +	lyso-PAF (%)	PAF (%)	alkyl-acyl GPC (%)
SLO (1 HU)	64.8	9.3	25.9
theta-Toxin (1 HU)	72.1	7.5	20.4
alpha-Toxin (2 HU)	77.8	4.2	18.0
delta-Toxin (2 HU)	73.4	4.9	21.7
SET (10 ug)	73.7	6.9	19.4
CAMP (10 ug)	71.6	9.2	19.2
PBS-buffer	100	0	0

As is apparent a metabolism from lyso-PAF to the highly active PAF is observed with all studied toxins. A time and dose-dependent release was observed for SLO, alpha-, delta- and theta-Toxin from Cl.perfringens. With scarlet erythrogenic toxin (SET) and CAMP from Streptococcus an effect was only observed with high concentrations. In the presence of sphingomyelinase however, CAMP proved to be highly active for histamine release.

In summary our studies show that bacterial toxins activate leukotriene generation in PMN as well as the metabolism of platelet-activating factor. Since these factors are highly active mediators of inflammation and interfere with various cells of specific and unspecific immunity further studies will help to clarify their role in bacterial infection.

LITERATURE

1. Bremm,KD, König,W, Pfeiffer,P, Rauschen,I, Theobald,K, Thelestam,M & Alouf,JE (1985). Infect.Immun.,50,844.
2. Hanahan,DJ (1986). Ann.Rev.Biochem.,55,483.

Fehrenbach et al. (Eds.), Bacterial Protein Toxins, Zbl. Bakt. Suppl. 17
© Gustav Fischer, Stuttgart, New York, 1988

Identification of the Carbohydrate Receptor for Shiga-like Toxin 2 from Escherichia Coli and Development of a Toxin Receptor Binding Immunoassay

J. E. Brown, R. J. Neill, A. D. O'Brien and A. A. Lindberg

Afrims, Bangkok 10400, Thailand
Wrair, Washington, DC, 20307-5100, USA
USUHS, 4301 Jones Bridge Road Bethesda, MD 20814-4799, USA.
Huddinge Univ. Hosp., S-141 86, Huddinge

ABSTRACT

Shiga toxin from Shigella dysenteriae 1 binds to cell surface receptors containing galactose $\alpha 1 \longrightarrow 4$ galactose (galabiose). To study the receptor specificity of E. coli Shiga-like cytotoxins (SLT's), we have examined the ability of galabiose-conjugated BSA to interfere with cytotoxic action of these toxins. In addition to inhibiting the cytotoxicity of pure Shiga toxin and SLT-1 in bacterial lysates, the glycoconjugate protected HeLa cell monolayers from cytotoxicity of Shiga-like toxin 2 in sonicates of E. coli 395 (Ø933W). The glycoconjugate was used to develop a receptor-binding microtiter plate assay, using anti-Shiga toxin monoclonal antibodies.

KEYWORDS

Shiga toxin, Shiga-like toxin, Vero toxin, receptor, Shigella dysenteriae 1, receptor binding assay.

INTRODUCTION

Bacillary dysentery, caused mainly by Shigella species, is responsible for 10-20% of acute diarrheal disease worldwide. Shigella dysenteriae type 1, considered the most virulent species, produces large amounts of a protein cytotoxin, Shiga toxin. Similar cytotoxins, termed Shiga-like toxins (SLTs), have been reported in pathogenic isolates of E. coli, Vibrio cholerae and V. parahemolyticus. E. coli 0157:H7 strain 933, an agent of hemorrhagic colitis, produces two distinct cytotoxins similar to Shiga toxin, which have been termed SLT-1 and SLT-2 (Strockbine and co-workers, 1986). Shiga toxin (Mr = 70,000), composed of one enzymatic subunit and five binding subunits, acts to inhibit protein synthesis.

We have proposed that the cell surface receptors for Shiga toxin are glycolipids containing the disaccharide Gal α1-4 Gal β(galabiose) in a terminal position (Lindberg and co-workers, 1987). Pure toxin has

been shown to bind specifically to glycolipids containing this
disaccharide. Binding of pure 125I-toxin to cell monolayers was
inhibited by galabiose covalently linked to BSA but not by free
oligosaccharide containing galabiose. Cytotoxic-associated binding
was also inhibited by galabiose-BSA in a concentration-dependent
manner.

To study the receptor specificity of E. coli Shiga-like toxins, we
have examined the ability of galabiose-conjugated BSA to prevent
cytotoxic action of these toxins. Monolayers were incubated in
HEPES-buffered medium at $0^{o}C$ with mixtures of bacterial lysate
and galabiose-BSA for 1 hour. Cells were then washed at $0^{o}C$ and
fresh medium was added. Plates were incubated overnight at $37^{o}C$
and examined for cytotoxicity. Galabiose-BSA prevented cytotoxicity
in a concentration-dependent manner with lysates of E. coli strains
H19, S/22/1, and 933, which all produce large amounts of Shiga-like
toxin 1. To test whether Shiga-like 2 has similar receptor
affinity, E. coli K12 substrain 395 was lysogenized with phage 933W,
which encodes for SLT-2. The glycoconjugate protected Hela cell
monolayers from cytotoxic effects of these lysates, although the
sonic lysates contained at least 100 fold less cytotoxic activity

The glycoconjugate was used to develop a receptor-binding microtiter
plate immunoassay. Plates were coated with 0.1 ml
galabiose-conjugated BSA (2 ug/ml) overnight and monoclonal antibody
specific for Shiga toxin was used to detect bound toxin. Pure toxin
could be detected at concentrations as low as 0.05 ug/ml.
Monoclonal antibodies specific for the toxin A subunit were more
sensitive than antibodies for the B subunit. Using this
enzyme-linked immuno-receptor assay, the amount of toxin in
bacterial lysates was determined. Lysates from high toxin producing
Shigella and E. coli contained 0.5-5 ug toxin/mg total protein.

These results indicate that Shiga toxin, SLT-1, and SLT-2 have
similar binding specificities. Therefore a receptor-based assay may
be useful as a clinical test for their detection. Detection of
SLT-2 in lysates will require an enrichment step to come within the
level of sensitivity of this assay.

REFERENCES

Lindberg, A.A., J.E. Brown, N. Stromberg, M. Westling-Ryd, J.E.
Schultz nd K.-A. Karlsson (1987). Identification of the carbohydrate
receptor for Shiga toxin produced by Shigella dysenteriae type 1.
J.Biol.Chem. 262: 1778-1785.

Strockbine N.A., L.R.M. Marques, J.W. Newland, H.W. Smith, R.K.
Holmes, and A.D. O'Brien (1986). Two toxin-converting phages from
Escherichia coli 0157:H7 strain 933 encode antigenicity distinct
toxins with similar biological activities. Infect.Immun. 53:
135-140.

Fehrenbach et al. (Eds.), Bacterial Protein Toxins, Zbl. Bakt. Suppl. 17
© Gustav Fischer, Stuttgart, New York, 1988

Clostridial Neurotoxins Prevent ³H-Noradrenaline Release from Primary Nerve Cell Cultures and Broken Brain Cells

E. Habermann, H. Müller and M. Hudel

Buchheim-Institut für Pharmakologie, Justus-Liebig Universität, Frankfurter Str. 107, D-6300 Gießen

Keywords: Tetanus toxin - botulinum neurotoxins - noradrenaline release - cell culture - brain.

Tetanus and botulinum A toxin are known to prevent the release of numerous neurotransmitters, among them noradrenaline (Bigalke and others 1981; Habermann 1981). The intention of the work presented was to develop (1) a cell culture system which allows long term exposure to the toxins, followed by neurochemical analysis, (2) a conventional and convenient broken cell preparation, both for quantitative comparisons between clostridial toxins, their derivatives and between antitoxin preparations.

(1) <u>Primary brain cultures</u> from 14 day old mouse embryos were grown in vitro for 14 days, and poisoned for 20 h (2-72 h) with clostridial toxins (1-1000 ng/ml). Then they were labeled by 1 h exposure to ³H-noradrenaline together with noradrenaline (1), iproniazid (10), ascorbic acid (20) all in µmol/l , and thoroughly washed with Krebs-Henseleit solution containing Hepes. Basal release was monitored by two 5 min exposures to 1 ml salt solution. Subsequent stimulation with 45 mmol/l K^+ (3 times for 5 min each) released part (about 30 %) of the radioactivity which consisted mainly of noradrenaline. The remainder was extracted with 2 % sodium dodecyl sulfate. Release of radioactivity was given in percent of total. It depended strictly on the presence of free Ca^{2+}. Pretreatment with amphetamine or reserpine diminished the subsequent noradrenaline uptake.

Tetanus toxin, as well as the neurotoxins from Cl. botulinum A and C1 partially prevent the release of ³H-noradrenaline, the botulinum toxins being about 10 times more potent. The detection limit was below 10^{-10} mol/l for tetanus toxin, and below 10^{-11} mol/l for botulinum A toxin. Even with the highest toxin concentrations complete inhibition was never achieved.

Both higher content and lesser release contribute to the decrease of percentual release due to the toxins. Inhibition increases with time for up to 20 h. Antitoxin prevents but does not revert the effect of tetanus toxin. Neuraminidase treatment of the cultures partially prevents the effect of tetanus toxin.

(2) <u>Superfused broken brain cells</u> were prepared as described by Bigalke and others (1981) but additionally homogenised by hand with a loose fitting Potter homogenizer. After 15 min exposure to ^{3}H-noradrenaline (with the additives mentioned above) and washing, the 2 % (w/v) preparation was incubated with the toxins for 2 hours at 37° C and filled into Millipore Swinnex filter holders (13 mm Ø) over two layers of Whatman GF-C glass fibre filters. After 30 min superfusion with 0.5 ml/min Krebs-Ringer solution buffered with Hepes, 1 min fractions were collected. A 2 min pulse of K^+ (31 mmol/l) was then given, which releases nearly 50 % of the radioactivity. The remainder was quantitatively eluted by final superfusion for 3 min with 0.5 N acetic acid. Absolute and percentual release was then calculated. It was made sure that pretreatment with tetanus or botulinum A toxin did not change the velocity of ^{3}H noradrenaline uptake.

Dependent on dosage, both tetanus and botulinum A neurotoxin partially (up to 50 %) prevent the release of noradrenaline. Like in cell cultures, both increased content and decreased absolute release of noradrenaline contribute to the inhibition by the toxins. The toxins are equipotent between 1.7 and 0.05 µg/ml. In this respect the present results differ from those obtained by Bigalke and others (1981) where botulinum A toxin had been 10 times less potent than tetanus toxin. Preincubation with different concentrations of antibodies (but not with V. cholerae neuraminidase) dose-dependently inhibits the effect of a tetanus toxin standard. The functional in vitro assay gives a quantitative measure of antibody content and may replace the conventional animal experiments.

Despite some qualitative differences in detail, both systems respond in a basically similar manner to tetanus and botulinum neurotoxins. Differences may be explained by the duration of exposure to the toxins, to neuraminidase, and to antibodies. The cell culture is more tedious, and prone to variations between individual culture plates but advantageous for long-term studies. The broken cell preparation is simple and sufficient for experiments not exceeding six hours. Both systems were used for comparison between monochainal and bichainal tetanus toxin with essentially the same result (Weller and others 1987).

REFERENCES

Bigalke, H., I.Heller, B.Bizzini and E.Habermann (1981). Tetanus toxin and botulinum A toxin inhibit the release and uptake of various transmitters, as studied with particulate preparations from rat brain and spinal cord. <u>Naunyn-Schmiedebergs Arch. Pharmacol.</u>, <u>316</u>, 244-251

Habermann, E. (1981). Tetanus toxin and botulinum A neurotoxin inhibit and at higher concentrations enhance noradrenaline outflow from particulate brain cortex in batch. <u>Naunyn-Schmiedebergs Arch. Pharmacol.</u>, <u>318</u>, 105-111.

Weller, U., F.Mauler and E.Habermann (1987). Monochainal tetanus toxin. Preparation, protoxin properties, and proteolytic conversion into isotoxins. <u>Proc. Third European Workshop on Bacterial Protein Toxins</u>, Überlingen 1987, p. - .

Fehrenbach et al. (Eds.), Bacterial Protein Toxins, Zbl. Bakt. Suppl. 17
© Gustav Fischer, Stuttgart, New York, 1988

Quantitation of the Binding of Bacillus thuringiensis Delta-Endotoxin to Brush Border Membrane Vesicles of Pieris brassicae

C. Hofmann and P. Lüthy

Institute of Microbiology, Swiss Federal Institute of Technology, Universitätsstr. 2, CH-8092 Zürich

Keywords: Binding, Iodination, Bacillus thuringiensis, Delta-endotoxin, Brush border membrane vesicles.

Binding of the insecticidal delta-endotoxin of Bacillus thuringiensis to cultured insect cells was visualized previously by light microscopy (Hofmann and Lüthy, 1986). Also binding to brush border membrane vesicles (BBMV) derived from the larval midgut of Pieris brassicae was qualitatively shown (Wolfersberger and others, 1986). In this communication quantitation of binding of the delta-endotoxin to BBMV will be presented.

Activated toxin, designated here simply as toxin, was prepared as previously described (Hofmann and Lüthy, 1986). Iodination of toxin with ^{125}I using Iodo-Gen was performed according to the manufacturers' instruction (Pierce). Iodinated toxin was still active against P. brassicae larvae and the immunological reaction with monoclonal antibodies was unchanged. The binding of the iodinated toxin to immobilized antibodies was competitively inhibited by non-labelled toxin. BBMV of P. brassicae were prepared as described by Wolfersberger and others (1987). The amount of BBMV was assessed by protein concentration. BBMV of the small intestine of rat were prepared according to Stieger and Murer (1983) and were kindly supplied by H. Murer (University, Zürich). 0.035mg BBMV were incubated with 10ng ^{125}I-toxin (1.67nM) in 0.1ml phosphate buffered saline (pH 7.5, 10mM, 150mM NaCl) containing 0.1% bovine serum albumin (PBS-BSA) at room temperature for 10min. Unbound ^{125}I-toxin was removed by centrifugation and the BBMV were subsequently washed twice. Competition was performed by incubating the BBMV with ^{125}I-toxin in the presence of increasing amounts of non-labelled toxin. ^{125}I-toxin and ^{127}I-toxin were mixed in different ratios before beeing added to the BBMV, in order to determine the dissociation constants (K_D), the Hill coefficient (h), the number of individual binding site populations, and the amount of binding sites (B_{max}) for each population. The amount of total bound iodinated toxin was derived from the amount of bound ^{125}I-toxin. The binding data were analyzed according to Pliska and others (1986). The dissociation constant for non-iodinated toxin was estimated using the data of competition experiments with non-iodinated toxin and the K_D, B_{max}, and h of iodinated toxin. The ligands (non-iodinated and iodinated toxin) were regarded as heterologous.

Binding of ^{125}I-toxin to the BBMV of P. brassicae was linear from 1 to 80 microgram per 0.1ml and was completed within 10min. Non-iodinated toxin and ^{127}I-toxin were able to compete for the binding of ^{125}I-toxin, indicating specific interaction of toxin with P. brassicae BBMV. When the competitors were present in a

tenfold excess the amount of bound ^{125}I-toxin started to decrease. The decrease
of binding correlated with the increase of amount of non-radioactive toxin.
Finally 83 and 74% of the total binding was inhibited by 1000-fold excess of
^{127}I-toxin and non-iodinated toxin, respectively. A further increase in the competitor concentration did not result in a further decrease of binding. When BBMV
were first incubated with ^{125}I-toxin and then with a 400-fold excess of non-labelled toxin no decrease of bound ^{125}I-toxin was obtained even after 2h.
On the other hand the delta-endotoxin did not bind specifically to BBMV of the
small intestine of rat, which is not a target. Binding of the tracer was not competitively inhibited by non-labelled toxin.
The analysis of the binding data of iodinated toxin and P. brassicae revealed two
binding site populations with K_D of 46nM and 490nM and B_{max} of 0.075nM and 10.5nM
for the high and the low affinity site, respectively. Both sites had a Hill coefficient approaching 1 and were saturable. Furthermore a third binding site population with a K_D of about 0.01mM appeared. However, this site must be due to a
non-specific attachment of the toxin to the vesicles, since the linearity of the
Scatchard plot in this ligand concentration range was too low.
The estimation of the K_D for non-iodinated toxin showed only one binding site
with a dissociation constant of 235nM. The higher affinity site obtained with the
iodinated toxin is very likely due to the iodine which is known to increase the
hydrophobic properties of proteins. The K_D values obtained in this study are comparable to values of other toxins, although they may fluctuate within 1 to 3 orders of magnitude (LeVine and Cuatrecasas, 1981).

References:

Hofmann, C., and Lüthy, P. (1986). Binding and activity of Bacillus thuringiensis
    delta-endotoxin to invertebrate cells. Arch. Microbiol., 146, 7-11.
Pliska, V., Heiniger, J., Müller-Lhotsky, A., Pliska, P., and Ekberg, B. (1986).
    Binding of oxytocin to uterine cells in vitro: Occurrence of several binding
    site populations and reidentification of oxytocin receptors. J. Biol. Chem.,
    261, 16984-16989.
Stieger, B., and Murer, H. (1983). Heterogeneity of brush-border-membrane vesi-
    cles from rat small intestine prepared by a precipitation method using Mg/EGTA.
    Eur. J. Biochem., 135, 95-101.
Wolfersberger, M.G., Hofmann, C., and Lüthy, P. (1986). Interaction of Bacillus
    thuringiensis delta-endotoxin with membrane vesicles isolated from lepidop-
    teran larval midgut. In: P. Falmagne, J.E. Alouf, F.J. Fehrenbach, J.
    Jeljaszewicz, M. Thelestam, (Eds.), Bacterial Protein Toxins. Zbl. Bakt.
    Hygiene, Suppl. 15, Gustav Fischer Verlag, Stuttart, New York. pp. 237-238.
Wolfersberger, M., Lüthy, P., Maurer, A., Parenti, P., Sacchi, F.V., Giordana, B.,
    and Hanozet, G.M. (1987). Preparation and partial characterization of amino
    acid transporting brush border membrane vesicles from the larval midgut of
    the cabbage butterfly (Pieris brassicae). Comp. Biochem. Physiol., 86A, 301-
    308.
LeVine, H., and Cuatrecasas, P. (1981). An overview of toxin-receptor interac-
    tion. Pharmac. Ther., 12, 167-207.

Fehrenbach et al. (Eds.), Bacterial Protein Toxins, Zbl. Bakt. Suppl. 17
© Gustav Fischer, Stuttgart, New York, 1988

Proteolytic Activation of Anthrax Toxin Bound to Cellular Receptors

S. H. Leppla, A. M. Friedlander and E. M. Cora

Bacteriology and Airborne Diseases Divisions, U. S. Army Medical Research Institute of Infectious Diseases Frederick, Maryland 21701-5011 USA

Anthrax toxin is one of several toxins in which the receptor recognition and effector activities (the "B" and "A" domains, respectively) are located on separate proteins (Leppla, 1982; Leppla and co-workers, 1985). The protective antigen (PA), lethal factor (LF), and edema factor (EF) proteins [all having molecular masses of 80-90 kilodaltons (kDa)] are the products of separate, non-contiguous genes (Leppla and co-workers, 1986; Robertson and Leppla, 1986). Previous evidence indicated that PA binds to receptors to produce a system that facilitates entry of LF and EF. Reciprocal inhibition by the latter two proteins argues that LF and EF are alternate "A" moieties competing for the same entry mechanism.

New data have provided an understanding of the interactions of the toxin components on the surface of sensitive cells. Radioiodinated PA bound with high affinity (Kd = 1-10 nM) to most types of cultured cells tested. Receptor-bound PA was cleaved by a cell-surface protease (not identified) to yield 65- and 20-kDa fragments. The 65-kDa fragment remained bound to cells, while the 20-kDa fragment was released. Labeled LF bound to cells only after PA was cleaved, suggesting that LF is binding to the 65-kDa PA fragment.

We used in vitro studies to further characterize the interaction of the components. A low concentration of trypsin was found to cleave PA selectively at arginine 167, which is located in a cluster of four basic amino acids. The nicked PA retained its native structure, but was separated into its constituent 20- and 65-kDa peptides by chromatography at pH 9.0 on MonoQ resin (Pharmacia). The purified 65-kDa amino-terminal fragment, soluble at pH 9.0, was shown by gel filtration and electrophoresis to be a distinct, stable, high-molecular weight species (molecular weight > 300,000). LF and EF bound competitively and with high affinity (Kd = 0.01 nM) to this macromolecular species. The purified 65-kDa PA fragment retained the ability to form a toxic mixture with LF.

These data show that cleavage of PA on the cell surface exposes a high-affinity site to which LF and EF bind. The resulting complex probably enters cells by endocytosis, since previous studies showed that amines protect against the action of PA and LF (Friedlander, 1986). Like several other toxins, anthrax toxin has now been shown to require proteolytic activation.

References:

Friedlander, A.M. (1986). Macrophages are sensitive to anthrax lethal toxin through an acid-dependent process. J.Biol.Chem., 261, 7123-7126.

Leppla, S.H. (1982). Anthrax toxin edema factor: A bacterial adenylate cyclase that increases cyclic AMP concentrations in eukaryotic cells. Proc.Natl.Acad.Sci.USA, 79, 3162-3166.

Leppla, S.H., B.E.Ivins, and J.W.Ezzell, Jr. (1985). Anthrax Toxin. In: L. Leive (Ed.), Microbiology--1985, American Society for Microbiology, Washington, D.C., pp. 63-66.

Leppla, S.H., D.L.Robertson, S.L.Welkos, L.A.Smith, and M.H.Vodkin (1986). Cloning and analysis of genes for anthrax toxin components. In: P.Falmagne, J.E.Alouf, F.J.Fehrenbach, J.Jeljaszewicz and M.Thelestam (Eds.), Bacterial Protein Toxins, Gustav Fischer Verlag, Stuttgart - New York.

Robertson, D.L. and S.H.Leppla (1986). Molecular cloning and expression in Escherichia coli of the lethal factor gene of Bacillus anthracis. Gene 44, 71-78.

Fehrenbach et al. (Eds.), Bacterial Protein Toxins, Zbl. Bakt. Suppl. 17
© Gustav Fischer, Stuttgart, New York, 1988

Lack of Evidence for Ion Channels During Diphtheria Toxin Cell Intoxication

E. Papini[1], R. Rappuoli[2] and C. Montecucco[1]

[1]Centro C. N. R. Biomembrane e Dipartimento di Scienze Biomediche Sperimentali,
[2]Centro Ricerche Sclavo S. p. a., Siena, Italy

After binding to the cell surface, diphtheria toxin is collected into coated pits and subsequently it is found into endosomal vesicles (1). Several evidence suggest that the acidic pH reached in the endosome lumen, is the driving force for the membrane translocation of the toxin.

The lipid interaction of the toxin both at neutral and low pH has been studied with different approaches (1). Different laboratories have shown that diphtheria toxin at low pH forms voltage dependent ion channels across black lipid membranes (2-4). Kagan et al. (3) have found that the channel has a very large diameter and on this basis have proposed that the protomer B of the toxin penetrates in the lipid bilayer and forms the ion channel. Chain A is supposed to unfold and translocate inside the channel in an extended form.

A method has been set up to by-pass the endocytosis step that consists in the incubation of cells with diphtheria toxin at low pHs; under these circumstances the toxin is though to enter into the cell cytoplasm across the plasma membrane (5,6). This protocol allows one to test several parameters previously not accessible to investigation.

In the present work we have investigated the possibility that a ion channel is the plasma membrane crossing form of the toxin on cells incubated at low pH. The two methods used are: a) measurement of the membrane potential with a carbocyanine probe (7) and b) measurement of potassium efflux with a potassium selective electrode (8).

Different cell lines such as: mouse and guinea pig spleen lymphocytes, Vero, CHO and PC-12 cells were equilibrated with the dye and gramicidin or α -toxin of S. aureus were added to show the quenching of the membrane potential. Under these conditions no variations were seen upon addition of up to 10^{-8} M diphtheria toxin both at neutral and acidic pHs; gramicidin addition after the toxin clearly depolarized the cells. At this toxin concentration and under the same experimental conditions the toxin enters into cells as demonstrated by the complete block of protein synthesis.

The same finding was obtained also with the potassium electrode that showed that diphtheria toxin did not induce any appreciable leak of potassium at concentration that showed a maximal effect on protein synthesis. Under the same conditions both gramicidin and the α-toxin of S. aureus were very potent.

In conclusion the present studies failed to demonstrate the formation of highly conducting ion channels during diphtheria toxin cell intoxication. One possible explanation for these unespected findings is that the present experiments were carried out at a toxin to membrane surface ratio two orders of magnitude lower than those of the BLM. When we worked at those concentrations also the techniques used here clearly showed an effect (although uncomplete) of the toxin on the membrane potential and potassium efflux from cells.

The mechanism of diphtheria toxin membrane translocation remains to be clarified at a molecular level and more experiments are needed to demonstrate the relevance of ion channels in the intoxication process.

REFERENCES

1. Olsnes, S. and Sandvig, K. (1987) in "Immunotoxins", Fraenkel, A.E. Ed., Martinus Nijoff Publising, in press

2. Donovan, J.J., Simon, M.I., Draper, R.K. and Montal, M. (1981) Proc. Natl. Acad. Sci. U.S.A. **78**, 172–176.

3. Kagan, B.L., Finkelstein, A. and Colombini, M. (1981) Proc. Natl. Acad. Sci. U.S.A. **78**, 4950–4954

4. Misler, S. (1983) Proc. Natl. Acad. Sci. U.S.A. **80**, 4320–4324

5. Sandvig, K. and Olsnes, S. (1980) J. Cell Biol. **87**, 828–832

6. Draper, R.K. and Simon, M.I. (1980) J. Cell Biol. **87**, 849–854

7. Rink, T.J. Montecucco, C., Hesketh, T.R. and Tsien, R.Y. (1980) Biochim. Biophys. Acta **595**, 15–30

8. Boquet, P. and Duflot, E. (1982) Proc. Natl. Acad. Sci. U.S.A. **79**, 7614–7618

Fehrenbach et al. (Eds.), Bacterial Protein Toxins, Zbl. Bakt. Suppl. 17
© Gustav Fischer, Stuttgart, New York, 1988

Effects of Macromolecular Synthesis Inhibition on Diphtheria Toxin Cell Surface Receptors

B. Rönnberg and J. Middlebrook

U.S. Army Medical Research Institute of Infectious Diseases, Fort Detrick, Frederick, MD 21701 5011, U.S.A.

ABSTRACT

Treatment of Vero cells with cycloheximide (Cyc) reduced their diphtheria toxin (DT) binding capacity, while cells treated with actinomycin D (Act) did not lose their ability to bind DT. Vero cells depleted of toxin receptors by CRM 197, a nontoxic analog of DT, did not regain their ability to bind DT in the presence of Cyc. These data establish that continous protein synthesis is necessary for the presence of functional DT cell surface receptors and also suggest that DT receptors do not recycle after binding ligand.

KEYWORDS

Diphtheria toxin, receptors, regulation, Vero cells

INTRODUCTION

Intoxication of susceptible cells by DT involves binding of the toxin to specific cell-membrane receptors, clustering of toxin-receptor complexes over specialized clathrin-coated regions of the membrane and internalization in endosomes, followed by translocation of the enzymatically active fragment A into the cytoplasm. Fragment A then catalyzes the transfer of ADP-ribose from NAD to elongation factor 2, resulting in an inactive elongation factor 2 and the cessation of protein synthesis (Eidels, Proia and Hart, 1983; Middlebrook and Dorland, 1984). While the biosynthesis and regulation of hormone receptors on eucaryotic cells has been extensively studied, correspondingly little is known about microbial toxin receptors. A monkey kidney-derived cell line (Vero) expresses large numbers of DT binding sites (Middlebrook, Dorland and Leppla, 1978) and provides a suitable system to study biosynthetic regulation of the DT receptor.

MATERIALS AND METHODS

A detailed description of the preparation of radiolabeled DT and the toxin receptor binding assay has appeared previously (Middlebrook, Dorland and Leppla, 1978). Typically, incubations were carried out at $37^{o}C$ under the time and drug conditions stipulated. To measure DT binding capacity, cells were rapidly chilled to $4^{o}C$ and bound with radiolabeled DT for 5 h. Protein and RNA synthesis were measured by the incorporation of tritiated leucine and uridine, respectively. CRM 197 was the generous gift of Rino Rappuoli, Sclavo Research Center, Siena, Italy.

RESULTS AND DISCUSSION

The effects of macromolecular synthesis inhibitors on DT binding capacity were studied. Vero cell monolayers were incubated for 2 h at $37^\circ C$ with various concentrations of Cyc or Act. Cyc-induced inhibition of protein synthesis led to a dose-dependent reduction in DT binding capacity. The Cyc-induced loss of DT binding capacity was not due to nonspecific toxicity, because the effect was completely reversible upon washing; cells regained their toxin-binding capacity within 2 h. Puromycin, an inhibitor of protein synthesis with a different mechanism of action from Cyc, also causes a reduction in DT binding capacity (Middlebrook and Dorland, 1981). This suggests that the effect is due to the general inhibition of protein synthesis and is not an effect specific to one of the inhibitors. Inhibition of RNA synthesis in Vero cells by incubation with lower (0.5, 1, and 2 µg/ml) concentrations of Act did not reduce their ability to bind DT. Instead, we observed an increase in DT binding capacity that continued at least 2 h after the drug was removed. This "overshoot" often reached 150% or more of control values. At higher (5 and 10 µg/ml) concentrations of Act, an irreversible depletion of functional DT receptors occurred. We also examined the effect of protein and RNA synthesis inhibition on the ability of cells to restore DT binding capacity after binding ligand. Following preincubation (2 h) with receptor-saturating concentrations of CRM 197 (at which time receptors were depleted about 90%), the toxin analog was removed and incubation continued. Cells in medium alone regained their toxin-binding capacity within 3-4 h. Cyc (2 µg/ml) blocked this restoration almost completely. Cells in medium containing Act (0.5 µg/ml) not only regained, but "overshot" DT binding capacity, again up to 150% of controls. At these drug concentrations, protein and RNA synthesis are 90% inhibited. We did not employ higher concentrations of Act since its inhibition of RNA synthesis at 1 µg/ml was irreversible.

Since it was possible that receptor-coding message was synthesized during the initial incubation period with CRM 197, a second series of experiments were run wherein Act was present throughout. At an Act concentration of 0.2 µg/ml (during both preincubation with CRM 197 and after its removal), cells regained their DT binding capacity essentially as did cells in medium. At a concentration of 0.5 µg Act/ml, cells did not recover their toxin binding capacity on continued incubation with either Act or medium alone. Apparently, we were working right on the edge of irreversible Act inhibition.

These data establish that continuous protein synthesis is required for a cell to maintain its full complement of functional DT cell surface receptors and to restore receptors after ligand binding. A requirement for RNA synthesis during receptor restoration may exist, but becomes evident only when RNA synthesis is inhibited irreversibly. One explanation for our data could be that, after binding ligand, diphtheria toxin receptors do not recycle.

ACKNOWLEDGMENTS

We would like to thank Dennis Leatherman for his expert technical advice. B. R. holds a National Research Council-USAMRIID Research Associateship.

REFERENCES

Eidels, L., R.L. Proia, and D.A. Hart (1983). Membrane receptors for bacterial toxins. Microbiol. Rev., 47, 596-620.

Middlebrook, J.L., R.B. Dorland, and S.H. Leppla (1978). Association of diphtheria toxin with Vero cells. J. Biol. Chem., 253, 7325-7330.

Middlebrook, J.L., and R.B. Dorland (1981). Receptor-mediated internalization of diphtheria toxin. In: J.L. Middlebrook and L.D. Kohn (Ed.), Receptor-Mediated Binding and Internalization of Toxins and Hormones, Academic Press, New York, pp. 15-29.

Middlebrook, J.L., and R.B. Dorland (1984). Bacterial toxins: cellular mechanisms of action. Microbiol. Rev., 48, 199-221.

Fehrenbach et al. (Eds.), Bacterial Protein Toxins, Zbl. Bakt. Suppl. 17
© Gustav Fischer, Stuttgart, New York, 1988

Preparation of Monoclonal Antibodies Against Diphtheria Toxin Receptor

H. Stenmark, J. Jacobsen, S. Olsnes and K. Sandvig

Institute for Cancer Research at The Norwegian Radium Hospital, Montebello, Oslo 3, Norway

ABSTRACT

Spleen cells from mice immunized with Vero cells were fused with myeloma cells, and clones producing antibodies that protect Vero cells against diphtheria toxin were selected. Four different clones that form protecting antibodies were isolated. All the antibodies bind to a membrane glycoprotein with an apparent molecular weight of 120,000. The protective effect was highest at low chloride concentration.

KEY WORDS

Diphtheria toxin, monoclonal antibodies, receptor, anion transport, Vero cells.

ISOLATION AND PROPERTIES OF PROTECTING ANTIBODIES

In spite of considerable effort in several laboratories, the receptor for diphtheria toxin has not been identified (Eidels, Proia and Hart, 1983; Middlebrook and Dorland, 1984). Protease treatment indicated that the receptor is a protein. However, also treatment of cells with phospholipases reduced toxin binding. In attempts to isolate the receptor, we immunized mice with Vero cells, that are particularly rich in diphtheria toxin receptors, fused the spleen cells with myeloma cells and screened for clones that produced antibodies that protect Vero cells against intoxication.

Four hybridoma lines producing protecting antibodies were isolated. When Vero cells were treated with the monoclonal antibodies and then with increasing concentrations of diphtheria toxin, approximately 3 times more toxin must be added to obtain the same intoxication as in the absence of antibody.

The protecting antibody 2E7-10 inhibited the binding of ^{125}I-diphtheria toxin to Vero cells to approximately the same extent as it protected against intoxication.

Cells were surface-labelled with ^{125}I and lactoperoxidase and then lysed with Triton X-100. Immunoprecipitation with monoclonal antibodies adsorbed to Protein A-Sepharose showed that a protein migrating corresponding to a molecular weight of 120,000 was specifically precipitated (Fig. 1).

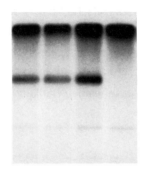

Fig. 1: Immunoprecipitation of ^{125}I-labelled surface protein. Protein A-Sepharose was reacted with the indicated monoclonal antibody or with medium alone. Then, after washing, a Triton X-100 lysate from ^{125}I-labelled Vero cells was added. The Sepharose was washed and the bound proteins were analyzed by polyacrylamide gel electrophoresis and autoradiography. Lane 1, 5H4-7; lane 2, 2E7-10; lane 3, 1A7; lane 4, medium alone.

All four antibodies were found to react with the same protein. The protein was bound to immobilized ricinus agglutinin, wheat germ lectin and concanavalin A and could be eluted with the specific sugars. This indicates that it is a glycoprotein. Labelling with $^{32}PO_4^{3-}$ indicates that it is a phosphoprotein. Experiments with Triton X-114 showed that it partioned into the detergent phase, indicating that it has hydrophobic regions exposed. Finally, the protein was bound to a column with immobilized Cibacron blue and could be eluted with 0.1 mM 4,4'-diisothiocyanostilbene 2,2'-disulfonic acid.

Recent experiments have indicated that an anti-idiotypic antiserum against anti-diphtheria toxin antibodies protects Vero cells against the toxin. This antiserum immunoprecipitates the same protein as the monoclonal antibodies.

REFERENCES

Eidels, L., Proia, R.L., and Hart, D.A. (1983). Membrane receptors for bacterial toxins. Microbiol.Rev., 47, 596-620.

Middlebrook, J.L., and Dorland, R.B. (1984). Bacterial toxins: Cellular mechanisms of action. Microbiol.Rev., 48, 199-221.

Fehrenbach et al. (Eds.), Bacterial Protein Toxins, Zbl. Bakt. Suppl. 17
© Gustav Fischer, Stuttgart, New York, 1988

The Inhibition by Tetanus Toxin of Catecholamine Release by Adrenal Cells

S. Van Heyningen, J. H. Phillips and A. Brown

Department of Biochemistry, University of Edinburgh, Hugh Robson Building,
George Square, Edinburgh EH8 9XD, Great Britain

ABSTRACT

Bovine adrenal medullary chromaffin cells secrete adrenaline and
noradrenalin in response to nicotine. This secretion is inhibited
about 25% by tetanus toxin. The inhibition is increased somewhat
by preincubating the cells with ganglioside GDlb, and increased to
over 80% by preincubating the toxin with ganglioside before adding
it to the cells.

KEYWORDS

Tetanus, ganglioside GT1, adrenal cells, adrenaline,
evoked-response

Although the action of tetanus toxin in vivo is entirely
on neuronal cells, its action in vitro may be relatively non-
specific. We are studying the action of the toxin on primary
cultures of bovine adrenal medullary chromaffin cells. These cells
have many similarities to sympathetic neurones. They secrete
catecholamines in response to a wide variety of agents, e.g.
potassium ions or nicotine. Knight et al. (1985) have shown that
this evoked secretion was inhibited by botulinus toxin type D, but
in their experiments there was no effect of tetanus toxin. However
Penner et al. (1986) were able to show that tetanus toxin directly
injected into these cells produced measurable changes in their
membranes.

Our suggestion is that externally added toxin may be able
to act on these cells only when it can bind to them. Chromaffin
cell membranes probably contain very little of the toxin-binding
ganglioside, GDlb and GT1, and so are inefficient at binding or
internalizing added toxin. If the cells are preincubated with
these gangliosides, they would become dissolved in the outer
membrane, and the cells should be better able to bind and take up
the toxin.

A primary culture of adrenal cells was incubated for 24h in the presence and absence of 10 ug/ml toxin. In some experiments, the cells or the toxin or both had been preincubated with 50 ug/ml ganglioside GT1 for 1.5h. After the incubation with the toxin, the release of adrenalin and noradrenalin evoked by nicotine was measured by a fluorimetric assay. The table shows the result of these experiments.

Cells and toxin	evoked release (% of cell content)
native cells, no toxin	16.2
native cells, treated with toxin	11.9
cells preincubated with ganglioside, no toxin	14.2
cells preincubated with ganglioside, then with toxin	10.5
toxin preincubated with ganglioside cells untreated	1.1
toxin and cells both preincubated with ganglioside	1.4

Toxin inhibits the evoked release by about 25% even when the cells have not been preincubated. Preincubating the cells with ganglioside has comparatively little effect: presumably these cells already have some toxin-binding sites (maybe other gangliosides which bind toxin more weakly). However treating the cells with a preformed ganglioside-toxin complex has a dramatic effect, inhibiting the release by over 80%. This complex must be taken up by the cells relatively well, and remain active.

These experiments show a marked effect of tetanus toxin on adrenal cells. The system is likely to prove a very useful one for future study of the action of tetanus toxin (and of the mechanism of secretion by adrenal cells), because it is relatively amenable to investigation.

ACKNOWLEDGEMENT
We are grateful to the Medical Research Council and the Wellcome Trust for grants towards this research.

REFERENCES
Knight, D.E., Tonge, D.A. & Baker, P.F. (1985). Inhibition of exocytosis in bovine adrenal medullary cells by botulinus toxin type D. Nature, London, 317, 719-721.

Penner, R., Neher, E. & Dreyer, F. (1986). Intracellularly injected tetanus toxin inhibits exocytosis in bovine adrenal chromaffin cells. Nature, London, 324, 76-78.

Fehrenbach et al. (Eds.), Bacterial Protein Toxins, Zbl. Bakt. Suppl. 17
© Gustav Fischer, Stuttgart, New York, 1988

Monochainal Tetanus Toxin: Preparation, Protoxin Properties and Proteolytic Conversion into Isotoxins

U. Weller, F. Mauler, E. Habermann

Buchheim-Institut für Pharmakologie, Justus-Liebig-Universität, Frankfurter Str. 107, D-6300 Gießen

Key words:Tetanus toxin, protoxin, isotoxins, trypsin, synapses

To elucidate the posttranslational processing of the primary product of the tetanus toxin gene, monochainal toxin (M) was extracted from bacterial cell bodies (strain Massachusetts) grown in Latham medium for 24h according to Ozutsumi and co-workers (1985). It was purified by $(NH_4)_2SO_4$ precipitation (40% saturation) followed by preparative HPLC gel-chromatography using a TSK G-3000 SWP column. The final product was homogenous in SDS-disk gel electrophoresis.

Upon treatment with trypsin, toxin M was nicked into a bichainal derivative (toxin BT). The chains separated by SDS disk gel electrophoresis upon reduction of the connecting disulfide bond. The original light chain was further processed by trypsin to a derivative of still lower (by~1kD) molecular weight. This late tryptic derivative was indistinguishable from the bichainal extracellular derivative (toxin BE) prepared from culture supernatant. Cl. tetani is known to synthethize a set of proteases, among them nicking ones. Hydrophobic interaction chromatography allowed the discrimination of (in terms of decreasing hydrophobicity) toxins M, BE and BT. Toxin BE turned out to be inhomogenous (Figure).
Besides with trypsin, nicking can also be achieved with chymotrypsin, elastase, post-arginine cleaving enzyme from mouse submaxillary gland, and clostripain, resulting in light chains of different sizes. Thus the monochainal primary gene product (toxin M) is proteolytically converted into a series of bichainal isotoxins.
Toxin M was then compared with the bichainal toxins BT and BE in various pharmacological tests.
1. Upon subcutaneous injection in mice, toxin M had an LD_{50} of 4ng/kg, about twice that of toxin BT or BE. Moreover, time to death was considerably prolonged after 50-100 LD of toxin M as compared with the same amount of toxin BT or BE.
2. The isolated phrenic nerve-hemidiaphragm from mice is known to be paralyzed by tetanus toxin. Toxin BT was equipotent with BE and about 10 times more potent than toxin M.

3. The ^{3}H-noradrenaline release (Habermann and co-workers, 1987) from both primary nerve cell cultures (mouse) and superfused broken brain cell preparations (rat) is inhibited by tetanus toxin. In both systems toxin BE and BT were 10 times more potent than toxin M.

Since activation takes place in every system tested, however to a different degree, toxin M may be regarded as a protoxin. Further studies should clarify the question whether nicking also occurs by intracellular proteases.

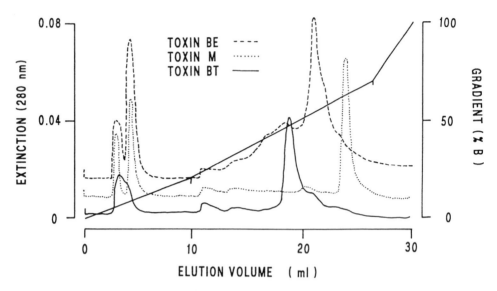

Figure. Hydrophobic interaction chromatography of toxin M (150 µg), BT (150 µg, immediatly after trypsin treatment, as described by Matsuda and Yoneda 1974) and BE (400 µg) on a LKB TSK Phenyl-5PW (7.5 x 75mm) HPLC column. Buffer A was 0.5M K-phosphate pH 8.0, buffer B was 0.025mM K-phosphate pH 8.0. Samples were mixed with the same volume of 2x buffer A and microfiltered. After loading the column was eluted with 0.5 ml/min for 20 min. Then flow was reduced to 0.05 ml/min. Peaks eluting with the first 10 ml were mainly benzamidine from the storage buffer (toxin M, toxin BE) or tris from the reaction mixture after trypsin treatment (toxin BT).

REFERENCES:

Habermann, E., H. Müller and M. Hudel (1987). Clostridial neuro-toxins prevent ^{3}H-noradrenaline release from primary nerve cell cultures and broken brain cells. Proc. 3rd Europ. Workshop Bact. Toxins (Überlingen).

Matsuda, M. and M. Yoneda (1974). Dissociation of tetanus toxin into two polypeptide fragments. Biochem. Biophys. Res. Com., 57, 1257-1262.

Ozutsumi, K., N. Sugimoto and M. Matsuda (1985). Rapid, simplified method for production and purification of tetanus toxin. Appl. Environm. Microbiol., 49, 939-943

Toxin Secretion and Internalization

Fehrenbach et al. (Eds.), Bacterial Protein Toxins, Zbl. Bakt. Suppl. 17
© Gustav Fischer, Stuttgart, New York, 1988

A Highly Coordinated Pathway for Enterotoxin Assembly and Secretion in Vibrio cholerae

T. R. Hirst[1], J. Holmgren[2], S. Johansson[2], J. Sanchez[2], M. Bagdasarian[3] and M. Sandkvist[3]

[1]Department of Genetics, University of Leicester, Leicester LE17RH, UK
[2]Department of Medical Microbiology, University of Goteborg, S-413 46 Goteborg
[3]Unit of Applied Cell and Molecular Biology, University of Umea, S-90187 Umea

ABSTRACT

Vibrio cholerae is able to secrete oligomeric toxins, such as cholera toxin and LT[1], across its cell envelope into the external milieu. 1. The component subunits of these toxins, transiently enter the periplasm as they traverse the envelope. 2. Oligomerization of the toxin subunits occurs in the periplasm prior to their secretion across the outer membrane. 3. The B subunit carboxyl-terminal domain plays a crucial role in A subunit – B subunit interaction. 4. The pathway of toxin assembly proceeds via A subunit association with B monomers or small oligomers, eg. dimers. 5. B subunits contain structural domains important for toxin translocation across the V. cholerae outer membrane. Our studies show that the events of toxin secretion are remarkably well-coordinated in ensuring the formation of a functional toxin that is successfully delivered across the bacterial cell-envelope.

KEYWORDS

Cholera toxin, E. coli heat-labile enterotoxin, protein export, secretion pathways, periplasm, outer membrane, subunit assembly, quaternary structure.

INTRODUCTION

Pathogenic factors, including toxins and surface adhesins are either located on the bacterial cell surface or released in the surrounding milieu. This means that efficient and often complex biological processes are necessary for ensuring the translocation of such pathogenic molecules from their site of biosynthesis in the cytoplasm, to the surface of bacteria and beyond. In Gram negative bacteria this is a formidable enterprise since the cell-envelope consists of two distinct membranes, interspersed by a protein-filled periplasm.

---

[1]LT, heat-labile enterotoxin from enterotoxinogenic strains of Escherichia coli.

We chose to investigate how proteins are translocated across bacterial cell envelopes by focussing on the events involved in the export and secretion of enterotoxins by Vibrio cholerae and certain diarrhoegenic strains of Escherichia coli. These organisms are responsable for a majority of the severe and at times fatal diarrhoeal diseases in man. Among the primary virulence factors produced by them are cholera toxin and heat-labile enterotoxin (LT). Both toxins have similar primary and quaternany structures, as well as identical modes of action (for reviews see; Holmgren, 1981, Sack, 1975). They are comprised of six polypeptide chains; a single A subunit (28 kDa) that activates adenylate cyclase, and five B subunits (12 kDa each) which bind to GMI-ganglioside (Dallas and Falkow, 1979; Gill and others, 1981; Holmgren, 1973; Mekalanos and others 1983; Moss and Richardson, 1978). Genes for the A and B subunits of LT (etxA and etxB)[2] are found on large conjugative plasmids, whereas the genes for cholera toxin (ctxA and ctxB) are located on the chromosome. The genes encoding LT and cholera toxin have been cloned and extensively analysed (Leong, Vinal and Dallas, 1985; Mekalanos and others, 1983; Yamamoto, Tamura, and Yokota, 1984).

The component subunits of LT and cholera toxin are initially synthesized as precursor polypeptides (pre A and pre B) with amino terminal signal sequences of 18 and 21 amino acids respectively (Dallas and Falkow, 1980; Mekalanos and others, 1983; Spicer and Noble, 1982). The mature subunits are generated by proteolytic removal of the signal sequences during export of the presursor polypeptides across the bacterial cytoplasmic membrane. When cholera toxin or LT are expressed in E. coli the mature A and B subunits assemble into holotoxin and these are located in the periplasm of the cell envelope (Hirst, Randall and Hardy, 1984; Hofstra and Witholt, 1984). In contrast, when either LT or cholera toxin are synthesized in V. cholerae they are secreted into the external milieu (Hirst and others, 1984; Neill, Ivins and Holmes, 1983). This remarkable difference suggests that V. cholerae possesses the capacity of translocating complex oligomeric proteins across its cell envelope; and this poses important and fundamental biological questions! How, for example, do the individual subunits traverse the envelope? Do they enter the periplasm prior to secretion across the outer membrane or are they secreted via zones of inner and outer membrane adhesion? At what stage during the secretion process are the subunits assembled into holotoxin? And what mechanisms, membrane components and toxin structural domains facilitate each step of the translocation event. In this paper we show that toxin secretion by V. cholerae is a beautifully coordinated process with each step combining to ensure the assembly and delivery of a functional toxin molecule into the extracellular milieu.

RESULTS

Pathway of Toxin Secretion in V. cholerae. Enterotoxin subunits enter the periplasm of V. cholerae as they traverse the cell envelope to reach the extracellular milieu. This was established by following the location of a pool of radiolabelled toxin subunits during their secretion from V. cholerae. For this purpose we used V. cholerae strain TRH7000 from which the cholera toxin genes had been deleted from the chromosome by site-directed mutagenesis and into which had been mobilized plasmid pWD600 that contained the cistrons for expressing LT (Dallas, 1983; Hirst and others, 1984; Hirst and Holmgren, 1987).

---

[2]LT genes from E. coli isolates of human and porcine origin have been given various mnemonic abbreviations, eg. elt, elt$_H$ elt$_P$, tox, elt307 etc. However since these genes are allelic we have selected etx as a unifying designation for all LT genes of E. coli.

V. cholerae TRH7000(pWD600) and its parental strain lacking the plasmid, were radioactively pulse-labelled with 200 μCi ^{35}S-methionine per ml for 0.5 min, and then chased with an excess of nonradioactive methionine. Samples of culture were chilled on ice, 0.5 and 14.5 min after the addition of the chase, and the radioactively labelled polypeptides in medium and periplasmic fractions analysed by SDS-polyacrylamide gel electrophoresis (Fig. 1).

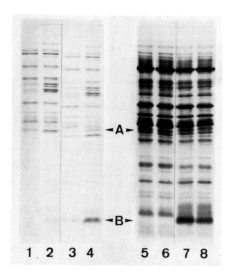

Fig. 1: Media and periplasmic fractions from V. cholerae TRH7000 and TRH7000(pWD600). Periplasmic fractions were obtained by resuspending labelled cells in 0.9% NaCl containing 2000 units per ml of polymixin B at 4°C for 15 min, and the cells removed by centrifugation as described by Hirst and Holmgren (1987). Lanes 1 and 2, media from TRH7000 chased for 0.5 and 14.5 min respectively; lanes 3 and 4, media from TRH7000(pWD600) chased for 0.5 and 14.5 min; lanes 5 and 6, periplasmic fractions for TRH7000 chased for 0.5 and 14.5 min; periplasmic fractions from TRH7000(pWD600) chased for 0.5 and 14.5 min. The migration position of A- and B-subunit standards are indicated.

As expected, the medium from the toxin-deleted control strain, TRH7000, lacked labelled polypeptides that could correspond to either the A or B subunits of LT (Fig. 1, lanes 1 and 2), whereas TRH7000 harbouring pWD600 secreted two polypeptides with molecular weights of 28,000 and 12,000 which comigrated with purified toxin A- and B- subunit standards (Fig. 1, lane 4). These two labelled polypeptides were clearly evident in the medium after 14.5 min of chase (lane 4) but were not present after the shorter chase time (0.5 min) (lane 3). This suggested that the subunits were still cell-associated after the shorter chase time. We therefore fractionated the cells to investigate if the subunit polypeptides were present in periplasmic fractions. Figure 3, lanes 7 and 8 show that a polypeptide having a molecular weight of 12,000 was present in periplasmic fractions from TRH7000(pWD600), but clearly absent from corresponding fractions from TRH7000 (lanes 5 and 6). We therefore conclude that this labelled polypeptide is the B subunit of LT, and that it passes through the periplasm as it traverses the cell-envelope of V. cholerae.

Kinetics of Toxin Efflux from V. cholerae. The turnover and rate of enterotoxin subunit efflux from the periplasm of V. cholerae TRH7000(pWD600) was analysed by radiolabelling a culture with ^{35}S-methionine for 0.5 min, and isolating periplasmic fractions throughout the subsequent chase period (Fig. 2, lanes 1 to 9).

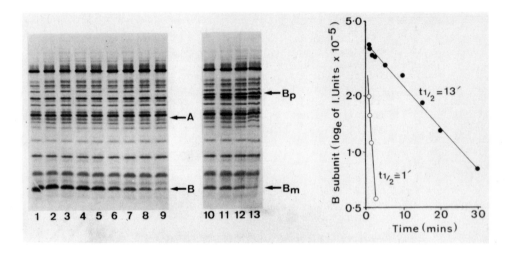

Fig. 2: Kinetics of enterotoxin assembly and secretion. Periplasmic fractions were obtained from a culture of V. cholerae TRH7000(pWD600) that had been radioactively pulse-labelled for 0.5 min and chased for different lengths of time. Equivalent amounts of each fraction were mixed with SDS-containing sample buffer and either boiled (lanes 1-9) or kept at 25° (lanes 10 to 13) before being analysed by SDS polyacrylamide gel electrophoresis and autoradiography. Reproductions of the autoradiograms are shown in which the times after the initiation of the pulse were: 0.75 min (lanes 1 and 10), 1 min (lanes 2 and 11), 1.5 min (Lanes 3 and 12), 2.5 min (lanes 4 and 13), 5 min (lane 5), 10 min (lane 6), 15 min (lane 7), 20 min (lane 8), 30 min (lane 9). The migration positions of LT A- and B- subunit standards (A and B) and of the B subunit monomers (Bm) and assembled pentamers (Bp) are indicated by arrows. The quantity of labelled B subunits migrating in the B subunit position (B)(0) in lanes 1 to 9 and in the B monomer position (Bm)(0) in lanes 10 to 13 were determined by densitometric scanning of the autoradiogram. The amounts given are in arbitrary integration units (Int. units) and are plotted against the time at which the samples were taken after the initiation of the pulse.

The amount of radiolabelled B subunits in the periplasm had reached a maximum level after the shortest chase time (0.25 min) (lane 1), indicating that the initial events in toxin secretion (ie, the biosynthesis and export of subunits to the periplasm) are rapid. The amount of labelled B subunits in the periplasm clearly decreased during the chase, and when the amounts were quntified by ensitometric scanning of the autoradiogram, the rate of decrease appeared to be governed by a 1st order, simple exponential process (Fig. 2). The half-time for turnover of labelled B subunits in the periplasm was calculated to be 13 min.

Location of toxin assembly in V. cholerae. We took advantage of an unusual property of the enterotoxin B subunits in order to investigate if the subunits which transiently enter the periplasm assemble into oligomers prior to their secretion across the V. cholerae outer membrane. Enterotoxin B subunit pentamers are stable in the presence of the ionic detergent, SDS, and migrate on SDS polyacrylamide gels as an oligomer with an apparent molecular weight of 45 kDa. Dissociation of B subunits pentamers into their component monomers occurs when they are heated to >70°C. Samples of periplasm obtained during the pulse-chase of V. cholerae TRH7000(pWD600) were mixed with SDS-containing sample buffer and either boiled for 5 min or kep at room temperature and then analysed by SDS polyacrylamide gel electrophoresis (Fig. 2, compare lanes 1 to 4 and 10 to 13). When the samples were boiled, the total quantity of labelled B subunits in each fraction migrated as 12kDa monomers (lanes 1 to 4). When, however, equivalent fractions were unheated before electrophoresis a single new protein species was identified that had an apparent molecular weight of 45kDa (lanes 10-13). In addition, a labelled polypeptide which migrated with an apparent molecular weight of 12kDa was present in the unheated samples, but its amount rapidly declined by approximately 75% during the first 2 min of the chase (lanes 10-13). We suggest that since experimental controls lacking the ability to produce enterotoxin did not produce any such 12kDa polypeptide, this molecule represents a transient intermediate in the assembly of B subunits. Measurements of the quantity of this intermediate revealed that it turned over with a half-time of ca.1 min (Fig 1). We conclude that enterotoxin B subunits enter the periplasm as 12kDa monomers that rapidly assemble and thus attain an SDS-resistant, stable quaternary structure before their efflux across the outer membrane.

Analyses of periplasmic fractions in a GM1-enzyme-linked immunosorbant assay (GM1-ELISA) using monospecific antibodies against the A subunit, demonstrated that the periplasmic pool contained fully assembled holotoxin (AB_5) which bound to GM1 and reacted with A subunit antibodies (data not shown). We therefore conclude that the periplasm is not only the site of B subunit pertamerization but also holotoxin formation.

Pathway of A- and B-subunit Assembly. Association of A and B subunit for form holotoxin could conceivably occur by either of the following pathways:-

$$(1)\ 5\ B_{monomers} \longrightarrow B_{pentamer} + A \longrightarrow AB_5$$

$$(2)\ 5\ B_{monomers} + A \longrightarrow AB_5$$

The first pathway is meant to implicate that A subunits only associate with preassembled B pentamers. Such a pathway has been previously suggested (Hirst and others, 1984), based on the finding that LT B subunit pentamers assemble and are secreted from V. cholerae irrespective of the presence or absence of A subunit synthesis. The second pathway however, is meant to imply that A subunits normally interact with B subunits at an earlier stage of B subunit oligomerization.

Evidence for the second pathway was obtained when the reassociation of purified cholera toxin subunits was analysed in vitro. Pure cholera toxin subunits were acidified and then either neutralized by the addtiion of alkali or by extensive dialysis against a buffer of neutral pH (Table1). Reassociation of acid-denatured B subunits occured spontaneously when neutral pH was restored. The extent of reassociation was monitored in a GM1-ELISA using monoclonal antibody LT-39, that bound to B pentamers but not B monomers. When acidified A and B subunits were mixed together and the mixture neutralized, fully assembled holotoxin was obtained. However, if acidified A and B subunits were neutralised independently[3] and then mixed together, a negligible amount of B subunits were found to be associated with the A subunits (Table 1). This indicated that the A subunit polypeptide associated either with B nonomers or small B subunit oligomers (eg dimers) during the pathway of holotoxin assembly and not with preformed B pentamers.

Table 1. Assembly pathway of cholera toxin in vitro: subunit A and subunit B association precedes B pentamer formation.

Experimental Approach	Toxin Detected by GMI-ELISA(%)	
	A subunit	B subunit
I. Neutralization with NaOH		
1. Acidified CT-A and acidified CT-B mixed and then neutralised	31	82
2. Acidified CT-A and acidified CT-B neutralized separately and then mixed	2	107
II. Neutralization by dialysis		
1. Acidified CT-A and acidified CT-B mixed and then neutralized	92	99
2. Acidified CT-A and acidified CT-B neutralized separately and then mixed	10	99
3. Acidified CT-A$_1$-fragment and acidified CT-B mixed and then neutralized	0.3	86

The carboxyl-terminal domain of the B subunit is important in A subunit- B subunit interaction. The gene encoding the B subunit of heat-labile enterotoxin was mutated at its 3' end by targeted addition of random nucleotide sequences. Two novel B subunits EtxB124 and EtxB138, with short carboxyl-terminal

---

[3]Acidification and neutralization of A subunits in the absence of B subunits does not adversely affect the tertiary structure of the A subunit polypeptide. (Hirst and others - manuscript in preparation).

extensions of 7 extra amino acids were found to be specifically defective in their ability to stably interact with A subunbits and form holotoxin[4] (Fig. 3).

<pre>
                         +103
                         GluAsn***
        pMMB68   GAAAACTAGT
                            SpeI
                         +102
                         GluLysLeuPheGlnProAspThrAsp***
        pMMB124   GAAAAGCTTTTTCAGCCTGATACAGATTAA
                            Hind III
                         +102
                         GluLysLeuAlaProGlnLysArgTrp***
        pMMB138   GAAAAGCTTGCCCCCCGAGAACGCTGGTGA
                            Hind III
</pre>

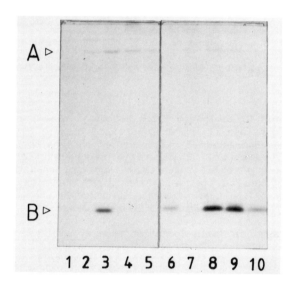

Fig 3: Inability of altered B subunits to associate with A subunits. Nucleotide sequences of the 3' portions of the engineered etxB genes and the wild-type, parental gene in plasmid pMMB68. Numbers above the predicted amino acid sequence indicate the number of the amino acid residue in the mature molecule of EtxB. E. coli strain CC118 (Manoil and Beckwith, 1985) containing plasmids indicated below were induced with IPTG and labelled with ^{35}S-methionine. Cells were disrupted, immunoprecipitated and subjected to SDS polyacrylamide gel electrophoresis. Samples in lanes 1 to 5 were precipitated with antiserum R833 directed against subunit A of cholera toxin and those in lanes 6 to 10

---

[4]EtxB124 and EtxB138 were "normal" with respect to a whole range of other properties, including export to the periplasm of E. coli, oligomerization into pentamers, recognition by anti-toxin antibodies, secretion from V. cholerae and binding to GM1-ganglioside.

with antiserum R420 against cholera holotoxin. Lanes 1
and 6, pMMB68, 2 and 7, pWD605; 3 and 8, pMMB68 and
pWD605; 4 and 9, pMMB124 and pWD605, 5 and 10, pMMB138
and pWD605.   Position of the A and B subunits are
indicated.

E. coli strains harbouring pWD605 (which encodes the A subunit of LT), together
with the plasmids that encode for authentic B subunit or EtxB124 or EtxB138 were
constructed in order to assess whether EtxB124 and EtxB138 interact with the LT
A subunit to form holotoxin.   Immunoprecipitates from cell extracts of these
strains were prepared using anti-cholera toxin A subunit antisera. (Fig. 3,
lanes 1 to 5) or anti-cholera toxin A/B subunit antisera (lanes 6 to 10).
Authentic EtxB encoded by pMMB68 was found to be immunoprecipitated by both
anti-A subunit and anti-A/B subunit antisera (compare lanes 3 and 8).   Therefore
authentic B subunits are assembled in vivo into a holotoxin complex that is
immunoprecipitable by antiserum raised against cholera toxin A subunit.

When similar analyses were performed on extracts containing both the A subuinit
and either EtxB124 or EtxB138, none of the B subunits were immunoprecipitated by
anti-A subunit antiserum (R833) (lanes 4 and 5) whereas they were precipitated
by anti-A/B subunit antiserum (R420) (lanes 9 and 10).   This shows that the
extra 7 amino acids on the carboxyl-termini of EtxB124 and EtxB138 prevent
stable interaction of these B subunits with the LT-A subunit.

Importance of B Subunit Oxidation in Toxin Assembly. Oxidation of cys and cys
to yield a disulphide bridge is a prerequisite for stable B subunit-B[9] subunit
interaction.   This was demonstrated with purified cholera toxin, which had been
acidified as described above.   Ordinarily, neutralization results in the
spontaneous association of the B subunits.   However, when the reducing agent
dithiothreitol was added to the acidified toxin subunits, this completely
abolished the ability of the toxin subunits to assemble when they were restored
to neutral pH (Hirst and other - manuscript in preparation).

Role of A and B Subunits in Toxin Secretion from V. cholerae. When strains of
V. cholera were constructed which harboured either plasmid pWD605 (encoding the
A subunit of LT) or plasmid pWD615 (encoding the B subunit of LT) it was found
that approximately 90% of the B subunits were secreted from V. cholerae
TRH7000(pWD615) whereas none of the A subunits expressed by TRH7000(pWD605) were
secreted (Hirst and others, 1984).   This shows that the B subunits of the toxin
contain structural information which enable the molecule to translocate across
the V. cholerae cell envelope and that comparable information is absent from the
A subunit.

DISCUSSION

Secretion of proteins across bacterial envelopes is a fascinating biological
phenomenon which is especially tantalizing for multimeric proteins which must
assemble at some stage of their biosynthesis.   The events of toxin secretion by
V. cholerae not only illustrate the diversity of steps involved in protein
movement across biological membranes but also the general principles governing
the assembly and translocation of multimeric proteins.

In this paper we show that toxin assembly is a beautifully coordinated process
which leads to the formation of a "native" toxin molecule that can be
successfully delivered to its site of action in the external milieu (Fig. 4).
In addition these observations challenge the currently held paradigm that
polypeptides traverse biological membranes as unfolded chains which lack

Pathway of Toxin Secretion in Vibrio cholerae

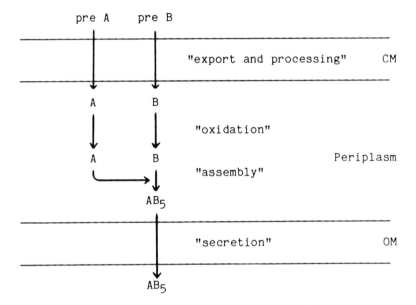

"native' tertiary structures (Eilers and Schatz, 1986; Randall and Hardy, 1986). Our data suggest that toxin secretion across the outer membrane of V. cholerae involves translocation of the molecule after it has folded and adopted a stable quaternary conformation.

ACKNOWLEDGEMENTS

We thank Margaret Law for help in preparing the manuscript. TRH is the recipient of a Wellcome Trust Senior Research Fellowship in Basic Biomedical Sciences. This work was in part supported by grants from The Wellcome Trust of Great Britian, the Swedish Board for Technical Development and the World Health Organization.

REFERENCES

Dallas, W.S., and S. Falkow (1979). The molecular nature of heat-labile enterotoxin (LT) of Escherichia coli. Nature, 277, 406-407.
Dallas, W.S., and S. Falkow (1980). Amino acid sequence homology between cholera toxin and Escherichia coli heat-labile toxin. Nature, 288, 499-501.

Dallas, W.S. (1983). Conformity between heat-labile toxin genes from human and porcine enterotoxinogenic Escherichia coli. Infect. Immun., 40, 647-652.

Eilers, M., and G. Schatz (1986). Binding of a specific lingand inhibits import of a purified presursor protein into mitochondria. Nature, 322, 228-232.

Gill, D.M., J.D. Clements, D.C. Robertson, and R.A. Finkelstein (1981). Subunit number and arrangement in Eschericia coli heat-labile enterotoxin. Infect. Immun., 33, 677-682.

Hirst, T. R., L.L. Randall, and S.J.S. Hardy (1984). Cellular location of heat-labile enterotoxin in Escherichia coli. J. Bacteriol., 157, 637-642.

Hirst, T.R., J. Sanchez, J.B. Kaper, S.J.S. Hardy, and J. Holmgren (1984). Mechanism of toxin secretion by Vibrio cholerae investigated in strains harbouring plasmids that encode heat-labile enterotoxins of Escherichia coli. Proc. Natl. Acad. Sci., 81, 7752-7756.

Hirst, T.R., and J. Holmgren (1987). Transient entry of enterotoxin subunits into the periplasm occurs during their secretion from Vibrio Cholerae. J. Bacteriol., 169, 1037-1045.

Hofstra, H., and B. Witholt (1984). Kinetics of synthesis, processing and membrane transport of heat-labile enterotoxin, a periplasmic protein of Escherichia coli. J. Biol. Chem., 259, 15182-15187.

Holmgren, J. (1973). Comparison of the tissue receptors for Vibrio cholerae and Escherichia coli enterotoxins by means of gangliosides and natural cholera toxoid. Infect. Immun., 8, 851-859.

Holmgren, J. (1981). Actions of cholera toxin and the prevention and treatment of cholera. Nature, 227, 680-685.

Leong, J., A.C. Vinal, and W.S. Dalls (1985). Nucleotide sequence comparison between heat-labile toxin B subunit cistrons from Escherichia coli of human and porcine origin. Infect. Immun., 48, 73-77.

Manoil, C., and J. Beckwith (1985). TnPhoA: A transposon probe for protein export signals. Proc. Natl. Acad. Sci., 82, 8129-8133.

Mekalanos, J.J., D.J. Swartz, G.D.C. Pearson, N. Harford, F. Groyne, and M. de Wilde (1983). Cholera toxin genes: nucleotide sequence, deletion analysis and vaccine development. Nature, 306, 551-557.

Moss, J. and S.H. Richardson (1978). Activation of adenylate cyclase by heat-labile enterotoxin. J. Clin. Invest., 62, 281-285.

Neill, R.J., B.E. Ivins, and R.K. Holmes (1983). Synthesis of the plasmid-coded heat-labile enterotoxin of Escherichia coli in Vibrio cholerae. Science, 221, 289-291.

Randall, L.L., and S.J.S. Hardy (1986). Correlation of competence for export with tack of tertiary structure of mature species: a study in vivo of maltose-binding protein of E. coli. Cell, 46, 921-928.

Sack, B. R. (1975). Human diarrhoeal disease caused by enterotoxigenic Escherichia coli. Ann. Rev. Microbial., 29, 333-353.

Spicer, E.K., and J.A. Noble (1982). Escherichia coli heat-labile enterotoxin. Nucleotide sequence of the A subunit gene. J. Biol.Chem., 257, 5716-5721.

Fehrenbach et al. (Eds.), Bacterial Protein Toxins, Zbl. Bakt. Suppl. 17
© Gustav Fischer, Stuttgart, New York, 1988

Mechanisms Involved in Intracellular Routing and Membrane Penetration of Protein Toxins

K. Sandvig[1], S. Olsnes[1], O. W. Petersen[2] and B. van Deurs[2]

[1]Institute for Cancer Research at The Norwegian Radium Hospital, Montebello, Oslo 3, Norway
[2]Department of Anatomy, The Panum Institute, University of Copenhagen, DK-2200, Copenhagen N

ABSTRACT

All known protein toxins with intracellular targets bind to cell surface receptors, are endocytosed, and enter the cytosol from an intracellular compartment. In spite of their structural similarities, the toxins described here, diphtheria toxin, pseudomonas exotoxin A, modeccin, volkensin, abrin and ricin use different mechanisms for transfer of the enzymatically active part into the cytosol. The uptake of the toxins, the intracellular routing and the final penetration of the toxins into the cytosol will be discussed in the present paper.

KEYWORDS

Toxic proteins, endocytosis, trans-Golgi network, membrane transport, intracellular routing.

INTRODUCTION

The protein toxins described here all have two functionally separated domains, one that binds to cell surface receptors and one that has the ability to enter the cytosol and inhibit protein synthesis enzymatically (for review, see Olsnes and Sandvig, 1985). With the exception of pseudomonas toxin which consists of a single polypeptide, the toxins consist of two polypeptides connected by a disulfide bond. This bond must be reduced to obtain maximal enzymatic effect.
Studies of these protein toxins are of interest for several reasons. They can be used to examine in which way large proteins are transferred across biological membranes. The transfer into the cytosol of even a few molecules can be monitored as inhibition of protein synthesis. Some of the toxins were originally studied because of their cancerostatic effect, and recently toxins have become widely used to make immunotoxins. Immunotoxins are molecules where either the whole toxin or a part of the molecule containing the enzymatically active polypeptide is coupled covalently to an antibody that reacts with antigens on the cell surface.

ENTRY OF DIPHTHERIA TOXIN AND PSEUDOMONAS TOXIN
INTO CELLS

The bacterial toxins diphtheria toxin and pseudomonas toxin both
require low pH for entry into the cytosol. Thus, a number of
compounds that increase the pH of intracellular compartments
protect against these toxins (Olsnes and Sandvig, 1985). Both
toxins are internalized via the coated pit/coated vesicle pathway
(Morris and co-workers,1983,1985), and after entry into the
cytosol they inhibit protein synthesis in cells by ADP-
ribosylation of elongation factor 2 (Middlebrook and Dorland,
1984). There is now good evidence that diphtheria toxin enters
from the early acidic vesicles called endosomes. One function of
the low pH is to induce a conformational change in diphtheria
toxin leading to exposure of the hydrophobic regions of the
molecule. This is reflected in the ability of the toxin to bind
Triton X-114 at low pH (Fig. 1).

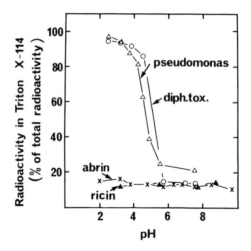

Fig. 1: Effect of pH on the ability of diphtheria
toxin, pseudomonas toxin, abrin and ricin to bind
Triton X-114. ^{125}I-labelled toxins were incubated with
a mixture of Triton X-114 (100 µl) and buffer
containing 0.14 M NaCl (300 µl) for 15 min at 0°C. The
samples were then heated to 37°C to induce phase
separation, and the radioactivity in the two phases was
measured.

Also pseudomonas toxin acquires the ability to bind Triton X-114
at low pH, although lower pH values are required than in the case
of diphtheria toxin. In spite of this similarity, there are data
suggesting that pseudomonas toxin enters the cytosol after fusion
of the endosomes with another cellular compartment (Morris and
Saelinger, 1986). Thus, at temperatures below 20°C where such

fusion processes are strongly inhibited, also the effect of
pseudomonas toxin was strongly inhibited, while the toxic effect
of diphtheria toxin which enters directly from the endosomes is
reduced to a much lesser extent. Furthermore, in the case of
diphtheria toxin it is possible to induce rapid entry of surface
bound toxin into the cytosol by exposing the cells to low pH,
thus mimicking the conditions in the endosomes. However, in the
case of pseudomonas toxin such direct entry cannot be induced. In
the case of diphtheria toxin it is therefore easier to study the
requirements for transport across the membrane and the
consequences of this transport for membrane functions.
At present, most details are known about the entry of diphtheria
toxin. Different lines of evidence suggest that not only is low
pH required to induce a change in the diphtheria toxin molecule,
but a pH gradient of about 1.5 pH units across the membrane is
required for entry to occur. When the pH in the medium is lowered
by addition of a weak acid like acetic acid or by preincubating
the cells with ammonium chloride, diphtheria toxin entry can no
longer be induced by medium with low pH (Sandvig and co-workers,
1986).

When diphtheria toxin entry is induced by low pH there seems to
be a proton flux into the cytosol. As shown in Fig. 2 the pH in
cells exposed to diphtheria toxin and low pH decreases to a
greater extent than in cells which were exposed to low pH only.

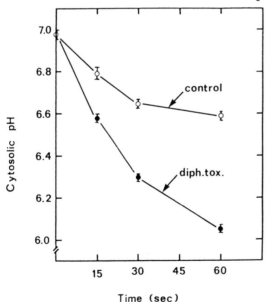

Fig. 2: Insertion of diphtheria toxin into the membrane
is associated with acidification of the cytosol. Vero
cells were incubated with diphtheria toxin (10 µg/ml)
for 10 min at 37°C to obtain toxin binding to cell
surface receptors. The cells were then exposed to a
buffer containing 0.14 M KCl, 2 mM $CaCl_2$, 20 mM

MES/tris, 10 mM gluconate, pH 5.0 for 15, 30 or 60 sec
before the buffer was removed and the same buffer
adjusted to pH 7.0 and containing ^{14}C DMO was added.
The distribution of DMO between cells and buffer was
measured, and the cytosolic pH was calculated (Sandvig
and co-workers, 1987).

Since studies involving diphtheria toxin and artificial lipid
membranes revealed that insertion of diphtheria toxin into these
membranes induced pore formation (Kagan and co-workers,1981;
Donovan and co-workers, 1981), we also tested whether entry of
diphtheria toxin into cells had an effect on the permeability for
calcium ions. As shown in Fig. 3, the $^{45}Ca^{2+}$ transport into Vero
cells is actually increased by entry of diphtheria toxin. Both
the proton flux (Fig. 2) and the $^{45}Ca^{2+}$-flux seem to last for a
longer period of time than required for entry of the diphtheria
toxin A-fragment, suggesting that they are not associated with
the entry of this protein, but occurs as a result of the
interaction with the membrane.

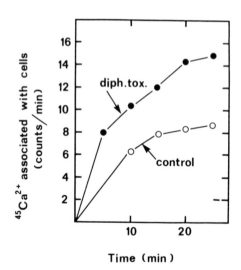

Fig. 3: Effect of diphtheria toxin entry on $^{45}Ca^{2+}$
uptake. Vero cells were incubated with or without
diphtheria toxin and exposed to low pH as described in
the legend to Fig. 2. Uptake of $^{45}Ca^{2+}$ was then
measured by incubating the cells in the low pH buffer.

We have earlier found that permeable anions are required both for
binding and for entry of diphtheria toxin, and that inhibitors of
this transport block diphtheria toxin entry (Sandvig and Olsnes,
1986). Furthermore, when diphtheria toxin is pulsed into the
membrane at low pH, anion transport is inhibited (Olsnes and
Sandvig,1986). Thus, both binding and entry seem to be located in

close proximity to the anion exchanger in the cells, and it is possible that the diphtheria toxin receptor and the anion exchanger is the same molecule. We are now investigating this possibility.

MECHANISMS INVOLVED IN THE ENTRY OF MODECCIN AND VOLKENSIN

The plant toxins modeccin and volkensin are found in two closely related plants (Stirpe and co-workers, 1985), and the toxins are immunologically related. Thus, anti-modeccin protects cells against volkensin. Also, both toxins are protected by amines and by low concentrations of monensin (0.1 uM). These low concentrations of monensin affect the Golgi apparatus (Tartakoff, 1983), whereas they have no effect on endosomal pH, suggesting that transfer of the toxins to the Golgi compartment is required for entry into the cytosol. Similarly to pseudomonas toxin, also the effect of modeccin is strongly reduced below 20°C supporting the view that a fusion process is required (Sandvig and co-workers, 1984; Draper and co-workers, 1984). In spite of the similarity between modeccin and volkensin it is evident from Table 1 that volkensin is more toxic on most cell lines than modeccin.

TABLE 1   Ability of Protein Toxins to Inhibit Protein Synthesis in Different Cell Lines

Cells growing in 24 well disposable trays were incubated with increasing concentrations of toxin for 24 hours and then the rate of protein synthesis was measured. The toxin concentration required to reduce protein synthesis to 50% of the control level was then estimated.

Cell line	Abrin	Ricin	Modeccin	Volkensin
		ID_{50} (ng/ml)		
Vero	0.30	0.34	0.29	0.004
A431	0.25	3.5	0.84	0.031
Hep 2	0.25	3.9	0.5	0.008
L	0.02	2	0.25	0.005
HeLa S$_3$	0.2	3	0.4	0.02
3T3	0.035	0.32	0.3	0.01
MCF7	0.25	0.4	19	0.2

TRANSPORT OF ABRIN AND RICIN INTO CELLS

In contrast to the other toxins described in this paper abrin and ricin do not require low pH at any step during their internalization. Also, abrin and ricin do not bind Triton X-114 at any pH value tested (Fig. 1). Again, when the toxic effect on different cell lines is studied, it is clear that they differ. Abrin is more toxic than ricin (Table 1). Similarly as observed for the other toxins it takes some time (about 1 hour in the case of abrin and ricin) before added toxin has any effect on protein synthesis. This time period probably represents the time it takes for the toxin to be endocytosed, transported to the right intracellular compartment, possibly modified by intracellular enzymes and then transported across the membrane and into the cytosol. Studies with gold-labelled ricin revealed that the conjugate was found both in coated pits and in uncoated invaginations of the membrane (van Deurs and co-workers, 1985; Sandvig and co-workers, 1987). It is so far not clear whether endocytosis occurs exclusively from coated pits or whether an alternative pathway involving uncoated areas of the membrane also exists. Experiments involving potassium depletion to induce depolymerization of clathrin suggest that endocytosis from uncoated areas occurs. Thus, endocytosis was found to occur even after the clathrin coats were removed (Moya and co-workers, 1985; Madshus and co-workers, 1987).

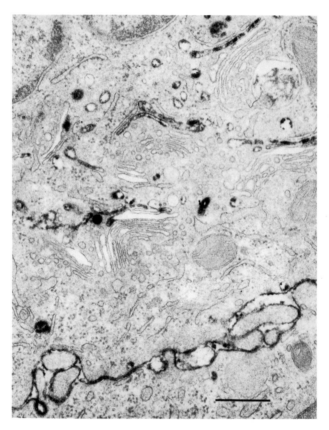

Fig. 4: Localization of ricin-horse radish peroxidase conjugate in Vero cells. Bar 0.5 µm.

We have recently discovered that acidification of the cytosol inhibits endocytosis of transferrin and EGF which are normally taken up by the coated pit/coated vesicle pathway (Sandvig and co-workers, 1987), while entry of ricin is much less affected by this treatment. This supports the idea that endocytosis by a second pathway does take place. Not only is ricin endocytosed under such conditions but the endocytosed toxin will also intoxicate the cells.

Normally, after entry of ricin, the toxin is found in endosomes, in the Golgi complex (Fig. 4) and in lysosomes (van Deurs and co-workers, 1985, 1986, 1987). In the case of abrin and ricin the low concentrations of monensin known to affect the Golgi apparatus (Tartakoff, 1983) will not protect, but sensitize the cells against these toxins, again suggesting a role for Golgi in toxin entry.

Furthermore, both cycloheximide and puromycin sensitize to these toxins suggesting that transport of newly synthesized proteins through the Golgi apparatus may interfere with the entry process of abrin and ricin. Also inhibitors of glycoprotein processing like swainsonine have a similar effect (Sandvig, Tønnessen and Olsnes, 1986). The sensitizing compounds discussed here all induce morphological changes in the Golgi apparatus, and these changes could in some unknown way also alter the efficiency of abrin and ricin entry. At temperatures below $20^{\circ}C$, both transfer of ricin to Golgi, the sensitizing effect of monensin and cycloheximide as well as most of the toxicity of ricin are inhibited (Sandvig, Tønnessen and Olsnes, 1986; van Deurs and co-workers, 1987), supporting the view that this organelle and especially the trans Golgi network (van Deurs et al. in preparation) is involved in the transport of the toxin to the cytosol.

AKNOWLEDGEMENTS

We wish to thank Tove Lie Berle, Jorunn Jacobsen, Keld Ottosen and Kirsten Pedersen for technical assistance. This work was supported by the NOVO Foundation.

REFERENCES

Donovan, J.J., M.I. Simon, R.K. Draper, and M. Montal (1981). Diphtheria toxin forms transmembrane channels in planar lipid bilayers. Proc.Natl.Acad.Sci.USA, 78, 172-176.

Draper, R.K., D.O. O'Keefe, M. Stookey, and J. Graves (1984). Identification of a cold-sensitive step in the mechanism of modeccin action. J.Biol.Chem., 259, 4083-4088.

Kagan, B.L., A. Finkelstein, and M. Colombini (1981). Diphtheria toxin fragment forms large pores in phospholipid bilayer membranes. Proc.Natl.Acad.Sci.USA., 78, 4950-4954.

Madshus, I.H., K. Sandvig, S. Olsnes, and B. van Deurs (1987). Effect of reduced endocytosis induced by hypotonic shock and potassium depletion on the infection of Hep 2 cells by picorna viruses. J.Cell.Physiol., 131, 14-22.

Middlebrook, J.L., and R.B. Dorland (1984). Bacterial toxins: Cellular mechanisms of action. Microbiol.Rev., 48, 199-221.

Morris, R.E., A.S. Gerstein, P.F. Bonventre, and C.B. Saelinger (1985). Receptor-mediated entry of diphtheria toxin into monkey kidney (Vero) cells: Electron microscopic evaluation. Infect.Immun., 50, 721-727.

Morris, R.E., M.D. Manhart, and C.B. Saelinger (1983). Receptor-mediated entry of Pseudomonas toxin: Methylamine blocks clustering step. Infect.Immun., 40, 806-811.

Morris, R.E., and C.B. Saelinger (1986). Reduced temperature
alters Pseudomonas exotoxin A entry into the mouse LM cell.
Infect.Immun., 52, 445-453.

Moya, M., A. Dautry-Varsat, B. Goud, D. Louvard, and P. Boquet
(1985). Inhibition of coated pit formation in Hep 2 cells
blocks the cytotoxicity of diphtheria toxin but not that of
ricin toxin. J.Cell.Biol., 101, 548-559.

Olsnes, S., and K. Sandvig (1985). In: Pastan, I., and M.C.
Willingham, (Eds.), Endocytosis, Plenum Press, New York, pp.
195-235.

Olsnes, S., and K. Sandvig (1986). Interaction between diphtheria
toxin entry and anion transport in Vero cells. I. Anion
antiport in Vero cells. J.Biol.Chem., 261, 1542-1552.

Sandvig, K., T.I. Tønnessen, and S. Olsnes (1986). Ability of
inhibitors of glycosylation and protein synthesis to sensitize
cells to abrin, ricin, shigella toxin and pseudomonas toxin.
Cancer Res., 46, 6418-6422.

Sandvig, K., T.I. Tønnessen, O. Sand, and S. Olsnes (1986).
Diphtheria toxin entry into cells is inhibited by acidification
of the cytosol. J.Biol.Chem., 261, 11639-11644.

Sandvig, K., and S. Olsnes (1986). Interaction between diphtheria
toxin entry and anion transport in Vero cells. IV. Evidence
that entry of diphtheria toxin is dependent on efficient anion
transport. J.Biol.Chem., 261, 1570-1575.

Sandvig, K., A. Sundan, and S. Olsnes (1984). Evidence that
diphtheria toxin and modeccin enter the cytosol from different
vesicular compartments. J.Cell.Biol., 98, 963-970.

Sandvig, K., S. Olsnes, O.W. Petersen, and B. van Deurs (1987).
Acidification of the cytosol inhibits endocytosis from coated
pits. J.Cell Biol., In press.

Stirpe, F., L. Barbieri, A. Abbondanza, A.I. Falalsca, A.N.F.
Brown, K. Sandvig, S. Olsnes, and A. Pihl (1985). Properties of
volkensin, a toxic lectin from Adenia volkensii. J.Biol.Chem.,
260, 14589-14595.

Tartakoff, A.M. (1983). Perturbation of vesicular traffic with
the carboxylic ionophore monensin. Cell, 32, 1026-1028.

van Deurs, B., L. Ryde Pedersen, A. Sundan, S. Olsnes, and K.
Sandvig (1985). Receptor-mediated emndocytosis of a
ricin-colloidal gold conjugate in Vero cells. Intracellular
routing to vacuolar and tubule-vesicular portions of the
endosomal system. Exp.Cell.Res., 159, 287-304.

van Deurs, B., O.W. Petersen, S. Olsnes, and K. Sandvig (1987).
Delivery of internalized ricin from endosomes to cisternal
Golgi elements is a discontinious, temperature sensitive
process. Exp.Cell Res., In press.

van Deurs, B., T.I. Tønnessen, O.W. Petersen, K. Sandvig, and S.
Olsnes (1986). Routing of internalized ricin and ricin
conjugates to the Golgi complex. J.Cell.Biol., 102, 37-47.

Fehrenbach et al. (Eds.), Bacterial Protein Toxins, Zbl. Bakt. Suppl. 17
© Gustav Fischer, Stuttgart, New York, 1988

Colicin E3: a Model for Translocation of Proteins Across Biological Memnranes

M. Mock and V. Escuyer

Unité des Antigènes Bactériens (UA CNRS 557), Institut Pasteur, 28 rue du Docteur-Roux, 75724 Paris Cedex 15, France

ABSTRACT

Exposure to low pH triggers an increase in the hydrophobicity of the colicin E3 molecule and makes it able to insert into lipid membranes. At acidic pH whole colicin E3 segregated in the detergent phase of Triton X-114, a property which was shown to be associated with the N-terminal part of the colicin molecule. Nucleotide sequence changes caused by three missense mutations affecting colicin E3 activity and located in different domains of the molecule were determined.

KEYWORDS

Colicin E3, hydrophobic domains, photoactivatable probes, Triton X-114, liposomes, missense mutations.

INTRODUCTION

Colicin E3 is a bactericidal protein produced by strains of **E. coli** carrying the colicinogenic plasmid Col E3 (Hardy, 1975). This 57,963 dalton protein (551 aa) (Masaki and Ohta, 1985) exerts its lethal effect by causing a specific cleavage of the ribosomal 16S RNA, resulting in the arrest of cell protein synthesis (Senior and Holland, 1971; Bowman and co-workers, 1971). Colicin E3 is released by colicinogenic cells as an equimolecular complex with a 9,631-dalton acidic polypeptide (Mock and co-workers, 1983) called the immunity protein (Jakes and Zinder, 1974). This protein is tightly associated with the enzymic domain of colicin E3, located on the C-terminal end of the molecule and acts as a specific inhibitor of its RNase activity (Ohno and co-workers, 1977).
In order to act on its intracellular target, colicin E3 has to cross both the outer, and inner membranes to reach the bacterial cytoplasm. Very little is known regarding the mechanism of this translocation across the cell envelope. Several studies have established that colicin E3 has a structural organization similar to that found for some bacterial toxins acting on eukaryotic cells. As represented in Fig. 1 different functions of the colicin E3 can be assigned to physically distinct domains of the molecule (Ohno-Iwashita and Imahori, 1980).

In the work presented below, we have used both biochemical and genetical approaches to obtain more information on the structure-function relationships in the colicin E3 molecule.

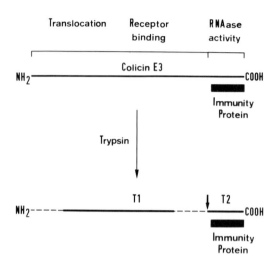

Figure 1. Schematic representation of the colicin E3–immunity protein complex
The different functional domains which have been localized on the colicin E3 molecule are indicated on a schematic drawing representing the whole molecule complexed to its immunity protein. The major colicin E3 polypeptides, T1 and T2, resistant to a limited trypsin digestion of the complex are represented in solid lines whereas dashed lines represent portions of the molecule which are totally digested. T2 (enzymatic peptide) (M_r = 11,000) is a well defined polypeptide corresponding to a precise nicking by trypsin as indicated by the arrow, and T1 (M_r about 35,000) represents a more heterogenous population of the N-terminal moiety of colicin E3.

RESULTS AND DISCUSSION

A series of recent studies have established that a low pH is required for the translocation of certain toxins through the cell membrane (Olsnes and Sandvig, 1984). An analogous requirement for acidic environment has been also demonstrated for the **in vitro** activity of colicins which alter bacterial inner membrane activity (E1 and A) (Davidson and co-workers, 1985; Pattus and co-workers, 1983). According to these observations we conducted experiments in order to establish if such a pH effect may also bear on the mechanism of entry of colicins acting on intracellular targets.

I. Interaction of Colicin E3 with Lipid Vesicles is pH-dependent and Allows Protection of Specific Colicin Polypeptides against Proteolysis

The use of artificial lipid vesicles can provide information on the mechanism whereby certain proteins, or part of them, interact with cell membranes in order to express their biological activities.

In preliminary experiments, direct binding of colicin E3 to asolectin vesicles was determined. ^{125}I-colicin E3 was found to bind to asolectin vesicles in a pH-dependent manner. At pH below 4.0, the major part of colicin E3 was recovered with the lipid vesicles whereas at pH 7.0 most of the labeled protein remained in solution.

The binding of colicin E3 to lipid vesicles and its insertion were then studied using liposomes containing radioactive photoactivatable phospholipid probes. The two probes, PCI and PCII, used in this work were previously described (Bisson and Montecucco, 1985). They both contain a nitrene photoactivatable group placed at two different levels of one fatty acid chain in order to probe the superficial (PCI) or the deeper regions (PCII) of the lipid membrane. The labeling of colicin E3 with the ^{3}H-PCI and ^{14}C-PCII probes was studied at different pH values. At pH 7.00 the molecule was only significantly labeled with the surface probe ^{3}H-PCI. When the pH was dropped down to 4.50 or 3.75 the colicin E3 labeling increased and the protein interacted with the deeper probe ^{14}C-PCII. The ratio of ^{3}H to ^{14}C labeling (i.e. surface/deep) decreased from 18 at pH 7.00 to 5.9 at pH 4.50 and 3.1 at pH 3.75. This pH dependent interaction of colicin E3 with the ^{14}C-PCII probe was shown to be reversible since raising the pH back from 3.75 to 7.00 before illumination gave a pattern of labeling similar to that observed at pH 7.00.

In order to determine if the interaction of colicin E3 with lipid vesicles at acidic pH allowed specific protection against proteolysis, the following experiments were then performed : ^{125}I-labeled colicin E3 was incubated at pH 3.0 in the presence or absence of asolectin vesicles (internal pH 7.0) and then digested with pepsin for 45 min. Three polypeptides M_r 16,000, 12,000, and 10,000 appeared particularly resistant to proteolysis and only when the vesicles were present.

No protection occurred when vesicle integrity was destroyed by the addition of the cytolytic toxin delta-lysin to the vesicles prior to colicin. In contrast, two of the three polypeptides (M_r = 12,000 and 10,000) were still protected when the lysin was added after the colicin. According to the mode of action of delta lysin, which removes large portions of lipid membrane, such an observation supports the notion that the two polypeptides could be inserted into the lipid membrane of closed vesicles rather than translocated inside their lumen.

Immunoprecipitation experiments using specific antisera directed against different parts of the colicin E3 indicated that all three protected polypeptides were located in the N-terminal region of the protein.

When the proteolysis experiment was performed at pH 7.0 (with trypsin instead of pepsin) no difference in the pattern of digestion was observed, in the absence or presence of lipid vesicles. This result showed that at neutral pH the interaction of colicin with the vesicles surface did not modify its trypsin sensitivity and that a low pH outside the vesicles was required for insertion and for obtaining protection of the M_r 16,000, 12,000 and 10,000 colicin E3 polypeptides.

II. Interaction of Colicin E3 and Immunity with the Nonionic Detergent Triton X-114

At supramicellar concentrations, Triton X-114 remains in solution at 0°C but separates into two phases at room temperature, with a detergent lower phase and an aqueous upper phase. This property was found to be very convenient for separating hydrophobic proteins (which partition in the detergent phase) from hydrophilic proteins (partitioning in the aqueous phase)(Bordier, 1981). In addition the property of partitioning in the Triton X-114 phase may also provide information on the surface hydrophobicity of proteins (Alcaraz and co-workers, 1984). Since an acidic pH seems to induce an increased hydrophobicity in colicin E3, we investigated the interaction of this protein with Triton X-114 as a function of pH. Figure 2 shows the partitioning of purified colicin E3-immunity protein complex between the upper and lower phases of Triton X-114.

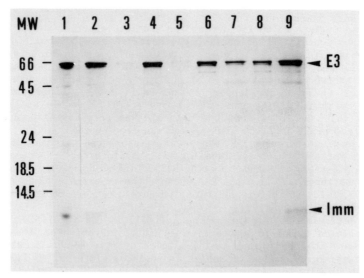

Figure 2. Phase partitioning of colicin E3 in Triton X-114 at various pH
Samples of colicin E3 preparation (80 ug of protein) were mixed with Triton X-114 at various pH and submitted to phase separation at 37°C. Aliquots of 35 ul from the aqueous upper phase (AP) and the detergent lower phase (DP) were analyzed by SDS-14 % polyacrylamide gel electrophoresis. Lane 1, colicin E3 (10 ug) before phase separation, lanes 2 and 3, respectively, the AP and DP after partitioning at pH 7.0 ; lanes 4 and 5, respectively, the AP and DP after partitioning at pH 4.2 ; lanes 6 and 7 respectively the AP and DP after partitioning at pH 3.8 ; lanes 8 and 9 respectively, the AP and DP after partitioning at pH 3.0.

Whereas at neutral pH colicin E3 and immunity protein segregated into the aqueous phase, at acidic pH, the proteins were found in the detergent phase, indicating an increase in surface hydrophobicity in these conditions. This effect was reversible as raising the acidic detergent phase to pH 7.0 allowed the two molecules to partition again in the aqueous phase.
As shown in figure 3, when the experiments were performed with trypsin digested colicin preparations, it became clear that the low pH induced hydrophobicity was not a property spread on the entire molecule but rather localized on defined domains. The catalytic peptide T2 remained hydrophilic at low pH and partitioned exclusively in the aqueous phase thereby totally dissociating from the immunity

protein. It should be pointed out that the enzymic peptide recovered in the aqueous phase was highly active **in vitro** ; therefore beside its interest in studying the structural organization of colicin E3 the detergent Triton X-114 also appears to be a convenient means of preparing the catalytic fragment of colicin E3. In contrast to T2, the N-terminal T1 peptide represents the portion of the colicin molecule which clearly becomes more hydrophobic at acidic pH. This is in agreement with the high content in non polar residues of the N-terminal portion of colicin E3 (Masaki and Ohta, 1985) and with our observation that the fragments protected against pepsin proteolysis after vesicle interaction were immunoprecipitated by antisera raised against the N-terminal part of the molecule.

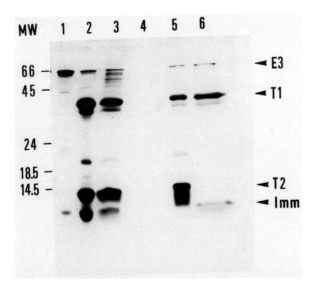

Figure 3. Phase partitioning of trypsin digested colicin E3 at neutral and acidic pH
Colicin E3 (400 ug) was submitted to limited trypsin digestion in 10 mM potassium phosphate buffer, pH 7.0. The colicin/trypsin ratio was 50:1 (wt/wt). The digestion was carried out at 37°C for 30 min and stopped by adding soybean trypsin inhibitor, the ratio of trypsin to trypsin inhibitor being 1:3 (wt/wt). The digestion mixture was divided in two parts which were submitted to phase separation in Triton X-114 either at pH 7.0 or at pH 3.0. The respective aqueous (AP) and detergent (DP) phases were concentrated 3 fold and aliquots (35 ul) were analyzed by SDS-14 % polyacrylamide gel electrophoresis. Lane 1, whole colicin E3 (10 ug) ; lane 2, trypsin digested colicin E3 (40 ug) before phase separation ; lanes 3 and 4, respectively, the AP and DP after partitioning at pH 7.0 ; lanes 5 and 6, respectively, the AP and DP after partitioning at pH 3.0. Whole colicin E3 (E3), immunity protein (Imm) and the T1 and T2 main tryptic peptides are indicated by arrows.

The data presented in these two sections establish for the first time that a low pH induces an increase hydrophobicity in the colicin E3 molecule and makes it able to insert into lipid membranes (Escuyer and co-workers, 1986).

We do not know at the present time if it is a low pH which triggers a change necessary for colicin E3 to penetrate into the bacterial cytoplasm **in vivo**. However, our observation that such an environment promotes the dissociation between the immunity protein and the enzymic domain of E3 **in vitro** (a phenomenon which is absolutely required **in vivo** for the activity of colicin E3) suggests that this mechanism might be relevant to the mode of action of colicin E3 on bacterial cell.

III. DNA Sequence Analysis of three Missense Mutations Affecting Colicin E3 Bactericidal Activity

In a previous study, we described the effects of mutations in the colicin E3 structural gene (Mock and Schwartz, 1980), three of which (**cea**C1, **cea**C2, **cea**C3) led to the production of inactive colicin molecules. Characterization of the mutants indicated that the **cea**C1 product is affected in cell envelope penetration whereas the **cea**C2 and **cea**C3 products are unable to inhibit protein synthesis **in vitro**.

We have determined the nucleotide sequence changes caused by these three mutations (Escuyer and Mock, 1987). The **cea**C1 mutation is caused by a serine to phenylalanine change at position 37 within the glycine-rich region at the N-terminal part of colicin E3.

This confirms the results described above suggesting a role of this domain in the colicin interaction with membranes. The **cea**C2 and **cea**C3 mutations, abolishing colicin E3 RNase activity, affect the C-terminal enzymatic domain of the molecule. In the **cea**C2 mutant, serine at position 529 was converted to leucine. The **cea**C3 mutation replaced a glycine residue at position 524 with an aspartic acid residue. The two mutations **cea**C2 and **cea**C3 which are five codon apart on the gene yield information on the amino acid residues involved in the RNase activity of colicin E3.

In conclusion, from the biochemical and genetical data presented in this work, the colicin E3 molecule appears to be a fruitful model for studying the structure-function relationships in proteins designed to cross biological membranes.

REFERENCES

Alcaraz, G., J.P. Kinet, N. Kumar, S.A. Wank and H. Metzger (1984). Phase separation of the receptor for immunoglobulin E and its subunits in Triton X-114. J. Biol. Chem., 259, 14922-14927.

Bisson, R. and C. Montecucco (1985). Use of photoreactive phospholipids for the study of lipid-protein interactions. In: Watts, A. and J.J.H.H.M. de Pont (Eds.), Progress in Protein-Lipid Interactions, Elsevier Science Publishers, pp. 259-287.

Bordier, C. (1981). Phase separation of integrated membrane proteins in Triton X-114 solution. J. Biol. Chem., 256, 1604-1607.

Bowman, C.M., J.E. Dahlberg, T.I. Kemura, J. Konisky and M. Nomura (1971). Specific inactivation of 16S ribosomal RNA induced by colicin E3 in vivo. Proc. Natl. Acad. Sci. U.S.A., 68, 964-968.

Davidson, V.L., K.R. Brunden and W.A. Cramer (1985). Acidic pH requirement for insertion of colicin E1 into artificial membrane vesicles: relevance to the mechanism of action of colicins and certain toxins. Proc. Natl. Acad. Sci. U.S.A., 82, 1386-1390.

Escuyer V., P. Boquet, D. Perrin, C. Montecucco and M. Mock (1986). A pH-induced increase in hydrophobicity as a possible step in the penetration of colicin E3 through bacterial membranes. J. Biol. Chem., 261, 10891-10898.

Escuyer V., and M. Mock (1987). DNA sequence analysis of three missense mutations affecting colicin E3 bactericidal activity. Mol. Microbiol. in Press.

Hardy, K.G. (1975). Colicinogeny related phenomena. Bacteriol. Rev., 39, 464-515.

Jakes, K.S. and N.D. Zinder (1974). Highly purified colicin E3 contains immunity protein. Proc. Natl. Acad. Sci. U.S.A., 71, 3380-3384.

Masaki, H. and T. Ohta (1985). Colicin E3 and its immunity gene. J. Mol. Biol., 182, 217-227.

Mock, M. and M. Schwartz (1980). Mutations which affect the structure and activity of colicin E3. J. Bacteriol., 142, 384-390.

Mock, M., C.G. Miyada and R.P. Gunsalus (1983). Nucleotide sequence for the catalytic domain of colicin E3 and its immunity protein. Evidence for a third gene overlapping colicin. Nucleic Acids Res., 11, 3547-3557.

Ohno S., Y. Ohno-Iwashita, K. Suzuki and K. Imahori (1977). Purification and characterization of active component and active fragment of colicin E3. J. Biochem. (Tokyo), 82, 1045-1053.

Ohno-Iwashita, Y. and K. Imahori (1980). Assignment of the functional loci in colicin E2 and E3 molecules by the characterization of their proteolytic fragments. Biochemistry, 19, 652-659.

Olsnes, S. and K. Sandvig (1984). Entry of polypeptide toxins into animal cells. In: Pastan, I. and M.C. Willingham (Eds.), Endocytosis, Plenum Publishing Corporation, pp. 195-234.

Pattus, F., M.C. Martinez, B. Dargent, D. Cavard, R. Verger and C. Lazdunski (1983). Interaction of colicin A with phospholipid monolayers and liposomes. Biochemistry, 22, 5698-5703.

Senior, B.W. and J.B. Holland (1971). Effect of colicin E3 upon the 30S ribosomal subunit of **Escherichia coli**. Proc. Natl. Acad. Sci. U.S.A., 68, 959-963.

Fehrenbach et al. (Eds.), Bacterial Protein Toxins, Zbl. Bakt. Suppl. 17
© Gustav Fischer, Stuttgart, New York, 1988

Electron Microscopic and Genetic Approaches to Colicin Release

C. Lazdunski, S. P. Howard, D. Cavard, V. Geli, R. Lloubès, A. Bernadac and D. Baty

Centre de Biochimie et de Biologie Moléculaire du C.N.R.S., 31 Chemin Jospeh-Aiguier, BP 71, F-13402 Marseille Cedex 9

ABSTRACT

Instead of a built-in signal for export, the release of colicins from colicinogenic cells is promoted by a small protein co-ordinately expressed with the colicin gene. Colicins are in a first step accumulated in the cytoplasm. Their release to the extracellular medium depends upon the expression of a small lipoprotein. This protein causes a non specific increase in the envelope permeability at least in part due to the activation of the detergent resistant phospholipase present in the outer membrane. The release process is non-specific with respect to the colicin itself which does not contain any topogenic export signal.

KEYWORDS

Colicin, lysis protein, bacterial release protein, phospholipase A, envelope-permeability.

INTRODUCTION

Colicins are toxic proteins produced by, and active against, *E. coli* and closely related bacteria. They are usually very large (40 kd to 90 kd) and yet can be excreted across both the inner and outer membranes of colicinogenic cells harbouring Col plasmids. The mechanism of colicin release to the extracellular medium has been the subject of many studies in recent years. Common features have emerged for the various colicins. Therefore in this report, we will illustrate these features by presenting the results obtained in our laboratory with colicin A.

RESULTS AND DISCUSSION

Most of the plasmids which encode colicins, also encode a small protein called "lysis protein" or "bacterial release protein", whose expression is required for colicin release (Pugsley, 1984; Cavard and co-workers, 1985; de Graaf and Oudega, 1986). The term lysis protein must be qualified since it has been shown that the release of colicin A is unaffected in *E. coli* mutants which display decreased levels of autolytic enzyme activities (Howard and co-workers, 1987). Furthermore the ultrastructure of colicinogenic cells is not grossly altered following full induction and colicin release (Cavard and co-workers, 1984).

Functional Organization of Colicin Operons

Lysis protein genes form with colicin genes an operon regulated by the SOS response and therefore repressed by the LexA protein (Little and Mount, 1982). The organization of the 3 genes *caa, cai* and *cal* encoding respectively colicin A (Caa), the immunity protein (Cai) and the pColA-lysis protein (Cal) has been analysed in detail (Lloubès and co-workers, 1986). The genes *caa* and *cal* form an operon, *cai* is

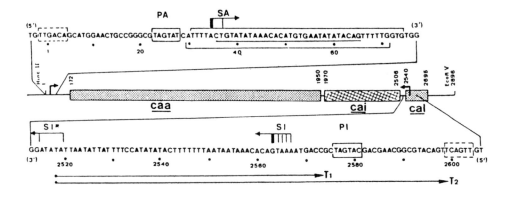

Fig. 1 : Organization of the *caa-cal* operon and the *cai* gene.
The nucleotide sequences for the promoters are presented : the recognition
and binding sequences for RNA polymerase are boxed with dotted lines (-35
sequence) and solid lines (Pribnow box). PA and SA indicate the Pribnow box
and transcriptional start site for the *caa-cal* operon while PI and SI indicate
those for the *cai* gene. SI* indicates the start site for *cai in vitro*. Arrows above
the start sites indicate the direction of transcription, the bold line indicates the
major band detected by SI mapping. In the case of SI*, one of the nucleotides
within the bracket corresponds to the start site. The binding site for LexA in
the operator region for *caa* is indicated by brackets overlining the protected
region for the sense-strand and brackets underlining the sequence (not
represented) for the anti-sense strand. The two overlapped consensus "SOS
sequences" are underlined. The sequence is numbered taking as the +1
nucleotide the cleavage site for *Hinc*II. Coding sequences for *caa*, *cai* and *cal*
are indicated by stippled and hatched boxes. Numbers above the boxes
indicate the first and last nucleotides of the coding sequence, and arrows
indicate the direction of transcription. Transcripts of *caa* and *caa-cal* are
indicated as well as the terminators T1 and T2.

located between these two genes and transcribed in the opposite direction from its own promoter (Fig.
1). Downstream of *caa*, there is a *rho*-independent terminor which arrests most of the transcripts initiated
at the promoter of the *caa-cal* operon (Lloubès and co-workers, 1986). This explains the coordinated
expression of Caa and Cal and the fact, previously reported (Cavard and co-workers, 1985), that much
more colicin A than Cal protein is produced after induction. This feature may be significant since it is
essential that a cell, once committed to the normally suicidal process of colicin production and release,
should maximise the amount of colicin it produces. We have observed that a critical concentration of Cal is
required to trigger colicin release and, deletion of the T1 terminator causes an early decrease in the
turbidity of the culture with concomitant loss of viability (data not shown).
Although cells which are excreting colicin do not show signs of extensive desintegration (Cavard and
co-workers, 1981; Cavard and co-workers, 1984), they do exhibit a number of features which indicate
that envelope functions are affected. They are no longer able to accumulate labelled substrates, they
release ions from the cytoplasm, and are sensitive to sucrose, which suggest that the inner membrane
has become permeable to small molecules (Pugsley and Schwartz, 1984). These effects can be almost
completely overcome by adding 20 mM Mg^{2+} to the medium. This treatment also prevents the decline in
culture turbidity but was reported to have no effect on colicin export (Pugsley and Schwartz, 1984; de
Graaf and Oudega, 1986). Some colicins are released as a complex with their immunity protein. However,
it has been demonstrated that the cloacin DF13 immunity protein was also produced and excreted in the
absence of cloacin molecules (de Graaf and Oudega, 1986).

```
-1   ↓  +1
AleCysGlnValAenAenValArgAepThrGlyGlySerValSerProSer

SerIleValThrGlyValSerMetGlySerAepGlyValGlyAenPro (33)
```

<u>Fig. 2</u> : Amino acid sequence of wild-type Cal. In AK31 mutant Cal, the underlined alanine (-1) has been substituted by a proline and in AL16 mutant, the underlined cysteine (+1) has been substituted by a threonine. The arrow indicates the site of cleavage. The mature Cal polypeptide chain is numbered 1 to 33.

The structures of the known bacterial release proteins feature a high degree of homology (Cavard and co-workers, 1985; de Graaf and Oudega, 1986). They all contain a signal peptide with a sequence, at the cleavage site, resembling the consensus lipoprotein modification sequence described by Wu and co-workers (1983). The polypeptide chain of the mature form is small, 33 amino acids for the colicin A lysis (Cal) protein and 28 amino acids for colicins E1, E2, E3 and cloacin DF13 lysis proteins.

For Cal, we have demonstrated that the precursor must be modified by a lipid before it can be processed and that the maturation is prevented by globomycin, an inhibitor of signal peptidase II (Cavard and co-workers, 1987). Using oligonucleotide-directed mutagenesis, the alanine (mutant AK31) and cysteine (mutant AL16) residues in the -1 and +1 positions of the cleavage site were replaced by proline and threonine residues, respectively, in two different constructs (Fig. 2). Both substitutions prevented the normal modification and cleavage of the parent protein (Fig. 3). It has also been demonstrated that the C-terminal nine amino acids are non essential for the quasi-lysis phenotype caused by the ColE2 lysis protein (Toba and co-workers, 1986).

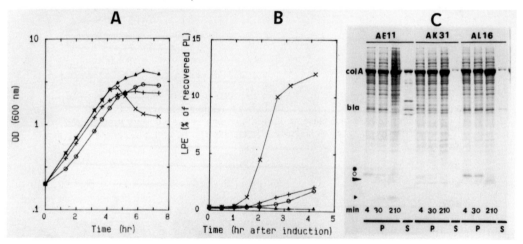

<u>Fig. 3</u> : Effect of mitomycin C (MTC) induction on growth and LPE content of cells containing wild-type and mutant Cal proteins. The growth curve (A) and the amount of LPE as a proportion of total phospholipids (B) are presented. The cells were grown to an optical density (OD) at 600 nm of approximately 1 and were either not induced or induced with MTC. The phospholipids were extracted and analyzed after further incubation. The plasmid contained and the induction conditions of the cells are as follows : X, W3110 (pAE11) wild-type induced; ▲ , W3110 (pAE11) non induced; + W3110 (pAK31) induced; o W3110 (pAL16) induced. (C) The modification and processing of wild type and mutant Cal protein, as well as the release of colicin A, were analyzed. The cells were induced with MTC for 90 min before labelling with S35-methionine. Then, at various times (as indicated), culture samples were centrifuged, the pellet (P) and supernatant (S) were analyzed by SDS/PAGE. A fluorogram is presented. The various Cal protein derivatives are indicated : ●, Cal modified precursor form; o, Cal unmodified precursor form;► Cal mature form; ► Cal signal peptide. The position of colicin A is indicated.

Although the detailed mechanism of release of colicins is not yet known, the increase in envelope permeability observed late after MTC induction, may be attributed, in part or totally, to the bacterial release protein-dependent activation of the detergent-resistant phospholipase A present in the outer membrane (Pugsley and Schwartz, 1984; Luirink and co-workers, 1985).

The marked activation of the detergent resistant phospholipase A observed with wild-type Cal was not observed with Cal mutants AK31 and AL16. Both Cal mutants were also defective for the secretion of colicin A (Fig. 3)(Cavard and co-workers, 1987). The increase in lysophosphatidyl ethanolamine (LPE), the product of the action of phospholipase A on phosphatidylethanolamine, the major membrane phospholipid, was not observed (Fig. 3). LPE may thus act as a membrane perturbant which could alter the permeability properties of the envelope and allow colicin to leak out of the cell. In addition, a subset of at least 20 proteins is also released to the extracellular medium (Fig. 3). Electron microscope studies with immunogold labelling of colicin A on cryosections of pldA and cal mutants indicated that the colicin remains in the cytoplasm and is not transferred to the periplasmic space (Cavard and co-workers, 1987). These results demonstrated that Cal must be modified and processed to activate the detergent-resistant phospholipase A and to promote release of colicin A. However, so far the mechanism of transfer of colicins across the inner membrane remains poorly understood. In particular, it is not known if any interaction between a given colicin and its lysis protein is involved, or if any specific regions or specific interactions between regions of the colicin polypeptide chain are required for this transfer. We have now addressed this question by constructing deletion mutants of colicin A and by a new approach using a cassette which contains a stop codon, a Shine-Dalgarno sequence and an initiation codon to separate the NH_2- and COOH-terminal regions of colicin A. Together, these deletions span the region from amino acid 15 to the end of the protein (Fig. 4).

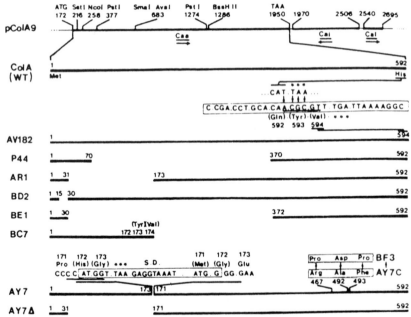

Fig.4 : Construction of recombinant plasmids. A part of the plasmid pColA9 is shown, as well as the constructions derived from it. The restriction sites are indicated above the number of the cleavage site. The oligonucleotides used for the constructions are boxed and the restriction sites created are underlined. Stars represent stop codons, S.D. the Shine-Dalgarno sequence. The amino acids in brackets were created during the construction. AY7 represents two proteins AY7N and AY7C. BF3 corresponds to the three mutations introduced into AY7C (Baty and co-workers, 1987a). AY7Δ contains the first 31 amino acids of AY7N (called AY7ΔN) and the AY7C protein.

None of these regions was found to be required for extracellular release or had any effect on the efficiency of this process. As well, the NH_2-terminal and central plus COOH-terminal domains could be demonstrated to be released to the same extent when produced as separate polypeptides as when produced as linked ones. The introduction into the COOH-terminal domain of mutations promoting cytoplasmic aggregation (Baty and co-workers, 1987a) prevented its release but had no effect on the secretion of the NH_2-terminal polypeptide (Baty and co-workers, 1987b).

These results demonstrated that no specific interaction between the NH_2- and the COOH terminal regions of the colicin A polypeptide chain is involved in the release of colicin A. We are led to conclude that there is no topogenic export signal in the polypeptide chain of colicin A involved in the release mechanism. Thus the process is non-specific with respect to the colicin itself and depends solely on the expression of the colicin A lysis protein.

REFERENCES

Baty, D., M. Knibiehler, H. Verheij, F. Pattus, D. Shire, A. Bernadac, and C. Lazdunski (1987a). Site-directed mutagenesis of the COOH-terminal region of colicin A : effect on secretion and voltage-dependent channel activity. Proc. Natl. Acad. Sci. USA, 84, 1152-1156.

Baty, D., R. Lloubès, V. Geli, C. Lazdunski, and S.P. Howard (1987b). Extracellular release of colicin A is non specific. EMBO J., in press.

Cavard, DP., A. Bernadac, and C. Lazdunski (1981). Exclusive localization of colicin A in cell cytoplasm of producing bacteria. Eur. J. Biochem., 119, 125-131.

Cavard, D., A. Bernadac, J.M. Pagès, and C. Lazdunski (1984). Colicins are not transiently accumulated in the periplasmic space before release from colicinogenic cells. Biol. Cell, 51, 79-86.

Cavard, D., R. Lloubès, J. Morlon, M. Chartier, and C. Lazdunski (1985). Lysis protein encoded by plasmid ColA-CA31 Gene sequence and export. Mol. Gen. Genet., 199, 95-100.

Cavard, D., D. Baty, S.P. Howard, H.M. Verheij, and C. Lazdunski (1987). Lipoprotein nature of the colicin A lysis protein : effect of amino acid substitutions at the site of modification and processing. J. Bacteriol., 169, 2187-2194.

De Graaf, F.K., and B. Oudega (1986). Production and release of cloacin DF13 and related proteins. Curr. top. in Microbiol. and Immunol., 125, 183-205.

Howard, S.P., M. Leduc, J. Van Heijenoort, and C. Lazdunski (1987). Lysis and release of colicin A in colicinogenic autolytic deficient Escherichia coli mutants. FEMS Microbiol. Lett., in press.

Little, J.W., and D.W. Mount (1982). The SOS regulatory system of Escherichia coli. Cell, 29, 11-22.

Lloubès, R., D. Baty and C. Lazdunski (1986). The promoters of the genes for colicin production, release and immunity in the ColA plasmid : effects of convergent transcription and LexA protein. Nucl. Acids Res., 14, 2621-2636.

Luirink, J., C. Van der Sande, J. Tommassen, E. Veltkamp, F.K. de Graaf, and B. Oudega (1985). Mode of action of protein H encoded by plasmid CloDF13 : effects of culture conditions and of mutations affecting phospholipase A activity on excretion of cloacin DF13 and on growth and lysis of host cells. J. Gen. Microbiol., 132, 825-834.

Pugsley, A.P. (1984). The ins and outs of colicins. Part I : production and translocation across membranes. Microbiol. Sci., 1, 168-175.

Pugsley, A.P., and M. Schwartz (1984). Colicin E2 release : lysis, leakage or secretion ? Possible role of a phospholipase. EMBO J., 3, 2392-2397.

Toba, M., H. Masaki, and O. Takahisa (1986). Primary structures of the ColE2-P9 and ColE3-CA38 lysis genes. J. Biochem., 99, 591-596.

Fehrenbach et al. (Eds.), Bacterial Protein Toxins, Zbl. Bakt. Suppl. 17
© Gustav Fischer, Stuttgart, New York, 1988

The Colicin A Lysis Protein: Structure and Function.

D. Cavard, S. P. Howard, D. Baty, H. M. Verheij and C. Lazdunski

C.N.R.S., Centre de Biochimie et de Biologie Moléculaire, 31, Chemin Joseph-Aiguier, BP 71, F-13402 Marseille Cedex 9

KEYWORDS : colicin, lysis protein, export, membrane, lipoprotein.

The colicin A lysis protein, Cal, is required for the release of colicin A to the medium by producing Escherichia coli. Colicin A is a toxin that specifically kills sensitive E. coli strains. It is synthesized and exported by E. coli cells carrying the plasmid pColA. Colicin A and its lysis protein are encoded by the genes caa and cal respectively, which form an operon.

In contrast to colicin A, the lysis protein Cal is produced in a precursor form. This precursor contains the sequence Leu-Ala-Ala-Cys at the C-terminal part of its signal peptide which corresponds to the consensus sequence Leu-X-Y-Cys for the modification and processing site of prolipoproteins in bacteria. Consequently, it must go through a series of post-translatinal modifications and processing reactions before it can be assembled and become functional. According to the pathway for the biosynthesis of murein lipoprotein in E. coli (Wu and Tokunaga, 1986), the precursor Procal form should : 1) be modified by a glyceride on the sulfhydryl group of the cysteine in the consensus sequence : 2) be processed by signal peptidase II between the alanine and cysteine residues of the consensus sequence to be released from the signal peptide ; 3) be acylated on the NH_2 group of the cysteine to generate a mature Cal lipoprotein. By labeling producing cells with ^{35}S-methionine in pulse-chase experiments, 4 forms of the Cal protein that are derived from each other as function of time have been identified. The first one synthesized, Procal, could not be labeled with ^{14}C-palmitate, in contrast to the two forms directly derived from it. The fourth one has just been demonstrated and is produced in very low amounts. The modification and processing reactions of Cal protein are very slow processes, in contrast to those of the major lipoprotein, and require approximately around one hour of chase to be complete.

By genetic recombination, a Cal overproducing plasmid, called pATI, has been constructed. It has been obtained by deletion, in the colicin A operon, of two thirds of the caa gene, the transcription terminator that follows the caa gene and two thirds of the intercistronic region between the caa and the cal genes. In this construct, the Cal protein is synthesized in the same amounts as the truncated colicin protein, that is in approximately 10 fold higher quantities than in the wild type strain. Pulse-chase experiments on the cells carrying this recombinant plasmid have confirmed the three steps of modification and processing of the Cal protein.

By oligonucleotide directed mutagenesis, two different amino acid substitutions in the lipoprotein consensus sequence have been made. In the first one, the -1 alanine was replaced by a proline to give Leu-Ala-Pro-Cys. In the second one, the +1 cysteine was changed to a threonine to obtain Leu-Ala-Ala-Thr. Both of these substitutions block the modifications of the Cal precursor and the normal processing of the signal peptide as demonstrated by labeling experiments with ^{35}S-methionine.

The Cal protein is responsible for both the "pseudo-lysis" that follows the induction of colicin A synthesis and the export of colicin A to the medium. It has been shown that in cells containing the overproducing plasmid, the pseudo-lysis of the cells is more rapid than in the wild type and that the export of the truncated colicin is faster than that of colicin A. In both of the cal mutants, neither pseudo-lysis nor the release of colicin A is observed.

It has been proposed by Pugsley and Schwartz (1984) that colicin lysis proteins act by activating the phospholipase A of the outer membrane of the producing bacteria, modifying the membrane's permeability and allowing the colicin to leave the cells. We have shown that phospholipase A is indeed activated after Cal synthesis only in the wild type cells and not in the cal mutant cells.

Pugsley, A.P. and M. Schwartz (1984) Colicin E2 release : lysis, leakage or secretion ? Possible role of a phospholipase. EMBO J. 3, 2393-2397.

Wu, H.C. and M. Tokunaga (1986) Biogenesis of lipoproteins in bacteria. Curr. Top. in Microb. and Immun. 125, 127-157.

Fehrenbach et al. (Eds.), Bacterial Protein Toxins, Zbl. Bakt. Suppl. 17
© Gustav Fischer, Stuttgart, New York, 1988

The Secretion of E. Coli Haemolysin

L. D. Gray[1], N. Mackman[2], K. Baker[3], J-M. Nicaud[4] and I. B. Holland[3]

[1]University of Newcastle upon Tyne, Department of Microbiology, Newcastle upon Tyne, England
[2]Scripps Clinic, Department of Immunology, La Jolla, California, U.S.A.
[3]University of Leicester, Department of Genetics, Leicester, England
[4]Institut National de Recherche Agronomique, Paris, France

ABSTRACT

The genetic organisation of the E.coli haemolytic determinant is described. An "ATP-binding site", conserved amongst several proteins, is identified in one protein which is esential for export, HlyB. This would be consistent with an energy transducing role for this polypeptide. The C-terminal 113 amino acids of HlyA are shown to be: (1) essential for secretion of the intact HlyA; (2) capable of their own secretion via the Hly export machinery when expressed independently; (3) capable of directing the secretion to the culture media of a polypeptide normally directed to the outer membrane via a periplasmic intermediate, OmpF. These data indicate that the entire information on HlyA required for interaction with the Hly export machinery is located within the C-terminal 113 amino acids. In addition, these results support our previous proposal that HlyA secretion does not proceed via a free periplasmic intermediate.

KEYWORDS

E.coli, haemolysin, secretion.

The haemolytic determinant of the human urinary tract isolate LE2001 comprises four or five polypeptides. HlyA is the secreted haemolysin but is not active unless modified by HlyC. The gene for HlyB may produce two polypeptides, HlyB1 and a smaller HlyB2 produced from an in frame initiation point within the open reading frame. This protein would be homologous with the C-terminal region of HlyB1. HlyB and HlyD, both located in the cell envelope, behave in fractionation experiments as though they form a trans-envelope structure. Both HlyD and HlyB are required for transport of HlyA. HlyA has no NH$_2$-terminal "signal" sequence and secretion is independent of secA.

Computer comparison of the amino acid sequence of HlyB with protein databases indicated significant similarities between HlyB and several other proteins. On inspection of the amino acids these were determined to comprise an "ATP-binding site" conserved amongst many proteins. This region was, however, encompassed by a broader domain conserved amongst several proteins involved in transport systems utilising a periplasmic binding protein. This domain, present on both HlyB1 and HlyB2, would be consistent with an energy transducing role for either or both of these polypeptides in HlyA translocation.

Deletion of 27 amino acids from the C-terminal of HlyA was shown by DNA sequence analysis and in vitro transcription-translation to produce a 104 kD truncated polypeptide. This polypeptide was observed to be haemolytically active but not secreted. Thus it was concluded that the C-terminal of HlyA is essential for its own secretion.

An EcoRI-HindIII fragment, encoding the C-terminal 23 kDa of HlyA was subcloned behind the tac promoter, utilising the ATG initiating codon of lacZ, on the high copy number plasmid pTTQ18. Expression from this DNA fragment produced a polypeptide corresponding to the C-terminal 23 kDa of HlyA. A small in frame BalI deletion made within this region reduced the size of the expressed polypeptide to 18.6 kDa. When complemented in trans with Hly export functions both of these polypeptides were effectively secreted. However, induction of expression in the absence of export function was lethal. The inserted DNA also encoded the N-terminal of HlyB and such lethality was ascribed to this truncated polypeptide or interactions between this truncated HlyB and the C-terminal of HlyA.

A DraI fragment, encoding solely the C-terminal 113 amino acids of HlyA, was subcloned to the high copy plasmid pUC12. Expression, initiated by the lac promoter, produced a 12 kDa polypeptide corresponding to the 6 first amino acids of lacZ and the 113 C-terminal amino acids of HlyA. This polypeptide was also secreted when complemented with Hly export functions. In the absence of export functions the 12 kDa polypeptide remained cytoplasmic. However, in this case presumably due to absence of the HlyB fragment, induction was not lethal.

A lacZ-ompF-hlyA gene fusion was constructed in pUC12 under the control of the lac promoter. The expressed polypeptide comprised the first 10 amino acids of a β-galactosidase moiety fused to 300 amino acids of OmpF (lacking the N-terminal secretory "signal" sequence and 30 C-terminal amino acids) followed by the 23 kDa of HlyA. This chimeric protein was shown by Western blottings using α-haemolysin antibody, to be effectively secreted to the culture medium when complemented with Hly export functions. This protein again was entirely cytoplasmic in the absence of HlyB,D.

These results confirmed that the C-terminal of 113 amino acids of HlyA contains all the information necessary for its secretion via the Hly secretory system. In addition, since OmpF in this hybrid was not incorporated into the outer membrane, these data support our previous proposal that HlyA secretion does not proceed via a free periplasmic intermediate. Rather the molecule is exported directly to the medium.

Fehrenbach et al. (Eds.), Bacterial Protein Toxins, Zbl. Bakt. Suppl. 17
© Gustav Fischer, Stuttgart, New York, 1988

Molecular Action of Cholera Toxin in Rabbit Intestinal Epithelial Cells

D. Longbottom and S. van Heyningen

Department of Biochemistry, University of Edinburgh, Hugh Robson Building, George Square, Edinburgh EH8 9XD, Great Britain

ABSTRACT

Both cholera toxin and sodium fluoride activated adenylate cyclase in the MPM fraction. The basal activity of the enzyme was very low and variable but gave a similar value, 0.5-1.0 pmoles cAMP produced.min^{-1}.mg $protein^{-1}$, for the three fractions (MPM, BLM and BBM). Both effectors increase the relative specific activity of adenylate cyclase in BLM and reduce it in BBM. When BLM were assayed for adenylate cyclase it was found that, with respect to MPM, the specific activity of fluoride-activated enzyme was 1.6-fold higher and for cholera toxin-activated enzyme it was 1.9-fold higher. These results indicate that the activation can be accounted for by an exchange of proteins between the BBM and the BLM.

KEYWORDS

Cholera toxin, MPM, BLM, BBM, adenylate cyclase.

ABBREVIATIONS

MPM, Mixed Plasma Membrane; BBM, Brush Border Membrane; BLM, Basal-Lateral Membrane.

INTRODUCTION

Although a great deal is known about the molecular mechanism of action of the ADP-ribosylating enterotoxin cholera toxin as an activator of adenylate cyclase, most of this work has been carried out on cells other than those found in the intestine where the toxin exerts its effect (van Heyningen, 1982). In the intestine the toxin binds to the BBM (Critchley, Magnani and Fishman, 1981) while adenylate cyclase appears to be located in the BLM (Murer and co-workers, 1976). Therefore it seemed appropriate to study this mechanism of activation. Initially MPM, BLM and BBM fractions were prepared from rabbit intestinal epithelial cells by a modification of the method of Schmitz and co-workers (1973). Marker enzyme assays were performed for BBM (sucrase and alkaline phosphatase) and BLM ((Na^+-K^+)ATPase) to determine the degree of separation. The activation of adenylate cyclase by sodium fluoride and cholera toxin was investigated in the three membrane fractions. The assay used is based on a method by Salomon (1979), using White's (1974) alumina-column procedure.

RESULTS

TABLE 1 Distribution of Adenylate Cyclase Activity in BBM and BLM
as Compared to Marker Enzymes.

Fraction	Relative enzymatic specific activity				
	Sucrase	Alkaline Phosphatase	(Na^+-K^+)ATPase	adenylate cyclase stimulated by	
				10mM F⁻	cholera toxin (20µg/ml)
H	0.4	0.4	0.5	N.D.	N.D.
MPM	1.0	1.0	1.0	1.0	1.0
BLM	0.5	0.6	2.2	1.6	1.9
BBM	4.1	2.7	0.4	0.7	0.7

N.D. = Not Determined, H=Homogenate
The specific activities of sucrase and alkaline phosphatase in the MPM are 1.77 and 0.2 µmoles substrate hydrolyzed.min^{-1}.mg protein^{-1} respectively and that of the (Na^+-K^+)ATPase is 7.3 pmoles.min^{-1}.mg protein^{-1}. The specific activities of adenylate cyclase in the MPM for activation by F⁻ and cholera toxin are 74 and 15 pmoles cAMP produced.min^{-1}.mg protein^{-1} respectively. The basal activity of adenylate cyclase in all three fractions was 0.5-1.0 pmoles cAMP produced.min^{-1}.mg protein^{-1}.

The results obtained, shown in Table 1, indicate that neither F⁻ or cholera toxin activate the enzyme in the BBM except as far as there is contamination by BLM. This means that the BBM probably does not contain catalytic subunits of adenylate cyclase. Therefore, an exchange of proteins between separated BBM and BLM could account for the activation in the BLM.

ACKNOWLEDGEMENTS

The authors wish to express their gratitude to Pfizer Central Research, Sandwich, Kent, England for providing all the cholera toxin and radiochemicals necessary for this work.

REFERENCES

Critchley, D.R., J.L.Magnani and P.H.Fishman (1981). Interactions of cholera toxin with rat intestinal brush border. J. Biol. Chem., 256, 8724-8731.
Murer, H., E.Ammann, J.Biber and U.Hopfer (1976). The surface membrane of the small intestinal epithelial cell . Localization of adenyl cyclase. Biochim. Biophys. Acta., 433, 509-519.
Salomon, Y. (1979). Adenylate cyclase assay. Adv. Cyc. Nucl. Res., 10, 35-55.
Schmitz, J., H.Preiser, D.Maestracci, B.K.Ghosh, J.J.Cerda and R.K.Crane (1973). Purification of the human intestinal brush border membrane. Biochim. Biophys. Acta., 323, 98-112.
van Heyningen, S. (1982). Cholera toxin. Review. Biosci. Rep., 2, 135-146.
White, A.A. (1974). Separation and purification of cyclic nucleotides by alumina column chromatography. Meth. Enzymol., 38, 41-46.

Fehrenbach et al. (Eds.), Bacterial Protein Toxins, Zbl. Bakt. Suppl. 17
© Gustav Fischer, Stuttgart, New York, 1988

Production of Cytotoxic Substances in Milk by Aeromonas Species

S. Notermans, J. Dufrenne and W. H. Jansen

National Institut of Public Health and Environmental Hygiene, P. O. Box 1, 3720 BA Bilthoven, Netherlands

Sixty-three percent of Aeromonas strains cultured in milk produced Vero-cell active substances other than hemolysins. Production of Vero-cell active substances by A.sobria isolated from human patients was more frequently observed than by environmental isolates of A.sobria. No A.caviae isolated from patients produced Vero-cell active substances but 50% of environmental isolates did. Two different Vero-cell active substances which were separable by $(NH_4)_2SO_4$ precipitation, were produced in milk: a heat-labile substance and a heat-stable substance ($20'/56^{o}C$).

Aeromonas species from environmental sources are increasingly being recognized as pathogens that may cause diarrea in humans. Although the role of Aeromonas species as enteric pathogens has not been proven conclusively, multiple virulent-associated biological activities have been detected in culture supernatants of Aeromonas species. Also production of different enterotoxic substances have been described (Asao and others, 1984; Chopra and others, 1986; Shimada and others, 1984; Ljung, Wretlind and Mölby, 1981). All these substances described show additionally cytotoxic or cytotonic activity. This report deals with production of heat-labile and heat-stable Vero-cell active substances produced in milk, where the production of hemolysin with cytotoxic activity rarely occurs.

The Aeromonas strains used in this study were isolated from drinking water, food and patients with a gastro-intestinal syndrome. For testing strains for production of Vero-cell active substances, strains were cultured in milk (15 ml of commercially sterilized skim milk in 100 ml erlenmeyer flasks) at $30^{o}C$ for 40 hrs with shaking (160 rev/min). Sterile culture fluids and sterile culture fluids heated at $56^{o}C$ for 20 min were tested for hemolytic activity (using rabbit erythrocytes) and for cytotoxic activity (using Vero-cells) as described earlier (Notermans and others, 1986). Hemolytic activity observed in the supernatants was neutralized by the addition of IgG anti-hemolysin purified as described by Asao and others (1984). The cytotoxic components were partially purified by $(NH_4)_2SO_4$ precipitation.

Production of hemolysins by the Aeromonas species was rarely observed in milk. If hemolysins were present, they were neutralized by the addition of IgG anti-hemolysin. Production of Vero-cell active substances, other than hemolysins, is presented in Table 1.

TABLE 1 Vero-cell Active Substances other than Hemolysins
Produced by Aeromonas Species in Milk at 30°C for 40 hrs.

| | Isolates from patients with a gastro-intestinal syndrome | | | Food and water isolates | | |
| | Number of strains with Vero-cell activity | | | Number of strains with Vero-cell activity | | |
	Total	Without* heating	With** heating	Total	Without* heating	With** heating
A.hydrophila	18	14 (78%)	8 (44%)	36	30 (83%)	16 (44%)
A.sobria	22	21 (96%)	14 (64%)	21	5 (24%)	3 (14%)
A.caviae	10	0 (0%)	0 (0%)	18	9 (50%)	5 (28%)

* Hemolysins with Vero-cell activity were neutralized by the addition
of IgG anti-hemolysin.
** 56°C for 20 min.

The median total Vero-cell titers for A.hydrophila isolated from environmental samples and patients were 100 and 400, respectively. For A.sobria these values were < 50 and 300, resp. For A.caviae these values were < 50 and < 50, resp. Vero-cell activity after heat-treatment was equal or lower than the total Vero-cell activity before heating. It has been noted that nearly all A.sobria strains isolated from patients produced Vero-cell active substances while no A.caviae strains did. $(NH_4)_2SO_4$ precipitation experiments showed that the heat-labile and heat-stable Vero-cell active substances precipitated at 20% and 80% saturated $(NH_4)_2SO_4$ concentration, resp., indicating that they are two different entities. In a previous study (Notermans and others, 1986) Aeromonas species were grown on Evans synthetic medium and 54% of A.hydrophila produced a cytotoxic entity without hemolytic activity, while none of the A.sobria and A.caviae produced such a substance. These findings show the effect of the composition of media on the production of biologically active substances by Aeromonas species. The existence of a heat-labile cytotoxic substance without hemolytic activity has not been described so far. In almost all studies cytotoxic activity was tested without neutralization of the hemolytic activity (Barer, Millership and Tabaqchali, 1986; Turnbull and others, 1984). Whether the production of Vero-cell active substances, as described here, are involved in the gastro-intestinal symptoms needs further investigation.

Asao, T., Y.Konoshita, S.Kozaki, T.Uemura, and G.Sakachigi (1984). Purification and some properties of Aeromonas hydrophila hemolysin. Infect.Immun., 46, 122-127.

Barer, M.R., S.E.Millership, and S.Tabaqchali (1986). Relationship of toxin production to species in the genus Aeromonas. J.Med.Microbiol., 22, 303-309.

Chopra, A.K., C.W.Houston, C.T.Genaux, J.D.Dixon, and A.Kurosky (1986). Evidence for production of an enterotoxin and cholera toxin cross-reactive factor by Aeromonas hydrophila. J.Clin.Microbiol., 24, 661-664.

Ljungh, A., B.Wretlind, and R.Mölby (1981). Separation and characterization of enterotoxins and two hemolysins from Aeromonas hydrophila. Acta Path.Microbiol.Scand.Sect.B, 89, 387-397.

Notermans, S., A.Havelaar, W.Jansen, S.Kozaki, and P.Guinée (1986). Production of "AH-1-toxin" by Aeromonas strain isolated from faeces and drinking water. J.Clin.Microbiol., 23, 1140-1142.

Shimada, T., R.Sakazaki, K.Horigome, Y.Uesaka, and K.Niwano (1984). Production of cholera-like enterotoxin by Aeromonas hydrophila. Jpn.J.Med.Sci.Biol., 37, 141-144.

Turnbull, P.C.B., J.van Lee, M.D.Meliotis, S.van de Walle, H.J.Koornhof, L.Jeffery, and T.N.Bryant (1984). Enterotoxin production in relation to taxonomic grouping and source of isolation of Aeromonas species. J.Clin.Microbiol., 19, 175-180.

Fehrenbach et al. (Eds.), Bacterial Protein Toxins, Zbl. Bakt. Suppl. 17
© Gustav Fischer, Stuttgart, New York, 1988

Production and Cellular Compartmentation of Protein B (CAMP-Factor) from Group B Streptococci

Takaisi Kikuni N. B. and F. J. Fehrenbach

Robert Koch-Institut des Bundesgesundheitsamtes, Abteilung für Mikrobiologie, Nordufer 20, D-1000 Berlin 65

KEYWORDS: Protein B, CAMP-factor, cellular compartmentation, group B streptococci

Protein B (CAMP-factor) of group B streptococci (GBS) is an extracellular polypeptide which acts as cocytolysin (1) and which binds in addition in a non-immune reaction immunoglobulins of different classes and from different mammalian species (2). Optimal growth conditions for the production of protein B by GBS were established using a 2 % maltose-containing TPY medium and a CO_2 gas atmosphere (0.1 l/h). Protein B was produced mainly during mid to late logarithmic growth phase and released into the supernatant without evidence of bacterial autolysis. GBS harvested at that time contained a major pool of protein B in the cytoplasm and a smaller pool in the cell envelopes.

The production of protein B from GBS (strain NCTC 8181, type IIb) and its cellular compartmentation were studied during aerobic and microaerophilic (CO_2: 0.1 l/h) growth at 37 °C in 800 ml shaker-flask cultures (120 rpm) using trypticase peptone-yeast extract (TPY) or Todd Hewitt broth (THB) supplemented with 2 % (w/v) maltose or glucose. Cocytolytic activity of protein B was measured in the different fractions as reported earlier (3).

In 2 % maltose-containing TPY medium, GBS grew exponentially for 4 - 6 h with a doubling time of approximately 45 - 50 min. Protein B was released during the logarithmic and post-logarithmic growth phase. The highest amount of extracellular protein B was obtained under microaerophilic culture conditions (500 HU/ml). Thus, the differential rates of protein B release (HU/µg bact. dry wt.) were 0.18 for aerobic and 0.33 for microaerophilic growth, respectively. The yield of protein B found in aerated cultures was thus about 50 % of that found under microaerophilic conditions (CO_2: 0.1 l/h).

TABLE 1: Protein B Production and Compartmentation during Growth of GBS Type IIb under Different Culture Conditions

culture conditions	fractions	protein B activity		
		hemolytic activity* (HU)	specific activity HU (mg protein)$^{-1}$	% of total** hemolytic activity
TPY plus 2 % glucose	CS	1.3×10^5	4.4×10^2	99.1 ± 0.5
	CP	7.7×10^2	0.1×10^2	0.6 ± 0.5
	CE	3.2×10^2	0.03×10^2	0.3 ± 0.1
TPY plus 2 % glucose CO_2 (0.1 1/h)	CS	1.8×10^5	6.4×10^2	99.7 ± 0.3
	CP	4.1×10^2	0.03×10^2	0.2 ± 0.1
	CE	1.7×10^2	0.02×10^2	0.1 ± 0.1
TPY plus 2 % maltose	CS	2.14×10^5	8.3×10^2	92.7 ± 3.5
	CP	1.32×10^4	0.7×10^2	5.7 ± 2.0
	CE	3.8×10^3	0.4×10^2	1.6 ± 1.0
TPY plus 2 % maltose CO_2 (0.1 1/h)	CS	4.2×10^5	1.5×10^3	96.3 ± 3.0
	CP	1.26×10^4	0.7×10^2	2.9 ± 1.5
	CE	3.3×10^3	0.3×10^2	0.8 ± 0.7
THB plus 2 % maltose	CS	2.1×10^5	8.3×10^2	94.3 ± 0.8
	CP	9.3×10^3	0.7×10^2	4.2 ± 1.4
	CE	3.4×10^3	0.4×10^2	1.5 ± 0.3
THB plus 2 % maltose CO_2 (0.1 1/h)	CS	2.9×10^5	1.2×10^3	95.7 ± 1.5
	CP	9.7×10^3	0.9×10^2	3.2 ± 1.0
	CE	3.4×10^3	0.4×10^2	1.1 ± 0.6

Table 1 demonstrates the influence of different media, carbon sources and gas atmospheres on the cellular distribution of protein B in GBS type IIb. Cells were grown to the late logarithmic phase in the individual culture medium. The highest protein B concentration was found using a 2 % maltose-containing TPY medium. The release of protein B was increased in the presence of CO_2. About 95 % of protein B produced were usually recovered from the culture supernatant. Higher concentrations of intracellular protein B were found in the cytoplasm and less in the cell envelopes.

REFERENCES

1. Fehrenbach, F.J., C.M.Schmidt, B.Sterzik, and D.Jürgens (1984). Interaction of amphiphilic bacterial polypeptides with artificial membranes. In: J.E.Alouf, F.J.Fehrenbach, J.H.Freer, J.Jeljaszewicz (Eds.) Bacterial Protein Toxins. Academic Press Inc. Ltd., London, pp. 317-324

2. Jürgens, D., B.Sterzik, and F.J.Fehrenbach (1987). Unspecific binding of group B streptococcal cocytolysin (CAMP-factor) to immunoglobulins and its possible role in pathogenicity.J.Exp.Med., 165, 720-732

3. Huser, H., L.Goeke, G.Karst, and F.J.Fehrenbach (1983). Fermenter growth of Streptococcus agalactiae and large-scale production of CAMP-factor. J.Gen.Microbiol, 129, 1295-1300

Genetic Aspects of Toxinogenesis

Fehrenbach et al. (Eds.), Bacterial Protein Toxins, Zbl. Bakt. Suppl. 17
© Gustav Fischer, Stuttgart, New York, 1988

Coordinate Regulation of Virulence Determinants

S. Calderwood, S. Knapp, K. Peterson, R. Taylor and J. Mekalanos

Department of Microbiology and Molecular Genetics Harvard Medical School, 25 Shattuck Street, Boston, Mass. 02115, U.S.A.

ABSTRACT

We have isolated a series of TnphoA gene fusions that are regulated by physiological signals that also control production of toxins in V. cholerae, B. pertussis, and E. coli. This method facilitates the identification of genes that encode additional virulence factors. The molecular basis for this observation is that a central virulence regulatory gene, (toxR, vir, and fur, respectively) is found to be responsible for the coordinate regulation of multiple virulence determinants in these organisms.

KEYWORDS

Cholera toxin, pertussis toxin, Shiga-like toxin, pilus colonization factors, transcriptional regulation.

INTRODUCTION

Virulence can be defined as the degree of pathogenicity. Within a given experimental infection model, one can clearly establish that virulence is also a multifaceted property for the pathogen as well. This can be most dramatically demonstrated by bacterial pathogens that infect mucosal surfaces. For example, it is thought that Vibrio cholerae utilizes motility and chemotaxis to penetrate the mucus gel overlaying the intestinal epithelium, bacterial surface pili and hemagglutinins to adhere to intestinal receptors, neuraminadase and protease production to degrade the mucus gel and provide growth substrates, and cholera enterotoxin and possibly other toxins (e.g., shiga-like toxin and hemolysins) to ultimately cause the cholera secretory diarrhea (1,2).
These virulence properties or determinants are not simply expressed in a haphazard manner but are usually carefully regulated by most pathogenic microbes. The most trivial reason

for this may be that organisms such as V. cholerae must naturally persist in non-animal environments where the production of virulence determinants offer only a metabolic drain on the organism. The expression of a given virulence determinant in laboratory media requires careful attention to media composition, growth phase, and physical parameters such as incubation temperature and pH. Nutritional parameters that have been implicated in the regulation of virulence determinants run the full gamut from specific ions to complex organics molecules.

A remarkable observation has recently emerged from the study of virulence gene expression. There is accumulating evidence that the regulation of one virulence factor is often coupled with the regulation of other virulence factors. Indeed, there are now well documented examples a single regulatory locus that orchestrates the coordinate transcriptional regulation of multiple virulence determinants. Understanding the molecular basis for this coordinate regulation of virulence determinants offers a number of applications the most important of which is improved vaccine production.

RESULTS

We have developed an experimental approach for the genetic analysis of bacterial virulence determinants and their regulation that involves the following steps: 1. Analysis of nutritional and physical parameters that regulate a virulence factor; 2. Isolation of TnphoA gene fusions that are regulated by these parameters; 3. Characterization of virulence defects associated with these TnphoA insertion mutations; 4. Identification of the regulatory gene controlling the expression of these TnphoA gene fusions. Using this system, we have examined the genetic basis for the coordinate regulation of bacterial virulence determinants utilizing three experimental organisms-Vibrio cholerae, Bordetella pertussis and Escherchia coli.

V. cholerae ToxR-mediated Regulation

Miller, Taylor and Mekalanos (1984, 1987) have shown that the toxR gene of V. cholerae encodes a transmembrane, DNA binding protein that activates the promoter of the cholera toxin operon (ctxAB). Osmolarity, pH, temperature, and the presence of certain amino acids all influence the production of cholera toxin and a set of other proteins produced by V. cholerae in a coordinate fashion. This regulation may reflect a shift in protein expression that marks a transition from growth in the environmental to colonization of the small intestine. We wanted to determine whether this physiological coordinate expression was determined at the genetic level by toxR-mediated transcriptional regulation. Our published results (Taylor and colleagues, 1987) indicated that null mutations in toxR did indeed eliminate the production of a proteins that were previously known to be physiologically regulated similar to cholera toxin. This result prompted us to develop a more general system for detecting toxR-regulated genes and identifying their function.

We have developed a pair of broad host range vectors for delivery of TnphoA (Manoil and Beckwith, 1986) into V. cholerae and other Gram-negative organisms. TnphoA is a derivative of transposon Tn5 that can produce on insertion gene fusions between a target gene and the gene for alkaline phosphatase (phoA). These fusions produce hybrid proteins that display alkaline phosphatase activity only if the target gene produces a secreted or membrane protein.

Approximately 40 TnphoA insertion mutations were isolated in V. cholerae 0395 using vectors pRT291 or pRT733, screened for PhoA activity, and then further characterized. SDS-polyacryamide gel analysis of one of these fusion strains (RT110.21) showed that it had lost a protein that in the wild-type strain appeared to be physiologically expressed in a manner that indicated it was toxR-regulated. This protein (TcpA) was eventually identified as the major subunit of a pilus colonization factor (the toxin coregulated pilus) produced by V. cholerae (Taylor and co-workers, 1987). DNA sequence analysis confirmed that the TnphoA insertion carried by RT110.21 was located in the structural gene for TcpA.

These results prompted us to isolate over 600 gene fusion events that produce a PhoA+ phenotype in V. cholerae. Characterization of each fusion strain in six different expression media that allow high or low expression of toxR-activated genes has allowed the identification of 30 fusions (ca. 10-12 genes) that are apparently toxR-regulated (Table 1). All the fusions that appeared toxR-regulated in terms of phsiological parameters were made toxR- by insertion of plasmid pVM55 (13) into the toxR gene. This genetic test proved that all these presumptive toxR-regulated gene fusions were indeed toxR-controlled at some level. Additional characterization by SDS-PAGE, western blot, ELISA, and Southern blot indicated that many of these fusions were in genes already known to be toxR-regulated (i.e., tcpA, ctxA, and ctxB). Other toxR-regulated gene fusions affect the production of the TcpA pilus but are not inserted in the tcpA gene and do affect the level of expression of this pilin subunit. These data are consistant with V. cholerae having at least 12 different toxR-activated genes or transcriptional units many of which are involved in virulence.

TABLE 1
Characteristics of Selected toxR-Regulated TnphoA
Fusions in Vibrio cholerae

STRAINS		ALKALINE PHOSPHATASE ACTIVITY (Units)			TYPE
			CULTURE CONDITIONS		
		LB pH 6.5/8.4	TRY+ NaCl 66/0 mM	M9+Asn/-Asn	
2-47		499/42	324/23	307/24	ctxA
2-47	toxR55	18/17			
3-8		769/60	507/65	550/61	unknown
3-8	toxR55	41/50			
3-12		141/10	84/9	72/8	unknown
3-12	toxR55	13/9			
8-11		252/25	126/13	141/13	unknown
8-11	toxR55	50/61			
2-44		971/54	640/35	680/36	tcpA

Coordinate Regulation by vir in B. pertussis

Weiss and Falkow (1983) have shown that the vir gene of B. pertussis is required for expression of the genes for pertussis toxin (ptx), filamentous hemagglutinin (fha), hemolysin (hly), dermonecrotic toxin (dnt), extracellular adenylate cyclase toxin (cyc), and other potential virulence factors of B. pertussis. The expression of these same virulence factors is regulated at the phsiological level by the concentration of Mg+2 or nicotinic acid (modulators) in the growth medium.

We have used our broad host range vectors for TnphoA to produce gene fusions in B. pertussis strain 18323. Over 110 fusion strains were then individually screened for alkaline phosphatase activity in media containing high and low modulator concentrations. This analysis identified 17 fusions that were expressed physiologically in a manner that suggested that they were vir-regulated (see Table 2). In addtion to fusions activated by vir+ growth conditions (low Mg/nicotinate, Stanier Scholte medium), we also found fusions that were repressed by vir+ growth conditions and activated by vir- growth conditions (high Mg/nicotinate). Characterization of fusions of both types have so far identified mutants that have altered protein phenotypes (e.g., hly- mutants, outermembrane proteins, and pili- mutants). Characterization of these mutatnts for virulence defects is currently in progress.

TABLE 2
Characterization of Selected vir-regulated
TnphoA Fusions in B. pertussis

STRAINS	ALKALINE PHOSPHATASE ACTIVITY		
	Stanier Scholte	+20 mM MgSO4	+5 mM Nicotinate
Wild-type background:			
18323	1	2	2
vir-activated:			
M8	744	70	21
M16	1024	104	86
M25	25	3	2
M34	1350	35	53
M49	1001	46	34
M75	187	18	12
M91	1088	43	29
vir-repressed:			
M6	17	284	505
M18	23	178	199
M24	34	329	182
M73	12	219	347

One of the TnphoA gene fusions that showed repression by vir+ growth conditions (M6) was cloned in E. coli by selecting for its kanamycin resistant phenotype. This fusion was then subcloned into the vector pRK290 and mobilized into B. pertussis strains 347 and 348. Strain 347 carries a Tn5 insertion in the vir gene while strain 348 carries a Tn5 insertion in the hly gene. The PhoA activity of the vir-repressed gene fusion (M6) was high (409 units) as expected in 347 (a vir- strain) and low (152 units) in 348 (a vir+ strain) when grown in then absense of Mg+2 or nicotinic acid. These data confirmed that the vir locus does indeed repress the expression of some genes and we have designated these vrg loci for "vir repressed genes."

Subcloning of the vir-negatively regulated fusion M6 was used to localize the promoter control expression of the phoA fusion protein. A subclone was obtained that had less than 500 bp upstream of the fusion junction and yet when mobilized back into B. pertussis, this subclone was still regulated. We determined the complete DNA sequence of this 500 base pair region including the TnphoA fusion junction. We then used exoIII digestion to introduce a set of upstream deletions into the presumptive promoter region. Each one was sequenced, subcloned and introduced into B. pertussis strains 348 and 347. This analysis demonstrated that a stacked promoters of varying strengths existed in this upstream region. Most important, the regulatory site where vir represses expression of the M6 fusion protein is apparently near the start or within the structural gene mutated in the M6 fusion. Within the coding sequence for the gene product encoded by the M6 fusion, we found a near perfect 20 bp dyad repeat. This repeat is quite homologous to repeats located upstream of the ptx transcriptional start site. This homology between repeated sequences located in a vir-activated and vir-repressed promoter suggests that we may have defined sequences at which form the binding site for the vir gene product.

Regulation of Shiga-like Toxin Gene Expression by fur.

Shiga-like toxin (SLT) is a cytotoxin structurally related to the Shiga toxin produced by S. dysenteriae. O'Brian and co-workers (1984) have shown that certain strains of E. coli, V. cholerae, and V. parahemolyticus produce this toxin primarily in media with reduced iron concentrations. Calderwood and co-workers (1987) have cloned the genes for Shiga-like toxin encoded by phage H19B and determined their nucleotide sequence. The genes are organized in what appears to be a single

TABLE 3
Regulation of an sltA::TnphoA Gene fusion by Iron
and the fur gene of E. coli

STRAINS	IRON ADDED	ALKALINE PHOSPHATASE ACTIVITY (Units)	INDUCTION RATIO
DHB24 (fur+) pSC105	0	547	
	10 uM	45	12.7
SBC24 (fur-) pSC105	0	576	
	10 uM	487	1.0

transcriptional unit, sltAB with only 12 bp separating the two reading frames. Both subunits have hydrophobic N-terminal signal sequences and the amino sequence of mature SltB is identical to the amino acid sequence of the B subunit of Shiga toxin from S. dysenteriae.

We have constructed a gene fusion between phoA and sltA (the gene encoding the A subunit of Shiga-like toxin of E. coli) and have used alkaline phosphatase activity encoded by this fusion to study the molecular aspects of iron regulation of slt expression. As can be seen in Table 3, slt expression is repressed by iron but this effect is dependent on a gene called fur (ferric uptake regulation) Braun (1984).

We have also used the TnphoA fusion to sltA to measure the effect of 5' deletions on the activity and regulation of the slt promoter by iron. This deletion analysis defined sequences involved in the slt promoter function and a 23 bp region involved in iron repression of slt transcription. Within this iron regulatory region is an 18 bp sequence of near perfect dyad symmetry that overlaps the presumptive -10 box of the slt promoter. The slt dyad shared considerable homology to dyad sequences found in other iron regulated promoters involved in siderophore production and uptake. The fur gene product has been postulated to encode an iron responsive repressor that inhibits transcription of these iron regulated genes in E. coli. We have showed that fur null mutations produce an iron constitutive phenotype for the slt promoter (Table 3) suggesting that the Fur-Fe complex may bind to the dyad repeat we identified in the region of the slt promoter involved in iron regulation. Because siderophore-based iron uptake systems are frequently virulence factors for a variety of pathogenic bacteria, the regulation of slt and these iron uptake genes by the fur gene product represents yet another example of coordinate regulation of virulence genes by a single regulatory gene.

DISCUSSION

In three different systems discussed here, virulence genes regulated in physiologically similar fashion appeared to be controlled by the same regulatory gene. These coordinate regulatory systems can be studied conveniently using TnphoA fusion technology. Our work predicts that by isolating gene fusions that are regulated physiologically like a given virulence factors (e.g., cholera toxin), one can identify other previously unknown virulence genes (e.g., tcpA). This approach should facilitate the genetic analysis of bacterial virulence and thus eventually make a contribution to vaccine development.

REFERENCES

Braun, V. 1984. Regualtion of iron uptake in Escherichia coli, p. 301-305. in D. Schlessinger (ed.), Microbiology-1983. American Society for Microbiology, Washington, D.C.

Betley, M.J., Miller, V.L., and Mekalanos, J.J. 1986. Genetics of Bacterial Enterotoxins, Ann. Rev. Microbiol. 40,577-605.

Calderwood, S.B., Auclair, F., Mekalanos, and Keusch, G.T. 1987. Nucleotide sequence of the iron-regulated shiga-like toxin genes of Escherichia coli. Proc. Natl. Acad. Sci. USA, 84,4364-4368.

Manoil, C., Beckwith, J. 1985. TnphoA: a transposon probe for protein export signals. Proc. Natl. Acad. Sci. USA 82,8129-8133.

Miller, V.L. and Mekalanos, J.J. 1984. Synthesis of cholera toxin is positively regulated at the transcriptional level by toxR. Proc. Natl. Acad. Sci. USA 81,3471-3475.

O'Brien, A.D., Lively, T.A., Chen, M.E., Rothman, S.W. and Formal, S.B. 1983. Escherichia coli 0157:H7 strains associated with haemorrhagic colitis in the United States produce a Shigella dyenteriae 1 (Shiga) like cytotoxin. Lancet 1:702.

O'Brien, A.D., Newland, J.W., Miller, S.F., Holmes, R.J., Smith, H.W. and Formal, S.F. 1984. Shiga-like toxin-converting phages from Escherichia coli strains that cause hemorrhagic colitis or infantile diarrhea. Science 226,694-696.

Taylor, R.K., Miller, V.L., Furlong, D.B., Mekalanos, J.J. 1987. Use of phoA gene fusions to identify a pilus colonization factor coordinately regulated with cholera toxin. Proc. Natl. Acad. Sci. USA 84,2833-2837.

Weiss, A.A. and Falkow, S. 1984. Genetic analysis of phase change in Bordetella pertussis. Infect. Immun. 43,263-269.

Fehrenbach et al. (Eds.), Bacterial Protein Toxins, Zbl. Bakt. Suppl. 17
© Gustav Fischer, Stuttgart, New York, 1988

Genetics of Shiga Toxin and Shiga-Like Toxins

Tsutomu Sekizaki[1,2] and K. N. Timmis[1]

[1]Department of Medical Biochemistry, University of Geneva, Switzerland
[2]Poultry Disease Laboratory, National Institute of Animal Health, Seki, Gifu 501-32, Japan

ABSTRACT

Shiga toxin and Shiga-like toxins are powerful cytotoxins elaborated by *Shigella dysenteriae* serotype 1 and other shigellae, and certain strains of *Escherichia coli* causing infant (or animal) diarrhoea or haemorrhagic colitis, respectively. Despite their pathogenic attributes, the toxins have not thus far been causally related to bacterial pathogenicity, largely as a result of the lack of availability of defined Shiga toxin-negative mutants and convenient animal models of infection. Recently, Shiga toxin-negative transposon insertion mutants of *S. dysenteriae* 1 were constructed and shown to be fully virulent in the Serény infection model (elicitation of keratoconjunctivitis in the guinea pig). Although Shiga toxin may not be a critical virulence factor of *S. dysenteriae* 1, it may nevertheless be a determinant of the severity of shigellosis and of the likelyhood of the development of serious complications such as haemolytic uraemic syndrome, a condition also observed in some cases of haemorrhagic colitis caused by Shiga-like toxin-producing strains of *E. coli*.

KEYWORDS

Shiga toxin, Shiga-like toxin, Vero toxin, *Shigella*, enterohaemorrhagic *E. coli* (EHEC), enteropathogenic *E. coli* (EPEC) dysentery, haemorrhagic colitis, Serény test, vaccines, transposon mutants

INTRODUCTION

Shiga toxin, a powerful toxin produced by *Shigella dysenteriae* serotype 1, was discovered in 1903 (Conradi, 1903). Since that time, its extremely high cytotoxic and lethal activities have been taken as an indication of the toxin's importance as a virulence factor of dysentery-producing shigellae. As a result, extensive studies have been undertaken to characterize the toxin's structure, function and mode of action (for excellent up-to-date reviews, consult Cantey, 1985; O'Brian and Holmes, 1987). These studies were recently stimulated and complemented by the discovery and characterization of toxins having similar activities and that are produced by some diarrhoea-producing enteropathogenic strains of *E. coli* (EPEC) and strains isolated from cases of haemorrhagic colitis (enterohaemorrhagic *E. coli* or EHEC). Konawalchuk and others (1977) first described the 026::H11 EPEC strain H-30 that produced a toxin which was cytotoxic to Vero cells, and which they designated Vero toxin. O'Brian and co-workers (1982; 1984) independently reported that some strains of EPEC and EHEC produce cytotoxins for HeLa cells that can be neutralized by rabbit anti-Shiga toxin antiserum, and designated them Shiga-like toxin (SLT). The Vero toxin originally described in EPEC strain H-30 appears to be the same SLT. Konawalchuk and colleagues (1978) also reported that some of the EPEC strains produced Vero toxins which were not neutralized by anti Shiga-toxin antiserum. The former toxin was designated SLT-I (or Vero toxin 1), and the latter SLT-II (or Vero toxin 2) (Scotland and co-workers, 1985; Strockbine and co-workers, 1986). Low level production of SLT-I has also been detected in some isolates of certain other Gram negative enteric pathogens, such as *Vibrio sp.*,

Salmonella typhimurium and *Campylobacter jejuni*. Significantly, the disease syndromes caused by the three principal types of toxin producers, *Shigella*, EPEC and EHEC, are distinct despite all being intestinal conditions, suggesting that the roles and/or relative importance of the toxins of these different pathogens may differ.

Shigellae provoke disease through invasion of and multiplication within the large bowel epithelium, causing localized destruction of the mucosa and a subsequent massive inflammatory reaction. This results in severe abdominal cramps and the frequent passage of bloody mucous stools (dysentery). The infection is generally self-limiting and clears up within a few days of the onset of symptoms. The ability to invade and multiply within epithelial cells is a crucial virulence factor of *Shigella* (Ogawa and colleagues, 1967; Gemski and colleagues, 1972), as are a number of other bacterial properties, such as the production of lipopolysaccharide O antigen (Watanabe and Timmis, 1984; Timmis and co-workers, 1985). Although the most severe form of shigellosis is caused by the high level Shiga toxin producing serotype *S. dysenteriae* 1, which also gives the highest frequencies of serious complications (e.g. HUS, see below), and although low level toxin producing mutants of *S. dysenteriae* 1 gave less severe infections in human volunteers than did the high level toxin-producing parental strain (Levine and others, 1973), the synthesis of Shiga toxin has not thus far been causally related to bacterial virulence. Man and some sub-human primates are the only animals known to be susceptible to shigellosis; the infection is typically one of young children but adults are also readily infected.

Disease caused by EPEC and EHEC strains does not involve invasion of the mucosa and results from bacterial colonization of the intestinal epithelial surface. Other than production of SLT, the only pathogenicity-related property detected so far in these groups of strains is that some EPEC strains, which typically infect infants, small children and pigs, adhere avidly to the small bowel epithelium and cause effacement of microvilli (e.g. Moon and colleagues, 1983). This, and the strong epidemiological correlation between production of substantial levels of SLT and the clinical condition from which the toxin producers were isolated - diarrhoea, haemorrhagic colitis or haemolytic uraemic syndrome (HUS) - suggests that SLT may be a major, perhaps the principal virulence factor of EHEC and some strains of EPEC (Scotland and colleagues, 1980; Smith and colleagues, 1983; Cleary and colleagues, 1985). However, as is the case for *Shigella* and Shiga toxin, no causal relationship has thus far been established between SLT production and bacterial virulence.

STRUCTURAL AND FUNCTIONAL PROPERTIES OF SHIGA TOXIN AND SLT

Shiga toxin is a protein consisting of two distinct types of subunit: the A subunit (Mr 32,000; single copy), although not toxic in its native form, contains the toxic region of the protein whereas the B subunit (Mr 7,700; 5 copies) contains the binding site for the toxin receptor on the epithelial cell surface (O'Brian and Holmes, 1987). Shiga toxin is thus similar in structure and function to many other A-B type toxins like cholera, diphtheria and pertussis toxins. Shiga toxin is thought to bind via its B subunits to a galactose $\alpha 1->4$ galactose-containing glycolipid or glycoprotein on the surface of susceptible cells and thence to be internalized by receptor-mediated endocytosis (O'Brian and Holmes, 1987). By a series of poorly characterized steps, the A subunit of the internalized toxin is proteolytically cleaved and its disulphide bridges reduced, thereby liberating a toxic fragment (A_1; Mr 27,000) which inactivates the 60S subunit of cytoplasmic ribosomes and causes the arrest of protein synthesis and cell death.

Shiga toxin exhibits several biological activities. When added to cells cultivated *in vitro*, it is an extremely powerful cytotoxin: the 50% cytotoxic dose (CD_{50}) is about 1 pg. When injected intravenously into mice or rabbits, Shiga toxin causes motor paralysis, microvascular haemorrhaging in the spinal cord and death, i.e. is lethal (LD_{50} about 200 ng), and superficially appears to have neurotoxic activity. When instilled into ligated ileal loops of the rabbit, it causes fluid secretion and was thus thought to have enterotoxic activity (50% enterotoxic dose about 20 ng). Shiga-like toxins also exhibit cytotoxic, enterotoxic, and lethal toxic activities, and are thus functionally similar to Shiga toxin. However, unlike the classical enterotoxins (cholera toxin and the heat stable and heat labile enterotoxins of *E. coli*), Shiga toxin kills absorptive epithelial cells and causes haemorrhaging of the ileal mucosa (Keenan and others, 1986)

SLT-I has structural and biological properties similar to those of Shiga toxin, and seems to adsorb to the same receptor. SLT-II is less well characterized but is known to have similar biological activities. Diarrhoea is induced by oral administration both of SLT-producing bacteria and of partially-purified toxin to infant rabbits (Pai and colleagues, 1986). In the latter case, the histopathological damage observed ressembles that caused by purified Shiga toxin.

The HUS syndrome, originally described by Gasser and co-workers (1955) as the association of haemolytic anaemia, thrombocytonaemia and acute renal failure, is epidemiologically correlated with infection by Shiga toxin- or SLT-I-producing bacteria (Cleary and colleagues, 1985). *S. dysenteriae* 1-associated HUS tends to be more severe than the *E. coli*-associated HUS (Koster and others, 1977), and HUS can occur even after infection with *S. dysenteriae* 1.

Some comparative characteristics of Shiga toxin and SLT are given in Table 1.

TABLE 1   Comparison of Shiga toxin and Shiga-like Toxins

Characteristics	Shiga toxin	Shiga-like toxins
Producing organism	S. dysenteriae 1	EPEC; EHEC; other strains of Shigella
Genetic location	chromosome	toxin-converting phage; chromosome
Disease caused	bacillary dysentery in humans;	diarrhoea in infants or animals; haemorrhagic colitis; HUS

GENETIC STUDIES ON SHIGA TOXIN

The principal difficulty in evaluating the biological role of Shiga toxin has been the lack of availability of Shiga toxin-negative mutants of *S. dysenteriae* 1. Attempts to isolate either spontaneous mutants (Gemski and others, 1972) or transposon mutants (K. Gamon and K.N. Timmis, unpublished data) were unsuccessful. A rational strategy to generate such mutants would have involved the molecular cloning of the toxin gene in *E. coli* K-12, followed by generation of specific deletion mutations *in vitro*, and substitution by homologous recombination of the mutant gene for the wild-type gene present in *Shigella*. The first step in this strategy, however, was effectively prohibited by successive pronouncements of the subcommittee of the NIH Recombinant DNA Advisory Committee charged with evaluating potential hazards of the cloning of toxin genes, despite the fact that the closely-related SLT's are produced by *E. coli*. It was therefore decided to generate toxin-negative mutants by *in vivo* genetic manipulations. This, however, required the accurate localization of the toxin determinant on the chromosome of *S. dysenteriae* 1.

To map the Shiga toxin gene, we constructed *Shigella* Hfr strains using a temperature-sensitive derivative of the conjugative plasmid, RP4 (Fig. 1). The derivative used, pMT999, is a Tn*501* transposon-containing derivative of pTH10 (Harayama and co-workers, 1980), which is itself a temperature-sensitive replication mutant of RP4. pMT999 specifies resistance to kanamycin, tetracycline, ampicilin and mercury and thus confers resistance to these antimicrobial agents upon host bacteria grown at 30°C. Since the plasmid fails to replicate at high temperature, however, bacteria grown at 42°C are sensitive to these agents. Kanamycin-resistant derivatives of *S. dysenteriae* 1

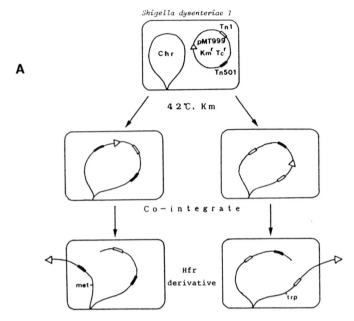

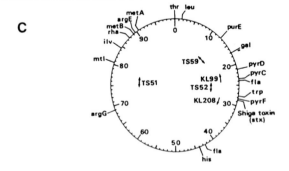

B Transfer properties of *Shigella* Hfr strains

Donor	No of transconjugants obtained/10^6 donor cells							
	PurE$^+$	Gal$^+$	Trp$^+$	His$^+$	ArgG$^+$	Ilv$^+$	Met$^+$	Leu$^+$
TS51	1	14	10	3	730	74000	30	1
TS52	10	290	530	27	210	170	5	4
TS59	1300	650	8	3	8	3	4	0.1

C

Fig. 1 Characteristics of Hfr derivatives of Shigella dysenteriae 1. A. Derivatives of Shigella dysenteriae 1 in which the temperature-sensitive RP4-derived plasmid pMT999 had inserted into the chromosome were selected by growth of bacteria at 42°C. B. The three derivatives TS51, TS52 and TS59 were mated with an appropriately-marked E.coli K-12 strain and transconjugants selected. The pattern of Shigella markers inherited by the E. coli recipient during these matings suggested the approximate sites of insertion of pMT999 in the chromosomes of TS51, TS52 and TS59, and thus their origins of chromosomal transfer. C. A genetic map of E. coli K-12 showing relevant loci and the equivalent locations in the Shigella chromosomes of the origins of transfer. The origins and orientations of transfer of two E. coli K-12 Hfr strains, KL99 and KL208, are also shown. The map location of the Shiga toxin gene stx, which was determined in the experiment summarized in Fig. 2, is shown.

A

$Shigella \xrightarrow{\quad fla^-\quad stx^+\quad} E.coli$

Donor X Recipient	Selected phenotypes	% Co-inheritance $purE^+$	gal^+	fla^-	trp^+	stx^+	fla^-	his^+	Recombinants examined
TS52	$PurE^+$	100	1.0	4.2	10.4	0	(4.2)	0	96
X	Gal^+	0	100	68.8	2.5	3.8	(68.8)	0	80
TS50	Trp^+	0	0	7.3	100	14.6	(7.3)	0	96
	His^+	0	0	(22.9)	1.0	1.0	22.9	100	96
TS59	Gal^+	0	100	11.3	0	ND	(11.3)	0	80
X	Trp^+	0	1.1	40.9	100	2.2	(40.9)	0	93
TS50	His^+	0	0	(28.0)	1.3	0	28.0	100	75

		$purE^+$	fla^+	trp^+	stx^-	fla^+	his^+	
KL99	Trp^+	0	(1.3)	100	96.3	1.3	0	80
X TS55	His^+	0	(67.5)	23.8	18.8	67.5	100	80

$E.coli \xrightarrow{\quad fla^+\quad stx^-\quad} Shigella\text{-}E.coli\ \text{hybrid}$

B

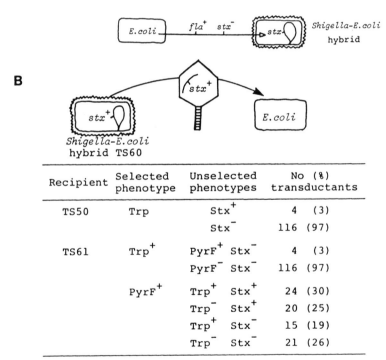

Shigella-E.coli hybrid TS60

Recipient	Selected phenotype	Unselected phenotypes	No (%) transductants
TS50	Trp	Stx^+	4 (3)
		Stx^-	116 (97)
TS61	Trp^+	$PyrF^+\ Stx^-$	4 (3)
		$PyrF^-\ Stx^-$	116 (97)
	$PyrF^+$	$Trp^+\ Stx^+$	24 (30)
		$Trp^-\ Stx^+$	20 (25)
		$Trp^+\ Stx^-$	15 (19)
		$Trp^-\ Stx^-$	21 (26)

Fig. 2 Mapping of stx. A. The matings performed are schematically shown above and below the table. TS50 is the appropriately marked E. coli K-12 recipient strain used in the first mattings. TS55 is an Stx$^+$ E. coli K-12 transconjugant (obtained from the TS52 x TS50 mating) that was used as a recipient in the second mating performed with an E. coli K-12 Hfr Stx$^-$ donor. B. The fine mapping phage P1 transductional analysis of stx was carried out using as donor strain E. coli K-12 TS60, an Stx$^+$ transconjugant obtained from the TS52 x TS50 mating. The results demonstrate close linakge of stx with pyrF (see Fig. 1).

(pMT999) were isolated following plating of bacteria at 42°C (Sekizaki and colleagues, 1987). The majority of such clones probably carried the pMT999 plasmid integrated into the bacterial chromosome via transposon Tn*501* or Tn*1* (Fig. 1) and would, as a result, be able to conjugally transfer chromosomal genes to recipient bacteria (i.e. be Hfr's). Three such derivatives, TS51, TS52 and TS59, were mated with the *E. coli* K-12 Rec$^+$ recipient TS50 and *E. coli* transconjugants having acquired individual *Shigella* chromosomal markers were selected. The chromosomal sites of insertion of pMT999, and thus the points of chromosome transfer of *Shigella* Hfr derivatives TS51, TS52 and TS59, seemed to reside near *ilv*, *trp* and *purE*, respectively (Fig. 1).

From previous observations, it seemed likely that the Shiga toxin gene would be located in the *mtl-argE* region of the chromosome of *Shigella flexneri* (Sansonetti and co-workers, 1983), and near *argE* (Timmis and co-workers, 1985) and *asnA* (and the lysine decarboxylase determinant: K. Gamon and T. Chakraborty, unpublished data) on the chromosome of *S. dysenteriae* 1. *E. coli* transconjugants having acquired *S. dysenteriae* 1 chromosomal markers of this region, i.e. *argG*, *ilv* and, *met* were therefore selected from a cross between *S. dysenteriae* 1 TS51 and *E. coli* K-12, and examined for production of cytotoxin. Some transconjugants having acquired *ilv* and/or *met* showed low cytotoxic activity (less than 10^2 CD$_{50}$ per ml of culture supernatant), but the distinction between weak activity and background was small and prevented further analysis. On the other hand, when the Hfr derivatives TS52 and TS59 were employed as donors, several transconjugants having acquired *gal*, *trp* or *his* loci showed high levels of cytotoxin production (greater than 10^4 CD$_{50}$ per ml of culture supernatant; Fig. 2). The gene which confers upon *E. coli* K-12 the ability to produce high levels of cytotoxin was designated *stx* (Shiga toxin). Genetical linkage of the *stx* and the *trp* loci was subsequently confirmed obvious by a further genetic cross between the Stx$^-$ *E. coli* K-12 Hfr strain KL99 and an Stx$^+$ *E. coli* K-12 transconjugant (96% co-inheritance; Fig. 2). Linkage analysis of these loci, and of the nearby marker *pyrF*, by transduction using bacteriophage P1, gave the gene order *trp-pyrF-stx* (Fig. 2); the distance between *pyrF* and *stx* was calculated to be 0.4 min (Sekizaki and colleagues, 1987).

The levels of cytotoxin produced by *E. coli* Stx$^+$ transconjugants and transductants were as high as that of the parental *S. dysenteriae* 1 strain, and these cytotoxic activities were completely neutralized by anti-Shiga toxin polyclonal and anti-SLT-I monoclonal antibodies (kindly provided by A. O'Brian).

The Stx$^+$ PyrF$^+$ *E. coli* transconjugant TS64 that was obtained in these experiments was mutagenized with transposon Tn-mini-*kan*, a kanamycin resistance derivative of transposon Tn*10* (Fig. 3). Over 10,000 independent Km-resistant transposon mutants of TS64 were pooled and used to propagate P1 phage. The phage lysate was then used to transduce the PyrF$^+$ and Km-resistance markers into the *E. coli* PyrF$^-$ Stx$^+$ strain TS70. The rationale of this strategy was that if there were *stx*::Tn-mini-*kan* mutations present in the pool of Km-resistant mutants of TS64, they should be co-transduced with PyrF$^+$ at a high frequency. Eighty-six independent PyrF$^+$ Km-resistant transductants obtained were tested for cytotoxin production and two were found to be negative. One such transductant, designated TS73, was used as a donor strain for transduction of the Km-resistance marker to Stx$^+$ *E. coli* transductants and transconjugants. All the transductants thus obtained were found to be cytotoxin negative. This means that the Tn-mini-*kan* transposon element in *E. coli* TS73 is inserted into the *stx* gene, or into neighbouring sequences essential for its expression. The mutant *stx* allele in TS73 was designated *stx-1*.

Since the mutant *stx-1* gene carries a positively-selectable Km-resistance marker, it can easily be transferred into other *E. coli* strains. Transduction of this mutant gene into *E. coli* Hfr strains KL99 and KL208 derivatives created two special *E. coli* Hfr strains, TS76 and TS77, respectively, which can donate by conjugation the mutant *stx-1* gene as an early marker to appropriate recipients (Fig. 3). A short (10 min.) interrupted mating between either TS76 or TS77 and *S. dysenteriae* 1 strains, followed by selection of Km-resistant transconjugants, resulted in substitution of the wild type *stx*$^+$ gene by the mutant allele *stx-1*. Whereas the parental *S. dysenteriae* 1 strain produced Shiga toxin at levels greater than 10^7 CD$_{50}$ per ml of culture supernatant, all Km-resistant *Shigella* transconjugants obtained from crosses with KL99 *stx-1* or KL208 *stx-1* produced no detectable cytotoxin (less than 10^2 CD$_{50}$ per ml of culture supernatant). This was repeated and confirmed with two other strains of *S. dysenteriae* 1 as recipients. The high frequencies of negative conversion of toxin production in short matings, using Hfr strains that transfer their chromosomes with opposite polarities, strongly supports the genetical location of the *stx* gene established in the *E. coli* transconjugants and transductants, and suggests that there is only one determinant for high level production of Shiga toxin in *S. dysenteriae* 1. Southern blot hybridization analysis of *stx*- and *stx-1*-containing bacteria, using as probe a DNA fragment derived from the cloned SLT-I gene (kindly provided by A. O'Brian), demonstrated that *stx* is the structural gene for Shiga toxin and that the *stx-1* mutation is located in the cistron of the A subunit of the toxin (G. Brazil, T. Sekizaki and K.N. Timmis, in preparation).

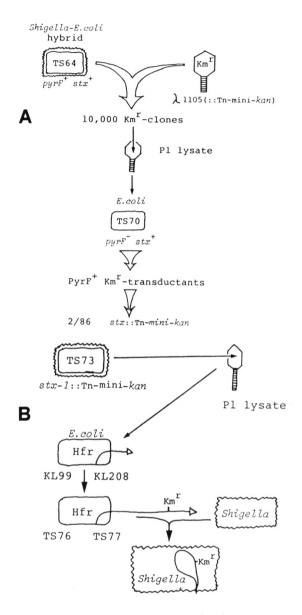

Fig. 3 Construction of stx insertion mutants of Shigella dysenteriae 1. A. The PyrF⁺ Stx⁺ E. coli K-12 derivative TS64 was mutagenized with transposon Tn-mini-kan, through infection with a lambda phage derivative carrying the transposon. 10,000 transposon mutants were pooled and a P1 lysate was prepared from a culture of this pool of mutants. The P1 lysage was then used to infect the PyrF⁻ Stx⁺ E. coli K-12 strain TS60, and PyrF⁺ kanamycin resistant transductants were selected. 86 such transductants were scored for production of Shiga toxin and 2 were identified as Stx⁻. The mutant stx allele present in one transductant, TS73, was designated stx-1. B. In order to be able to readily transfer the stx-1 allele into Shigella, the kanamycin resistance insertion mutant allele was transfered by P1 transduction from TS73 into the two Hfr derivatives KL99 and KL208 to produce TS76 and TS77, respectively. These derivatives conjugally transfer with opposite polarity the stx-1 allele as an early marker. Short matings of TS76 and TS77 with several S. dysenteriae 1 requirements resulted in the isolation of many kanamycin resistant transconjugants; all failed to produce Shiga toxin in significant amounts.

The transposon mutations in the *stx* locus described here constitute the first characterized mutations that inactivate Shiga toxin production. They will be of considerable utility in the evaluation of the role of Shiga toxin in shigellosis. Two models of bacterial virulence are frequently used to test the pathogenic potential of shigellae and enteroinvasive *E. coli* strains, namely the Serény test (induction of keratoconjunctivitis in the guinea pig) and invasiveness for tissue culture cells. Toxin-negative mutants of *S. dysenteriae* 1 strains AA17855 were fully virulent in the Serény test and invasive for HeLa cells (Sekizaki and colleagues, 1987). Moreover, recent experiments with *S. flexneri* indicate that the SLT produced by this bacterium does not play a role in the killing of invaded host cells (Sansonetti and Mounier, 1987). Therefore, a role for Shiga toxin in bacterial virulence has not been demonstrated with these models. Experiments with models that better reflect the natural infection are now required to reveal a more subtle role, if any, of the toxin in bacterial virulence.

GENETIC STUDIES ON SLT

SLT-I and SLT-II production by a number of EPEC and EHEC strains is determined by toxin converting phages, some of which have been shown to be related to bacteriophage lambda (Smith and co-workers, 1983; O'Brian and colleagues, 1984). *E. coli* K-12 can be lysogenized by these phages, and such lysogens synthesise high levels of SLT. The cloning in *E. coli* K-12 of genes determining high level production of SLT from these phages confirmed that the phages carry the structural gene of the toxin (Newland and others, 1985; Willshaw and others, 1985; Huang and others, 1986). The gene consists of two cistrons that encode the A and B subunits, organized in an operon, with the A cistron situated proximal to the operon promoter. The nucleotide sequences of two cloned SLT-I genes has been reported (Calderwood and colleagues, 1987; Jackson and colleagues, 1987). Comparison of the amino acid sequences with that of the B subunit of Shiga toxin, and DNA hybridization studies, have demonstrated a high degree of homology of SLT-I and Shiga toxin, and significant homology between STL-I and STL-II (Willshaw and colleagues, 1985; Strockbine and others., 1986; Calderwood and co-workers, 1987; O'Brian and Holmes, 1987).

VACCINE DEVELOPMENT

Shigellosis epidemics, particularly those caused by *S. dysenteriae* 1, are currently serious public health problems in some Developing Countries where hygiene and nutrition are inadequate and other infections are prevalent. The multiple drug resistance nature of current epidemic strains of *Shigella* renders difficult effective clinical management of infection with available antibiotics and contributes significantly to the high mortality of such infections. Efficacious vaccines are thus urgently required. Available evidence suggests that an efficacious vaccine will consist of an orally administered live organism that is able to colonize the intestinal mucosa and stimulate mucosal immunity to appropriate antigens. One type of organism currently being developed is an attenuated derivative of *S. dysenteriae* 1 (Mills and colleagues, 1988). In this case, however, high level production of Shiga toxin would be a potential hazard of the vaccine. The *E. coli* Hfr strains TS76 and TS77, which donate the transposon insertion mutant *stx-1* allele of Shiga toxin gene as early markers, constitute a convenient system to mutationally eliminate high level production of Shiga toxin in *S. dysenteriae* 1, and to enable construction of a safe vaccine.

ACKNOWLEDGEMENTS

We thank A. O'Brian and S. Harayama for stimulating discussions, helpful advice and important reagents, and F. Rey for expert secretarial assistance. Work carried out in the authors' laboratory was supported by grants from the Swiss National Science Foundation and the Diarrhoeal Diseases Control Programme of the World Health Organization.

REFERENCES

Calderwood, S.B., F. Auclair, A. Donohue-Rolfe, G.T. Keusch, and J.J. Mekalanos (1987). Nucleotide sequence of the Shiga-like toxin genes of *Escherichia coli*. Proc. Nat. Acad. Sci. USA 84, 4364-4368.

Cantey, J.R. (1985). Shiga toxin - an expanding role in the pathogenesis of infectious disease. J. Infect. Dis. 151, 775-782.

Cleary, T.G., J.J. Mathewson, E. Faris, and L.K. Pickering (1985). Shiga-like cytotoxin-production by enteropathogenic *Escherichia coli* serogroups. Infect. Immun. 47, 335-337.

Conradi, H. (1903). Ueber löslische, durch aseptische Autolyse, erhaltene Giftstoffe von Ruhr- und Typhusbazillen. Dtsch. Med. Wochenschr, 29, 26-28.

Gasser, C., E. Gantier, A. Steck, E. Siebenmann, and R. Oechslin, (1955). Hämolytisch-urämische Syndrome: bilaterale niereninden-nekrosen bei akuten erworbenen hämolytischen anamien. Schweiz. Med. Wochenshr. 85, 905-909.

Gemski, P., Jr. A. Takeuchi, O., Washington, and S.B. Formal (1972). Shigellosis due to *Shigella dysenteriae* 1: relative importance of mucosal invasion versus toxin production in pathogenesis. J. Infect. Dis. 126, 523-530.

Harayama, S., M. Tsuda, and T. Iino (1980). High frequency mobilization of the chromosome of *Escherichia coli* by a mutant of plasmid RP4 temperature-sensitive for maintenance. Mol. Gen. Genet. 180, 47-56.

Huang, A., S. DeGrandis, J. Friesten, M. Karmali, M. Petric, R. Congi, and J.L. Brunton (1986). Cloning and expression of the genes specifying Shiga-like toxin production in *Escherichia coli* H19. Infect. Immun. 166, 375-379.

Jackson, M.P., J.W. Newland, R.K. Holmes, and A.D. O'Brian (1987). Nucleotide sequence analysis of the structural genes for Shiga-like toxin encoded by bacteriophage 933J from *Escherichia coli*. Microbiol. Pathg. 2, 147-154.

Keenan, K.P., D.D. Sharpnack, H. Collins, S.B. Formal, and A.D. O'Brian (1986) Morphologic evaluation of the effects of Shiga toxin and *E. coli* Shiga-like toxin on the rabbit intestine. Am. J. Path. 125, 69-80.

Konowalchuk, J., N. Dickie, S. Stavric, and J.I. Speirs (1978). Comparative studies of five heat-labile toxic products of *Escherichia coli*. Infect. Immun. 22, 644-648.

Konowalchuk, J., J.I. Speirs, and S. Stavric (1977). Vero response to a cytotoxin of *Escherichia coli*. Infect. Immun. 18, 775-779.

Koster, F., J. Levin, L. Walker, K.S.K. Tung, R.H. Gilman, M.M. Rahaman, M.A. Majid, S. Islam, and Jr. R.C. Williams (1977). Hemolytic-uremic syndrome after shigellosis. Relation to endotoxemia and circulating immune complexes. N. Engl. J. Med. 298, 927-933.

Levine, M.M., H.L. Dupont, S.B. Formal, R.B. Hornick, A. Takeuchi, E.J. Gangarosa, M.J. Snyder, and J.P. Libonati (1973). Pathogenesis of *Shigella dysenteriae* 1 (Shiga) dysentery. J. Infect. Dis. 127, 261-270.

Mills, S.D., T. Sekizaki, and K.N. Timmis (1988). Analysis and manipulation of *Shigella* virulence determinants for vaccine development. In: A.A. Lindberg, E. Norrby and H. Wigzell (Eds) Nobel Symposium: The Vaccines for the Future, in press.

Moon, H.W., S.C. Whipp, R.A. Arzenio, M.M. Levine, and R.A. Gianella (1983) Attaching and effacing activities of rabbit and human enteropathogenic *Escherichia coli* in pig and rabbit intestines. Infect. Immun. 41, 1340-1351.

Newland, J.W., N.A. Strockbine, S.F. Miller, A.D. O'Brien, and R.K. Holmes (1985). Cloning of Shiga-like toxin structural genes from a toxin converting phage of *Escherichia coli*. Science 230, 179-181.

O'Brian, A.D., and R.K. Holmes (1987). Shiga and Shiga-like toxins. Microbiol. Rev. 51, 206-220.

O'Brian, A.D., G.D. LaVeck, M.R. Thompson, and S.B. Formal (1982). Production of *Shigella dysenteriae* type 1-like cytotoxin by *Escherichia coli*. J. Infect. Dis. 146, 763-769.

O'Brian, A.D., J.W. Newland, S.F. Miller, R.K. Holmes, H.W. Smith, and S.B. Formal (1984). Shiga-like toxin-converting phages from *Escherichia coli* strains that cause hemorrhagic colitis or infantile diarrhea. Science 226, 694-696.

Ogawa, H., A. Nakamura, R. Nakaya, K. Mise, S. Honjo, M. Takasaka, T. Fujiwara, and K. Imaizumi (1967). Virulence and epithelial cell invasiveness of dysentery bacilli. Jpn. J. Med. Sci. Biol. 20, 315-328.

Pai, C.H., J.K. Kelly, and G. Meyers (1986). Experimental infection of infant rabbits with Verotoxin-producing *Escherichia coli*. Infect. Immun. 51, 16-23.

Sansonetti, P.J., T.L. Hale, G.J. Dammin, C. Kapfer, Jr. H.H. Collins, and S.B. Formal (1983). Alterations in the pathogenicity of *Escherichia coli* K-12 after transfer of plasmid and chromosomal genes from *Shigella flexneri*. Infect. Immun. 39, 1392-1402.

Sansonetti, P.J., and J. Mounier (1987). Metabolic events mediating killing of host cells by *Shigella flexneri*. Microb. Pathogen. 3, 53-61.

Scotland, S.M., N.P. Day, and B. Rowe (1980). Production of a cytotoxin affecting Vero cells by strains of *Escherichia coli* belonging to traditional enteropathogenic serogroups. FEMS Microbiol. Lett. 7, 15-17.

Scotland, S.M., H.R. Smith, and B. Rowe (1985) Two distinct toxins active on Vero cells from *Escherichia coli* 0157. Lancet ii, 885-886.

Sekizaki, T., S. Harayama, G.M. Brazil, and K.N. Timmis (1987). Genetic manipulation *in vivo* of *stx*, a determinant essential for high level production of Shiga toxin by *Shigella dysenteriae* serotype 1: localization near *pyrF* and generation of Stx⁻ transposon mutants. Infect. Immun., in press.

Smith, W.H., P. Green, and Z. Parsell (1983). Vero cell toxins in *Escherichia coli* and related bacteria: transfer by phage and conjugation and toxic action in laboratory animals, chickens and pigs. J. Gen. Microbiol. 129, 3121-3137.

Strockbine, N.A., L.R.M. Marques, J.W. Newland, H.W. Smith, R.K. Holmes, and A.D. O'Brien (1986). Two toxin-converting phages from *Escherichia coli* 0157:H7 strain 933 encode antigenically distinct toxins with similar biological activities. Infect. Immun. 53, 135-140.

Timmis, K.N., C.L. Clayton, and T. Sekizaki (1985). Localization of Shiga toxin gene in region of *Shigella dysenteriae* 1 chromosome specifying virulence functions. FEMS Microbiol. Lett. 30, 301-305.

Timmis, K.N., S. Sturm, and H. Watanabe (1985). Genetic dissection of pathogenesis determinants of *Shigella* and enteroinvasive *Escherichia coli*. In: J. Holmgren, A. Lindberg, and R. Möllby, R. (Eds). Development of Vaccines and Drugs against Diarrhea. 11th Nobel Conference, Stockholm, pp. 107-126.

Watanabe, H., and K.N. Timmis (1984). A small plasmid in *Shigella dysenteriae* 1 specifies one or more functions essential for O antigen production and bacterial virulence. Infect. Immun. 43, 391-396.

Willshaw, G.A., H.R. Smith, S.M. Scotland, and B. Rowe, (1985). Cloning of genes determining the production of Vero cytotoxin by *Escherichia coli*. J. Gen. Microbiol. 131, 3047-3053.

Fehrenbach et al. (Eds.), Bacterial Protein Toxins, Zbl. Bakt. Suppl. 17
© Gustav Fischer, Stuttgart, New York, 1988

Genetic and Biochemical Studies of Type II Heat-Labile Enterotoxins of Escherichia Coli

R. K. Holmes, C. L. Pickett and E. M. Twiddy
Uniformed Services University of the Health Sciences, 4301 Jones Bridge Road, Bethesda, Maryland 20814-4799, U.S.A.

ABSTRACT

Heat-labile enterotoxins of Vibrio cholerae and Escherichia coli are related proteins with similar mechanisms of action that belong to two distinct serogroups. Cholera toxin (CT) and type I E. coli heat-labile enterotoxins (LTh-I and LTp-I) are members of serogroup I, whereas E. coli type II heat-labile toxins (LT-IIa and LT-IIb) belong to serogroup II. The structural genes for LT-IIa were cloned and sequenced, and prototype LT-IIa and LT-IIb toxins were purified and characterized. The genetic and biochemical characteristics of type II enterotoxins are summarized and compared with those of type I enterotoxins.

KEYWORDS

Escherichia coli, heat-labile enterotoxin, Vibrio cholerae, cholera toxin, ganglioside, receptor, adenylate cyclase, ADP ribosylation, immunochemistry.

INTRODUCTION

In recent years extraordinary progress has been made in defining the mechanisms of pathogenesis of bacterial diarrheal diseases (Levine and colleagues, 1983; Levine, 1987). The classic example of enterotoxin-mediated diarrheal disease is asiatic cholera, caused by intestinal infection with the toxinogenic but noninvasive bacterium Vibrio cholerae. Cholera toxin (CT) secreted by V. cholerae binds to ganglioside GM1 receptors on mucosal cells of the small intestine, ADP-ribosylates the G_s regulatory component of adenylate cyclase in the plasma membrane, stimulates adenylate cyclase activity, and causes secretion of fluid and electrolytes into the intestinal lumen.

Escherichia coli that cause diarrheal diseases in humans or animals are currently classified as enterotoxigenic, enteropathogenic, enteroinvasive, enterohemorrhagic, and enteroadherent, based on their mechanisms of pathogenesis (Levine, 1987). Enterotoxigenic E. coli (ETEC) are frequently associated with traveler's diarrhea and with infant diarrhea in developing countries. By definition ETEC produce heat-labile enterotoxin (LT), heat-stable enterotoxin

(ST), or both. Shiga-like toxin (SLT) (O'Brien and Holmes, 1987) is an enterotoxin that also has lethal and cytotoxic activities, and production of high levels of Shiga-like toxin is particularly associated with enterohemorrhagic E. coli (EHEC). Heat-labile enterotoxin of E. coli is the subject of the current paper.

The extensive literature about LT and CT is reviewed elsewhere (Betley, Miller, and Mekalanos, 1986; Eidels, Proia, and Hart, 1983; Finkelstein and colleagues, 1987; Levine and colleagues, 1983; Middlebrook and Dorland, 1984; Yamamoto, Gojobori, and Yokota, 1987; Yamamoto and colleagues, 1984). LT and CT have been purified to homogeneity and characterized, and their structural genes have been cloned and sequenced from representative strains of E. coli and V. cholerae. These studies established that LT and CT belong to the same family of molecules. They are composed of homologous polypeptide subunits, have common as well as unique antigenic determinants, bind to ganglioside GM1 as a receptor on plasma membranes, catalyze ADP-ribosylation of the G_s regulatory subunit of adenylate cyclase in target cells, and are encoded by homologous structural genes. ETEC isolates from humans and pigs were shown to produce antigenic variants of LT, designated LTh and LTp, respectively, but both were neutralized by polyclonal reference antisera against CT.

Recent studies in our laboratory have characterized a new serogroup of LT, designated type II heat-labile enterotoxin (LT-II). LT-II is not neutralized by antisera against CT or classical LT (LT-I), and antisera against LT-II do not neutralize CT or LT-I. The major purpose of this paper is to summarize current knowledge about LT-II and compare its properties with LT-I.

DISCOVERY OF LT-II

Among a collection of ETEC strains isolated in Thailand, Moseley and colleagues (1982) identified several strains from animals that caused rounding of Y1 adrenal cells but failed to be neutralized by antiserum against CT or to react in colony hybridization tests with an LT gene probe. They concluded that these strains produced a cytotoxin rather than LT. These atypical strains were also sent to our laboratory by Dr. Peter Echeverria, and strain SA53 from a water buffalo was chosen as the prototype for our studies.

E. coli SA53 produced cell-associated, heat-labile toxin that caused cultured Y1 adrenal cells to become rounded, induced increased vascular permeability in rabbit skin after intracutaneous injection, but was not neutralized by hyperimmune antisera prepared against purified CT, LTh or LTp (Green and colleagues, 1983; Guerrant and colleagues, 1985; Holmes and colleagues, 1986a and 1986b; Holmes, Twiddy, and Neill, 1985). Partial purification of the toxin by 870 to 940 fold was achieved in several experiments, but the material was heterogeneous and toxicity did not correspond with any of the major proteins. The partially purified toxin caused rounding of Y1 adrenal cells at a dose of about 25 ng, activated adenylate cyclase in Y1 cells, showed no evidence of cytotoxicity, did not bind to agarose, was not inactivated by ganglioside GM1, and had a lower isoelectric point (pI 6.5-6.8) than that of LTp (pI 7.4) or LTh (pI 8.0). Recognizing both the similarities of its toxic activities and the differences in its chemical properties when compared with LTp and LTh, the toxin was provisionally called LT-like toxin.

In an independent study initiated in Sao Paulo, Brazil, E. coli strains isolated from food were classified as ETEC based on toxicity tests (Franco, Guth and Trabulsi, 1985). Four such strains from food and two from patients, representing five different E. coli serotypes, were later found to be atypical because their toxicity was not neutralized by anti-CT and they gave negative responses in several immunologic tests for LT. After a reference antiserum against LT-II and a DNA probe for LT-II were developed (Pickett and colleagues, 1986), it became possible to demonstrate that the toxins produced by these strains belonged to the LT-II serogroup (Guth and colleagues, 1986a). E. coli strain 41 from Sao Paulo was subsequently shown to produce an LT-II that was antigenically cross-reacting but not identical with the LT-II from E. coli SA53 (Guth and colleagues, 1986b). The LT-II encoded by SA53 is now called LT-IIa, and the LT-II encoded by strain 41 is now called LT-IIb.

GENETIC STUDIES OF LT-II

Because synthesis of LT-I in E. coli is plasmid-determined, our initial studies focussed on plasmids in strain SA53 as possible carriers of the genetic determinants for production of LT-IIa (Green and colleagues, 1983). Two plasmids of 69.2 and 57.6 megadaltons were demonstrated in SA53. The larger plasmid hybridized in Southern blots with a DNA probe for LT-I structural genes, but strain SA53 did not produce either immunoreactive or biologically active LT-I. Furthermore, production of LT-IIa by derivatives of SA53 from which both plasmids had been eliminated occurred at the same level as for wild type SA53, and absence of plasmid DNA from the cured strains was confirmed in control experiments by Southern blots using radiolabeled plasmid DNAs as the probes. We concluded, therefore, that the genetic determinants for LT-IIa were not on plasmids and were most likely chromosomal. The possibility that LT-IIa genes could be part of a transposable element or a prophage was not excluded.

The structural genes for LT-IIa were cloned from a substrain of E. coli SA53 into various cosmid or plasmid vectors and expressed either in E. coli HB101 or in the minicell producing strain P678-54 (Pickett and colleagues, 1986). Initially, the bacterial DNA was partially digested with Sau3a, and large fragments were cloned into the BamHI site of the cosmid vector pHC79. The LT-IIa genes were subsequently subcloned into the temperature sensitive, runaway replication vector pMOB45 to construct strain HB101(pCP3837) which made several hundred times more toxin than the ancestral strain SA53. Smaller sub-clones in pBR322 vectors were also constructed and analyzed to map more precisely the physical location of the toxin genes and to identify the polypeptides synthesized in minicells that represented components of the toxin. By these methods the determinants for LT-IIa were shown to be located within a single 1.7 kilobase pair EcoRI-PstI fragment of DNA from SA53, and the subunits of LT-IIa were identified as polypeptides of approximately 11.8 and 28 kilodaltons. In Southern hybridizations radiolabeled DNA probes for LT-I and LT-IIa hybridized with samples of DNA from strains that made the corresponding toxin but failed to hybridize with DNAs coding for the heterologous toxin. These hybridizations were performed under conditions of low stringency and established that the genes for LT-I and LT-IIa were not highly homologous.

The organization of the LT-IIa operon was examined by constructing λplacMu operon fusions, and the nucleotide sequence of the LT-IIa structural genes was determined by dideoxy chain termination methods using appropriate subclones and synthetic oligonucleotide primers (Pickett, Weinstein, and Holmes, 1987). The results indicated that transcription originates from a promoter located adjacent to the toxin structural genes and proceeds first through the A gene and then through the B gene. Similarities between the operons for LT-I (Dallas, Gill, and

Falkow, 1979; Yamamoto and colleagues, 1984) and LT-IIa included a single promoter for transcription of the A and B genes, a probable Shine-Delgarno sequence adjacent to each of the structural genes, and a short overlap between the end of the A gene and the beginning of the B gene (4 nucleotides for LT-I and 11 nucleotides for LT-IIa) such that the A and B genes are translated from the polycistronic mRNA in different reading frames. The sequence coding for the A subunit of LT-IIa was 57% homologous with the sequence for the A subunit of LTh-I and 55% homologous with the sequence for the A subunit of CT. The nucleotide sequences coding for the A1 regions of LT-IIa and LTh-I were more highly homologous (62%), and the sequences coding for the A2 regions were significantly less homologous (36%). There was no significant homology between the B subunit gene of LT-IIa and the B subunit gene of LTh-I or CT. Translation of the coding sequences indicated that the A and B subunits of LT-IIa are most likely synthesized as precursors with hydrophobic leader sequences of 18 and 19 amino acid residues, respectively. The leader sequences are presumed to be removed by proteolysis during secretion from the cytoplasm to the periplasmic space, where assembly of the holotoxin is presumed to occur in a manner similar to that described for LT-I. The predicted sizes of the mature polypeptides were 241 amino acid residues (27,172 daltons) for the A polypeptide of LT-IIa and 104 amino acid residues (11,413 daltons) for the B polypeptide of LT-IIa.

Comparative molecular studies of the LT-II gene family will require, at a minimum, analysis of the nucleotide sequence of the LT-IIb genes. Toward this end the structural genes for LT-IIb were cloned from E. coli strain 41, and subcloning and nucleotide sequence analysis of the LT-IIb genes is in progress (Pickett and Holmes, unpublished data).

BIOCHEMICAL STUDIES OF LT-II

As noted above, our initial efforts to purify LT-IIa from sonic extracts of E. coli strain SA53 by traditional biochemical methods achieved purifications of about 870 to 940 fold. By modifying the methods and introducing additional procedures we improved the purification of toxin from SA53 to 12,300 fold (Holmes, Twiddy, and Pickett, 1986), but such preparations remained too impure to permit direct identification and characterization of the subunit structure of the toxin. At approximately the same time, however, we had constructed the genetically engineered, hypertoxinogenic E. coli strain HB101(pCP3837) described above. By combining the use of strain HB101(pCP3837) for toxin production with the improved purification procedures, it was possible to obtain small amounts of LT-IIa purified to homogeneity (Holmes, Twiddy, and Pickett, 1986).

The dose of the pure LT-IIa needed to induce rounding of Y1 adrenal cells in the microtiter assay was only 0.5 picograms, making LT-IIa approximately 25 to 50 times more potent on a weight basis in that assay system than either CT or LT-I (Holmes, Twiddy, and Pickett, 1986). The dose response curves for induction of cAMP accumulation in Y1 adrenal cell cultures confirmed that the potency of LT-IIa was greater than LT-I. In contrast, the purified LT-IIa did not induce secretory responses in ligated ileal segments of adult rabbits at doses sufficient to produce strongly positive responses with CT controls. This was in contrast to the weak but positive secretory responses that had been seen in ligated ileal segments inoculated either with LT-IIa producing bacteria or with relatively impure preparations of LT-IIa. Because of the small amounts of purified LT-IIa available for study, it has not yet been established if the lack of response in rabbit ileal segments challenged with highly purified LT-IIa reflected either a difference in species or tissue specificity between LT-IIa and the type I heat-labile enterotoxins or a difference in their possible importance as virulence factors in the gut.

The purified LT-IIa toxin was radioiodinated and analyzed by SDS-PAGE and autoradiography (Holmes, Twiddy, and Pickett, 1986). These studies confirmed the results of the minicell experiments described above and demonstrated that the toxin was composed of A and B polypeptides. The predicted molecular weights of the processed polypeptides reported above are consistent with the mobilities that were observed. The purified toxin was almost completely in the unnicked form, but treatment with trypsin and reduction of intrachain disulfide bonds converted the A polypeptide into fragments designated A1 (Mr about 21,000) and A2 (Mr about 7,000) in a manner analogous to trypsin treatment of LTh-I or LTp-I. The stoichiometry of the A and B polypeptides in LT-IIa holotoxin has not yet been determined by direct methods; however, if the ratio is 1 A and 5 B polypeptides (as established for CT and LT-I), then the predicted molecular weight of LT-IIa holotoxin based on the nucleotide sequence data presented above is 84,237 daltons.

Highly specific rabbit polyclonal antiserum was also prepared against purified LT-IIa (Pickett and colleagues, 1986), and the reciprocal failure of cross-neutralization of toxins in serogroups I and II by heterologous anti-LT-I or anti-LT-II antisera was confirmed with the pure toxins (Holmes, Twiddy, and Pickett, 1986). Finally, analysis of inhibition of toxicity by crude and purified gangliosides demonstrated that LT-IIa was much less susceptible to inhibition by GM1 and much more susceptible to inhibition by mixed gangliosides than was LT-I or CT, suggesting that the receptor for LT-IIa might be different than that for LT-I or CT (Holmes, Twiddy, and Pickett, 1986).

The LT-IIb toxin from E. coli strain 41 was obtained in highly purified form and characterized by Guth and colleagues (1986b). The mobilities of the polypeptide subunits and the cleavage of the A polypeptide into A1 and A2 fragments when LT-IIb was treated with trypsin were very similar to those observed previously for LT-IIa. The purified LT-IIb differed significantly from LT-IIa, however, in that it had a significantly lower isoelectric point (pI 5.2-5.6 vs. 6.8), was activated by treatment with trypsin (minimal dose of LT-IIb to induce rounding of Y1 cells decreased from 94 picograms before trypsin treatment to 3 picograms after treatment), formed a line of partial identity with LT-IIa in Ouchterlony type immunodiffusion tests with antiserum prepared against LT-IIa, and was much more resistant than LT-IIa to inhibition by ganglioside GM1 or mixed gangliosides. Solid phase radioimmunoassays confirmed that LT-IIa and LT-IIb were antigenically cross-reacting but not identical molecules and also demonstrated the existence of shared epitopes between enterotoxins in serogroups I and II. Experiments are in progress (Holmes and Twiddy, unpublished data) to isolate and characterize monoclonal antibodies against purified LT-IIa toxin and to construct strains that will produce larger amounts of LT-IIa or LT-IIb (Pickett, Perera, and Holmes, unpublished data). The availability of such monoclonal antibodies and the ability to prepare purified LT-IIa and LT-IIb in larger quantities will facilitate further biochemical studies of these toxins.

The activation of adenylate cyclase and the ADP-ribosyl transferase activity of LT-IIa was studied in more detail in human fibroblasts by Chang and colleagues (1987). Activation of adenylate cyclase in fibroblast membranes was enhanced by NAD, GTP, dithiothreitol, and by pretreatment of the toxin with trypsin. The proteins in fibroblast membranes that were ADP ribosylated by CT or LT-IIa were similar, and ADP-ribosylation of the G_s proteins by LT-IIa or CT was significantly decreased when membranes were prepared from cells pretreated with either toxin. These studies indicated that LT-IIa, like CT, increased adenylate cyclase activity of membranes, apparently by ADP ribosylating the G_s regulatory component of adenylate cyclase.

Finally, Fukuta and colleagues (1987) examined the carbohydrate-binding
specificities of CT, LTh-I, LT-IIa and LT-IIb by immunostaining thin layer
chromatograms of crude or purified gangliosides and by solid phase
radioimmunoassays with purified gangliosides. Each of the four toxins had a
different binding specificity. CT and LTh-I both bound strongly to GM1 and less
strongly to GD1b, but LTh-I also bound weakly to GM2 and to asialo GM1. The rank
order of gangliosides to which LT-IIa bound, starting with the strongest binding,
was GD1b, GD1a, GT1b, GQ1b, GM1, GD2, GM2 and GM3. LT-IIb bound to a subset of
the gangliosides to which LT-IIb bound. In decreasing rank order of binding
strength, LT-IIb bound GD1a, GT1b and GM3. Lack of binding of LT-IIb to GM1
explained the observation that binding of LT-IIb to mixed gangliosides was
inhibited by pretreating them with neuraminidase. Based on these observations,
the probable binding site for CT and LTh-I is the terminal sugar sequence
Galβ1-3GalNAcβ1-4(NeuAcα2-3)Gal... . LT-IIa binds to this same sugar sequence,
but the presence of a second N-acetylneuraminic acid as in GD1b and GD2
stimulates binding instead of preventing it, and attachment to the terminal
galactose of N-acetylneuraminic acid as in GD1a, GT1b, and GQ1b does not block
binding. Finally, LT-IIb probably recognizes the terminal sugar sequence
NeuAcα2-3Galβ1-4GalNAc... ; it binds to GD1a and GT1b but does not bind to GM1.

DISCUSSION

The studies summarized here demonstrate that the family of heat-labile enterotoxins of E. coli can be separated into two major groups, designated LT-I and
LT-II, which are antigenically distinct in neutralization tests. Each group
contains antigenic variants, i.e. LTh-I and LTp-I in serogroup I and LT-IIa
and LT-IIb in serogroup II. The ability to catalyze ADP ribosylation of G_s
and activate adenylate cyclase is a conserved function of the A subunits of the
toxins in both serogroups, although this activity has not yet been demonstrated
directly for LT-IIb. The B subunits of these toxins have receptor binding
activity, but the specificity for binding to particular sugar sequences of
gangliosides differs between serogroup I and serogroup II as well as between the
LT-IIa and LT-IIb toxins of serogroup II. Analysis of nucleotide sequences
demonstrated significant homology of the LTIIa A gene with the A genes of CT
and LTh-I but no significant homology of the B gene of LT-IIa with the B genes
of CT and LTh-I.

Yamamoto, Gojobori, and Yokota (1987) recently analyzed available data concerning
the evolution of the LT-I and CT structural genes. Based on analysis of
nucleotide substitutions between the CT and LT-I structural genes and comparison
of bacterial 5S rRNAs, they concluded that E. coli and V. cholerae diverged from
a common ancestor much longer ago (about 670 million years) than the divergence
of CT and LT-I genes from a common ancestor (about 130 million years ago). In
contrast, the divergence of LTh-I and LTp-I genes was estimated to have occurred
recently (about 0.9 million years ago). Considering the low G-C content of the
LT-I genes, their low frequency of usage of optimal codons for E. coli, and their
estimated evolutionary time of divergence from the CT genes, these authors
postulated that LT-I genes were introduced into E. coli as foreign genes after
E. coli and V. cholerae diverged.

Our analysis of the nucleotide sequence of LT-IIa indicated that gene families
corresponding to serogroups I and II of the heat-labile enterotoxins diverged
from a common ancestor before the divergence of CT from LT-I (Pickett,
Weinstein, and Holmes, 1987). In the case of LT-IIa, the G-C content of the A
and B genes was 40% and 39%, respectively, and their frequency of usage of
optimal codons for E. coli was .39 and .54, respectively. These numbers suggest

that LT-IIa genes may also have been introduced into E. coli as foreign genes from another source. It seems likely that the B gene of LT-IIa has evolved toward a more favorable codon usage for E. coli than has the A gene of LT-IIa.

Our studies of serogroup II enterotoxins have revealed that the cholera/E. coli family is more ancient in evolutionary terms and more diverse than previously recognized. Additional studies will be required to determine the prevalence of the various genes that belong to the cholera/E. coli enterotoxin family among bacteria of various genera isolated from different biological sources and geographic areas. It is clear that individual members of the heat-labile enterotoxin family have very different binding carbohydrate binding specificities, but the importance of these differences as possible determinants of cell or tissue tropisms, species specificities, or pathogenic potential of the individual toxins is just beginning to be studied.

ACKNOWLEDGMENTS

The studies reported here were supported in part by research grant 5 R22 AI14107 from the National Institutes of Health. We thank Barbara Holmlund for secretarial assistance. The opinions or assertions contained herein are the private ones of the authors and are not to be construed as reflecting the views of the Department of Defense or the Uniformed Services University of the Health Sciences. The experiments reported herein were conducted according to the principles set forth in the Guide for the Care and Use of Laboratory Animals, Institute of Laboratory Animal Resources, National Research Council, DHEW Pub. No. (NIH) 78-23.

REFERENCES

Betley, M.J., V.L. Miller, and J.J. Mekalanos (1986). Genetics of bacterial enterotoxins. Annu. Rev. Microbiol., 40, 577-605.
Chang, P.P., J. Moss, E.M. Twiddy, and R.K. Holmes (1987). Type II heat-labile enterotoxin of Escherichia coli activates adenylate cyclase in human fibroblasts by ADP ribosylation. Infect. Immun., in press.
Dallas, W.S., D.M. Gill, and S. Falkow (1979). Cistrons encoding Escherichia coli heat-labile toxin. J. Bacteriol., 139, 850-858.
Eidels, L., R.L. Proia, and D.A. Hart (1983). Membrane receptors for bacterial toxins. Microbiol. Revs., 47, 596-620.
Finkelstein, R.A., M.F. Burks, A. Zupan, W.S. Dallas, C.O. Jacob, and D.S. Ludwig (1987). Epitopes of the cholera family of enterotoxins. Revs. Infect. Dis., 9, 544-561.
Franco, B.D.G.M., B.E.C. Guth, and L.R. Trabulsi (1985). Isolamento e caracteristicas de cepas de Escherichia coli enteropatogenica isoladas de alimentos. Rev. Microbiol. (Sao Paulo), 16, 49-55.
Fukuta, S., J.L. Magnani, E.M. Twiddy, R.K. Holmes, and V. Ginsburg (1987). Enterotoxins of the Vibrio cholerae/Escherichia coli family: comparison of the carbohydrate-binding specificities of cholera toxin and E. coli toxins LTh-I, LT-IIa, and LT-IIb. Submitted for publication.
Green, B.A., R.J. Neill, W.T. Ruyechan, and R.K. Holmes (1983). Evidence that a new enterotoxin of Escherichia coli which activates adenylate cyclase in eucaryotic target cells is not plasmid mediated. Infect. Immun., 41, 383-390.
Guerrant, R.L., R.K. Holmes, D.C. Robertson, and R.N. Greenberg (1985). Roles of enterotoxins in the pathogenesis of Escherichia coli diarrhea. In: L. Leive (Ed.), Microbiology-1985, American Society for Microbiology, Washington, D.C., pp. 68-73.

Guth, B.E.C., C.L. Pickett, E.M. Twiddy, R.K. Holmes, T.A.T. Gomes, A.A.M. Lima, R.L. Guerrant, B.D.G.M. Franco, and L. Trabulsi (1986a). Production of type II heat-labile enterotoxin by Escherichia coli isolated from food and human feces. Infect. Immun., 54, 587-589.

Guth, B.E.C., E.M. Twiddy, L.R. Trabulsi, and R.K. Holmes (1986b). Variation in chemical properties and antigenic determinants among type II heat-labile enterotoxins of Escherichia coli. Infect. Immun., 54, 529-536.

Holmes, R.K., B.A. Green, E.M. Twiddy, R.J. Neill, and W.T. Ruyechan (1986a). Genetic and biochemical studies of a new heat-labile enterotoxin of Escherichia coli that activates adenylate cyclase. In: S. Kuwahara and N.F. Pierce (Eds.), Advances in Research on Cholera and Related Diarrheas, Vol.3, KTK Scientific Publishers, Tokyo, pp. 221-226.

Holmes, R.K., C.L. Pickett, B.W. Belisle, E.M. Twiddy, J.W. Newland, N.A. Strockbine, S.F. Miller, and A.D. O'Brien (1986b). Genetics of toxinogenesis in Escherichia coli relating to vaccine development. In: J. Holmgren, A. Lindberg and R. Mollby (Eds.), Development of Drugs against Diarrhea, 11th Nobel Conference, Stockholm 1985, Studentlitteratur, Lund, Sweden, pp. 68-73.

Holmes, R.K., E.M. Twiddy, and R.J. Neill (1985). Recent advances in the study of heat-labile enterotoxins of Escherichia coli. In: Y. Takeda and T. Miwatani (Eds.), Bacterial Diarrheal Diseases, Martinus Nijhoff Publishers, Boston, pp. 125-135.

Holmes, R.K., E.M. Twiddy, and C.L. Pickett (1986). Purification and characterization of type II heat-labile enterotoxin of Escherichia coli. Infect. Immun., 53, 464-473.

Levine, M.M. (1987). Escherichia coli that cause diarrhea: enterotoxigenic, enteropathogenic, enteroinvasive, enterohemorrhagic, and enteroadherent. J. Infect. Dis., 155, 377-389.

Levine, M.M., J.B. Kaper, R.E. Black, and M.L. Clements (1983). New knowledge on pathogenesis of bacterial enteric infections as applied to vaccine development. Microbiol. Revs., 47, 510-550.

Middlebrook, J.L., and R.B. Dorland (1984). Bacterial toxins: cellular mechanisms of action. Microbiol. Revs., 48, 199-221.

Moseley, S.L., P. Echeverria, J. Seriwatana, C. Tirapat, W. Chaicumpa, T. Sakuldaipeara, and S. Falkow (1982). Identification of enterotoxigenic Escherichia coli by colony hybridization using three enterotoxin gene probes. J. Infect. Dis., 145, 863-869.

O'Brien, A.D., and R.K. Holmes (1987). Shiga and Shiga-like toxins. Microbiol. Revs., 51, 206-220.

Pickett, C.L., E.M. Twiddy, B.W. Belisle, and R.K. Holmes (1986). Cloning of genes that encode a new heat-labile enterotoxin of Escherichia coli. J. Bacteriol., 165, 348-352.

Pickett, C.L., D.L. Weinstein, and R.K. Holmes (1987). Genetics of type IIa heat-labile enterotoxin of Escherichia coli: operon fusions, nucleotide sequence, and hybridization studies. Submitted for publication.

Yamamoto, T., T. Gojobori, and T. Yokota (1987). Evolutionary origin of pathogenic determinants in enterotoxigenic Escherichia coli and Vibrio cholerae. J. Bacteriol., 169, 1352-1357.

Yamamoto, T., T. Nakazawa, T. Miyata, A. Kaji, and T. Yokota (1984). Evolution and structure of two ADP-ribosylation enterotoxins, Escherichia coli heat-labile toxin and cholera toxin. FEBS Letters, 169, 241-246.

Fehrenbach et al. (Eds.), Bacterial Protein Toxins, Zbl. Bakt. Suppl. 17
© Gustav Fischer, Stuttgart, New York, 1988

Regulation of Virulence in Bordetella Pertussis

S. Stibitz[1], A. A. Weiss[2] and S. Falkow[3]

[1]Office of Biologics Research and Review, Food and Drug Administration, 8800 Rockville Pike, Bethesda, MD 20892, U.S.A.
[2]Department of Microbiology and Immunology, Box 678, Medical College of Virginia, Richmond, VA 23298, U.S.A.
[3]Department of Medical Microbiology, Stanford University, Stanford, CA 94305, U.S.A.

ABSTRACT

A region of the *Bordetella pertussis* chromosome containing the sites of Tn5-insertions having Vir⁻ or FHA-deficient phenotypes has been cloned. This plasmid directs the synthesis of FHA-cross-reactive material in *E. coli*. Tn5-mutagenesis defined four regions involved in the synthesis and/or export of this product. These are the FHA structural gene, two loci affecting the synthesis and/or export of the FHA product, and the *vir* locus. Further results show that the *vir* locus, in *trans*, can restore the virulent-phase phenotype to avirulent-phase strains, and that the *vir* locus contains the site involved in phase-variation in *B. pertussis*.

KEYWORDS

Regulation of virulence, *Bordetella pertussis*, virulence factors, coordinate regulation, filamentous hemagglutinin, FHA, DNA-cloning, Tn5-mutagenesis, *vir* locus, phase-variation.

INTRODUCTION

Bordetella pertussis, the causative agent of whooping cough is a highly successful pathogen of humans. Its success is evident when one examines the ability of this bacterium to be passed to an uninfected individual upon exposure to an infected individual. This attack rate has repeatedly been assessed at greater than 80% for unvaccinated household contacts (Broome and co-workers, 1981; Isomura, Suzuki, and Sato, 1985; Mertsola and co-workers, 1983). A number of molecular entities are produced by this organism which may be important in its ability to colonize the human host and to subsequently cause disease. Candidates for adherence factors include the filamentous hemagglutinin (FHA) (Urisu, Cowell, and Manclark, 1986), and pili. A number of toxins are also elaborated. Tracheal cytotoxin, a small molecule, causes paralysis of cilia in the mucociliary elevator of the respiratory tract and sloughing of the ciliated cells (Goldman, Klapper, and Baseman, 1982). Pertussis toxin has profound physiological effects on the host, among them the paralysis of phagocytic cells (Becker and co-workers, 1985; Meade and co-workers, 1984). Another toxin, the extracytoplasmic adenylate cyclase, has similar activity (Confer and Eaton, 1982; Friedman and co-workers, 1987).

B. pertussis reveals its sophistication not only in the diversity and range of its attack on host defenses, but by the fact that most of these virulence factors are coordinately regulated. This regulation takes two forms. In one, under certain environmental conditions, the synthesis of FHA, pertussis toxin, extracytoplasmic adenylate cyclase, hemolysin, and other factors is repressed. Such conditions include reduced temperature or increased concentration of Mg^{++} ions or nicotinic acid, and repression is reversible upon reversal of the culture conditions (Lacey, 1960; McPheat, Wardlaw, and Novotny, 1983). Another form of regulation, sometimes described as phase-variation, refers to the ability of the organism to spontaneously "switch off" the synthesis of the aforementioned factors. Such a change is stable upon passage of the organism, and we refer to such a derivative as being in the "avirulent phase". The ability to make the virulence determinants can be spontaneously regained by "switching on" thus reverting to the "virulent phase" (Weiss and Falkow, 1984). Interestingly, a class of Tn5-insertion mutations in *B. pertussis* mimic this phase-variation and define a genetic locus *vir*. Mutations in *vir* result in the loss of the ability to synthesize multiple virulence-associated determinants including FHA, pertussis toxin, adenylate cyclase, and hemolysin (Weiss and co-workers, 1983; Weiss and Falkow, 1984). The work we report here represents the first steps in our efforts to understand the molecular nature of the *vir* locus and its role in regulation of virulence in *B. pertussis*.

RESULTS AND DISCUSSION

Figure 1 shows a physical map of the plasmid pUW21-26. This plasmid contains a segment of the *B. pertussis* chromosome inserted into the cosmid cloning vector pHC79. This plasmid was selected from a gene bank by virtue of its hybridization to DNA probes from sequences surrounding the sites of Tn5-insertion mutations which were Vir⁻ or FHA-deficient. The sequences used for probes are shown in Fig. 1 above the restriction map of pUW21-26 and in relationship to the sites of four Tn5-insertions in the *B. pertussis* chromosome encompassed by this clone. pUW21-26, in *E. coli* HB101, directs the synthesis of a product immunologically cross-reactive with FHA. This product is detected on nitrocellulose filters upon which the HB101[pUW21-26] have been grown and then washed off. As this assay does not involve lysis of the bacterial cells, it is most likely detecting a secreted protein. When the *E. coli* are grown under conditions which cause phenotypic repression in *B. pertussis*, i.e. reduced temperature (26°), 0.625 mg/ml nicotinic acid, or 5.0 mg/ml $MgCl_2$, the FHA product is not detected (Stibitz, Weiss, and Falkow). As normal responses to environmental signals have been maintained in this system, we have used it to begin to define the genetic and molecular elements of the *B. pertussis* regulatory system in *E. coli*.

Below the restriction map of pUW21-26 in Fig. 1 are shown the sites of a number of Tn5-insertions which were isolated in this cosmid in *E. coli*. Those which affect the ability of the plasmid to direct the synthesis of a detectable FHA-cross-reactive product in *E. coli* are indicated by brackets. Such insertions fall into four groups which correspond to the loci we have termed *fhaA*, *fhaB*, *fhaC*, and *vir* as shown. These loci will be discussed in turn.

The position and extent of the *fhaA* locus is defined by a group of Tn5-insertions in pUW21-26 which all have the phenotype of apparent overproduction of FHA-cross-reactive material in *E. coli*. This region also contains the sites of insertion of the original Tn5-insertions which resulted in an FHA-deficient phenotype in the *B. pertussis* strains BP353 and BP354 (Weiss and co-workers, 1983). Other workers and ourselves have observed that these *B. pertussis* strains make much reduced amounts of apparently normal FHA (Brown and Parker, 1987; Urisu, Cowell, and Manclark, 1986). We therefore suggest that *fhaA* encodes a factor necessary for the proper expression and/or export of FHA in *B. pertussis* but is not a structural gene for FHA. *E. coli* may encode its own analog of *fhaA* and the introduction of *fhaA* might actually interfere with its functioning. Such a hypothesis could explain the dispensability of *fhaA* for FHA expression in *E. coli* as well as the increase in detection of FHA when *fhaA* is inactivated by insertion.

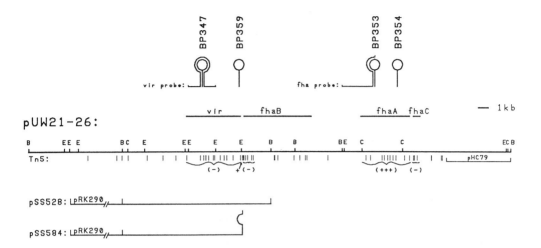

Fig. 1: Composite map of the *fha-vir* region. A restriction map of the cosmid pUW21-26 is shown. Symbols for restriction enzymes are B, *Bam*HI; C, *Cla*I; and E, *Eco*RI. Sites of insertion of Tn5 in the *B. pertussis* chromosome are shown for the strains BP347, BP353, BP354, and BP359. DNA sequences used as probes to isolate pUW21-26 are shown as well. Sites of Tn5-insertions isolated in the cosmid in *E. coli* are depicted by short vertical lines below the map. These insertions result in a normal (+) phenotype unless otherwise indicated by inclusion in brackets. Other plasmids derived from pUW21-26 are shown in register with the sequences they contain.

We believe the locus we have called *fhaB* is the structural gene for a major FHA protein. FHA has not been well defined biochemically and is usually observed as a number of polypeptides of varying size (Irons, Ashworth, and Wilton-Smith, 1983). The largest product seen in SDS polyacrylamide gels is about 200 kDa in size. It has not been clear however if this large product is the result of polymerization of smaller subunits or if the smaller products seen are breakdown products of a larger polypeptide. In part to examine this question we took a number of the Tn5-insertions isolated in *fhaB* on pUW21-26 and transferred them to the *B. pertussis* chromosome by recombination such that the wild-type locus was replaced. These strains were then examined by Western analysis for the synthesis of products reacting with antisera to FHA. Some recombinant strains synthesized FHA-cross-reactive products that were reduced in size. Figure 2 shows the size of the FHA product seen in these strains plotted versus the map position of the Tn5-insertion. It can be seen that there is a linear relationship between these two parameters and that one can extrapolate to a protein of zero size to arrive at a position which should correspond to the start of the FHA gene. The position of this start site corresponds to the leftmost boundary of a small group of Tn5-insertions having a negative phenotype in *E. coli*. Taken together our data suggest that an open reading frame of about 6 kb encodes an FHA-cross-reactive polypeptide of about 200 kDa which is transcribed from left to right on the map of pUW21-26. These data therefore support the notion that FHA is synthesized as a large protein and that smaller species are the result of cleavage or perhaps "premature" termination of transcription and/or translation during synthesis. The Tn5-insertions which we returned to the *B. pertussis* chromosome had no effect on the amount of FHA-product detected in *E. coli*. This reflects the fact that we are unable to detect a change in size of the product by the assay we are using, but also indicates that epitopes that are detected by FHA antisera are encoded early in *fhaB*. Given the rod-like structure of FHA (Blom, Hansen, and Poulsen, 1983) it is a reasonable hypothesis that such epitopes are repeated periodically along its length.

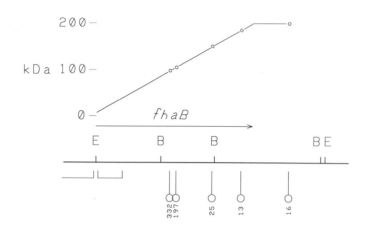

Fig. 2: Truncation of FHA-cross-reactive products formed in recombinant strains of *B. pertussis*. For the Tn5-insertions shown the size of the largest FHA-cross-reactive product seen by Western analysis is mapped versus the site of Tn5-insertion. Extrapolation to zero size gives a start site for a 200 kDa polypeptide near the *Eco*RI site. Brackets below the restriction map show regions identified by Tn5-mutagenesis of pUW21-26 (see Fig. 1).

A cluster of three Tn5-insertions in pUW21-26 defines a small region, *fhaC*, which, together with *vir* and *fhaB* allows the detection of FHA-cross-reactive material in *E. coli*. We suggest that this locus encodes a factor involved in the proper expression and/or export of FHA in *E. coli*. We have not yet introduced mutations in *fhaC* to the *B. pertussis* chromosome to assess the role of this locus in its native genetic background.

The last region we will discuss is the *vir* locus. The *vir* locus is just to the left of and nearly contiguous with *fhaB*, and spans approximately 5kb. *vir* is required for the expression of FHA in

E. coli and for the expression of multiple virulence-associated traits in *B. pertussis*. It was previously hypothesized that *vir* encodes a *trans*-acting positive regulatory element that acts at multiple virulence related loci (Weiss and Falkow, 1984). The data we will present here support that hypothesis.

The *vir* locus as shown in Fig. 1 encompasses the sites of Tn5-insertion in the *B. pertussis* strains BP347 and BP359. These strains were isolated as having a Vir⁻ phenotype, i.e. they had lost the ability to synthesize FHA, pertussis toxin, extracytoplasmic adenylate cyclase, and hemolysin. We have cloned the *Bam*HI fragment containing *vir* from pUW21-26 into the broad host range cloning vector pRK290. This plasmid, pSS528 (see Fig. 1), can be transferred via conjugation to Vir⁻ strains of *B. pertussis* with the result that they become Vir⁺ in phenotype, having simultaneously regained the ability to synthesize FHA, pertussis toxin, and hemolysin (adenylate cyclase was not assayed). When this experiment is repeated using a derivative of pSS528 in which *fhaB* has been deleted, pSS584 (see Fig. 1), the same result is obtained.

The strains upon which either of these plasmids will confer a Vir⁺ phenotype include those which are *vir*⁻ due to Tn5-insertion as well as those which have arisen spontaneously from *vir*⁺ strains (by phase-variation). The latter result demonstrates that the change in the DNA corresponding to the Vir⁺ to Vir⁻ transition is contained within this cloned region. To address this issue more fully we have cloned the *vir* locus from a series of B. pertussis strains derived sequentially by switching from Vir⁺ to Vir⁻ and Vir⁻ to Vir⁺ etc. When these *vir* loci are returned to avirulent phase strains in *trans* as described above for pSS528, it is found that those cloned from Vir⁺ organisms are capable of conferring the Vir⁺ phenotype while those from Vir⁻ strains are not. We therefore conclude that the *vir* locus contains the site of phase-variation. Interestingly, when these cloned genes are compared by restriction analysis no rearrangement, either deletion or inversion can be detected between the *vir*⁺ and *vir*⁻ forms of the locus.

We have recently mapped, by recombination between progressive deletions of the cloned *vir*⁺ form *of vir* and a *vir*⁻ allele in the *B. pertussis* chromosome, the position of the DNA alteration involved in phase-variation. This change maps within an approximately 1.3 kb deletion interval included in the region we have defined as *vir*. Although DNA-sequence analysis of this interval is not complete one sequence difference has been noted. This is the insertion of one nucleotide, a G residue in the *vir*⁻ form of the allele when compared to the *vir*⁺, and is presumably a frameshift mutation within a region encoding a functional part of Vir. This insertion has occured within a run of six G's, a condition known to favor the occurence of frameshift mutations (Streisenger and Owen, 1985). If our analysis of this region ultimately confirms that this is the only change in the DNA involved in the virulence phase transition, it will be, with one exception, unlike other mechanisms of phase-variation which have been described. Indeed, it raises the question of whether this can reasonably be called phase-variation at all. In other words, does it represent a means which has evolved to allow *B. pertussis* to change its complete character at a rate exceeding that of "natural" mutations? A precedent for such a mechanism does exist in the case of expression of pili in *Neisseria gonorrhoeae*. Piliated *N. gonorrhoeae* strains that have been made deficient in homologous DNA recombination are found to switch off their piliated phenotype via the introduction of a frameshift mutation in the pilin gene (Koomey and co-workers, 1987). This mutation is the loss of a C from a run of 8 C's, and reversion to a pili⁺ phenotype involves the reacquisition of a C to restore the reading frame.

An understanding of the regulation of pathogenic potential in *B. pertussis* is emerging. The studies we have presented demonstrate that a single genetic locus, *vir*, plays a central role, acting at many other genes to activate the synthesis of virulence-associated factors. The *vir* locus is thus a master-switch and its expression or non-expression determines the entire character of the bacterium. The level of expression of *vir* itself will, we believe, ultimately be shown to be modulated by the environmental influences already known to affect the pathogenic character of this organism. Further study will increase our understanding of this and other aspects of this system of regulation such as, the number and molecular nature of gene products encoded within the *vir* locus, the nature of the interaction between these products and the genes they regulate, and the nature of the control of expression of *vir* and/or these genes in response to environmental influences.

REFERENCES

Becker, E.L., Kermode, J.C., Naccache, P.H., Yassin, R., March, M.L., Munoz, J.J., and R.I. Sha'afi (1985). The inhibition of neutrophil granule enzyme secretion and chemotaxis by pertussis toxin. J. Cell Biol., 100, 1641-1646.

Blom, J., Hansen, G.A., and F.M. Poulsen (1983). Morphology of cells and hemagglutinogens of *Bordetella* species: resolution of substructural units in fimbriae of *Bordetella pertussis*. Infect. Immun., 42, 308-317.

Broome, C.V., Preblud, S.R., Bruner, B., McGowan, J.E., Hayes, P.S., Harris, P.P., Elsea, W.E., and D.W. Fraser (1981). Epidemiology of pertussis, Atlanta, 1977. J. Pediatr., 98, 362-367.

Brown, D.R, and C.D. Parker (1987). Cloning of the filamentous hemagglutinin of *Bordetella pertussis* and its expression in *Escherichia coli*. Infect. Immun., 55, 154-161.

Confer, D.L., and J.W. Eaton (1982). Phagocyte impotence caused by an invasive bacterial adenylate cyclase. Science, 217, 948-950.

Friedman, R.L., Fiederlin, R.L., Glasser, L., and J.N. Galgiani (1987). *Bordetella pertussis* adenylate cyclase: effects of affinity purified adenylate cyclase on human polymorphonuclear functions. Infect. Immun., 55, 135-140.

Goldman, W.E., Klapper, D.G., and J.B. Baseman (1982). Detection, isolation, and analysis of a released *Bordetella pertussis* product toxic to cultured tracheal cells. Infect. Immun., 36, 782-794.

Irons, L.I., Ashworth, L.A., and P. Wilton-Smith (1983). Heterogeneity of the filamenous haemagglutinin of *Bordetella pertussis* studied with monoclonal antibodies. J. Gen. Microbiol., 129, 2769-78.

Isomura, S., Suzuki, S., and Y. Sato (1985). Clinical efficacy of the Japanese acellular pertussis vaccine after intrafamiliar exposure to pertussis patients. Dev. Biol. Stand., 61, 531-537.

Koomey, J.M., Gotschlich, E.M., Robbins, K., Bergstrom, S., and J. Swanson (1987). Effects of *recA* mutations on pilus antigenic variation and phase transitions in Neisseria gonorrhoeae. Genetics, (in press).

Lacey, B. W. (1960) Antigenic modulation of *Bordetella pertussis*. J. Hyg. Camb., 58, 57-93.

McPheat, W.L., Wardlaw, A.C., and P. Novotny (1983). Modulation of *Bordetella pertussis* by nicotinic acid. Infect. Immun., 41, 516-522.

Meade, B.D., Kind, P.M., Ewell, J.B., McGrath, P.P., and C.R. Manclark (1984). In vitro inhibition of murine macrophage migration by *Bordetella pertussis* lymphocytosis promoting factor. Infect. Immun., 45, 718-725.

Mertsola, J., Ruuskanen, O., Eerola, E., and M.K. Viljanen (1983). Intrafamilial spread of pertussis. J. Pediatr., 103, 359-363.

Streisenger, G, and J.E. Owen (1985). Mechanisms of spontaneous and induced frameshift mutation in bacteriophage T4. Genetics, 109, 633-659.

Stibitz, S., Weiss, A.A., and S. Falkow. A genetic analysis of the *fha-vir* region of *Bordetella pertussis*. submitted for publication.

Weiss, A.A., Hewlett, E.L., Myers, G.A., and S. Falkow (1983). Tn5-induced mutations affecting virulence factors of *Bordetella pertussis*. Infect. Immun., 42, 33-41.

Weiss, A.A., and S. Falkow (1984). Genetic analysis of phase change in *Bordetella pertussis*. Infect. Immun., 43, 263-269.

Urisu, A., Dowell, J.L., and C.R. Manclark (1986). Filamentous hemagglutinin has a major role in mediating adherence of *Bordetella pertussis* to human WiDr cells. Infect. Immun., 52, 695-701.

Fehrenbach et al. (Eds.), Bacterial Protein Toxins, Zbl. Bakt. Suppl. 17
© Gustav Fischer, Stuttgart, New York, 1988

Genetics and Structure of Thiol-Activated Toxins

K. Kehoe[1], J. Walker[2], G. Boulnois[2], J. Shields[1] and L. Miller[1].

[1]Department of Microbiology, University of Newcastle upon Tyne, Medical School,
Framlington Place, Newcastle upon Tyne, NE2 4HH, UK
[2]Department of Microbiology, University of Leicester, Medical Sciences Building, University
Road, Leicester, LE1 7RH, UK

ABSTRACT

Cloned genes encoding the thiol-activated toxins streptolysin O (slo) and pneumolysin (ply) have been
sequenced and the primary sequences of the toxins have been predicted from the DNA sequences. The
N-terminus of the predicted SLO sequence contains 33 residues which possess the consensus features of
a signal peptide. A further 67 residues appear to be removed subsequent to secretion to produce a
52,655 low molecular weight form of the toxin. This can be aligned, without extensive gaps, with the
predicted pneumolysin sequence to reveal that 42% of the residues are identical and a further 23% of
the residues are structurally similar. Both toxins contain only one Cys residue located at identical
positions, within a common 12 residue sequence, close to the C-terminal ends of the molecules.
Mutants of the slo gene which terminate translation proximal to this sequence abolish toxin
activity. Mutants which remove the five C-terminal residues of SLO reduce toxin activity.

KEYWORDS

Thiol-activated toxins, streptolysin O, pneumolysin, listeriolysin, secretion, structure-function
relationships, mechanism of action.

INTRODUCTION

The thiol-activated toxins are produced by fifteen different species of pathogenic Gram positive
bacteria from four different generae, and are grouped together because they share a number of common
biological properties. All are cytolytic for a wide range of eucaryotic cell types, reversibly
sensitive to oxidation (thiol-activated), irreversibly inhibited by cholesterol and related 3B-
hydroxysterols, and share immunological crossreactivity (for reviews see 1,4). With the single
exception of pneumolysin, produced by Streptococcus pneumoniae, all are secreted by the producing
organisms. Their cytolytic activities and their abilities to inhibit polymorphonuclear functions at
sublytic concentrations (1,4) suggest that they may be important virulence factors for the producing
organisms. Streptolysin O (SLO), produced by group A streptococci, is the best studied thiol-
activated toxin and is often considered as the prototype of this group. There is good evidence that
SLO binds to cholesterol in the target cell membrane in a temperature independent manner, and that
binding is followed by a temperature dependent oligomerization of 20 -100 SLO monomers into large arc
and ring shaped structures which can be visualised by electron microscopy ( ). Freeze etch studies
have suggested that these oligomers may span the membrane (4). Studies on intact SLO oligomers
isolated from erythrocyte membranes have shown that they are essentially lipid free and capable of
reconstituting into cholesterol free liposomes, suggesting that cholesterol is required only for the
initial binding of SLO to the membrane (3). Formation of oligomers appears to result in the
production of functionally large pores which allow the release of large molecular weight cytoplasmic
molecules, leading to cell death (5). Because of their common biological and immunological
properties, other thiol-activated toxins are considered to have a very similar mechanism of action to SLO.

																			20
M	S	N	K	K	T	F	K	K	Y	S	R	V	A	G	L	L	T	A	A
L	I	I	G	N	L	V	T	A	N	A	E	S	N	K	Q	N	T	A	40 S
T	E	T	T	T	N	E	Q	P	K	P	E	S	S	E	L	T	T	E	60
K	A	G	Q	K	T	D	D	M	L	N	S	N	D	M	I	K	L	A	80 P
K	E	M	P	L	E	S	A	E	K	E	E	K	K	S	E	D	K	K	100 K
S	E	E	D	H	T	E	E	I	N	D	K	I	Y	S	L	N	Y	N	120 E
L	E	V	L	A	K	N	G	E	T	I	E	N	F	V	P	K	E	G	140 V

Figure 1 : The 140 N-terminal residues of the predicted SLO sequence.
   The data is from Kehoe et al (7). The 33 N-terminal residues corresponding to the predicted SLO signal sequence are highlighted by the closed box. The 67 residues which appear to be removed to generate the low molecular weight form of SLO are underlined. The open box depicts the predicted N-terminus of the low molecular weight form of SLO.

The common properties of thiol-activated toxins suggests that they may have originated from a common evolutionary source. However, hybridization studies employing a cloned SLO gene (slo) probe and low stringency hybridization conditions have failed to detect homology between slo and DNA from species expressing other thiol-activated toxins (6). This suggests that thiol-activated toxin genes have undergone a considerable degree of divergence and that functionally important structures might be identifiable as conserved regions in the primary sequences of toxins from taxonomically diverse species. To determine if this is the case we have determined the complete nucleotide sequences of two cloned thiol-activated toxin genes: the slo gene from S.pyogenes, and the pneumolysin gene (ply) from S.pneumoniae (7,10). In this chapter we summarise our studies on the structural relationships between the predicted primary sequences of SLO and pneumolysin which have allowed us to tentatively identify a number of functionally important regions in these thiol-activated toxins.

THE N-TERMINAL REGIONS OF SLO AND PNEUMOLYSIN:
The cloning and sequencing of the complete slo gene from S.pyogenes strain Richards are described in detail elsewhere (7). Fig. 1 shows the N-terminal 140 residues of the SLO sequence, which has been predicted from the DNA sequence (7). The first 33 residues, which are enclosed in a box in Fig. 1, possess all the consensus features of a signal peptide involved in protein export (8,9). A sequence containing five charged residues (K K T F K K Y S R) is followed by sixteen predominantly hydrophobic residues encompassing two glycines and ending with threonine at position 28. Within the next six residues there are two consensus cleavage sites for a signal peptidase (A N A or A E S). We predict that this sequence is recognised as a signal peptide and removed during SLO secretion.

Amino acid sequencing of SLO purified from culture supernatants of S.pyogenes strain S84 Kalbak, have tentatively identified the four N-terminal residues to be S-D-E-D- (P.Falmagne and J.Alouf, personal communication). This is quite distinct from the residues adjacent to the predicted SLO signal peptide, but very similar to residues 100 - 104 (S-E-E-D-) of the predicted SLO sequence (Fig. 1). The difference in the second residues (E instead of D) could be accounted for by a single base change in strains Richard and S84 Kalbak. The serine at position 100 is preceded by a lysine, suggesting a protease sensitive site. We suggest that the 67 residues between the end of the predicted signal sequence and Ser$_{100}$ are removed by proteolytic cleavage either during or after secretion of SLO, to produce a low molecular weight form of the toxin. This is consistent with our previous studies which detected two molecular weight forms of SLO, differing in M_r by ca. 8000, in E.coli minicells expressing the cloned slo gene (6). Two similar molecular weight forms have also been purified from S.pyogenes culture supernatants and no significant differences in their specific

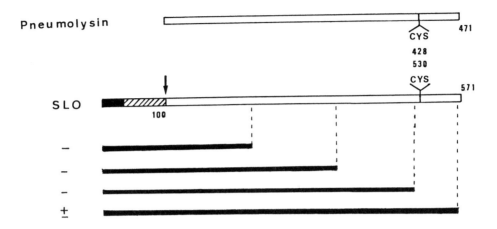

Figure 2 : Relative positions of the single Cys residues in SLO and pneumolysin.
          The relationships between the toxins are described in detail by Kehoe et al (7), and are summarised in the text.

hemolytic activities have been observed (2). This indicates that the 67 residues are removed after SLO secretion and that their removal is not required for toxin activation, at least in vitro. The possibility that these residues play some role in toxin activity or stability in vivo, or even that they facilitate some step in toxin export cannot be ruled out.

Unique among the thiol-activated toxins, pneumolysin is not secreted by the producing organism and, except for removal of the N-terminal methionine, does not undergo post-translational processing (10). The availability of the cloned and sequenced slo and ply genes will allow us to test this and our prediction of the SLO signal sequence, by isolating slo mutants and constructing slo-ply gene fusions.

STRUCTURAL HOMOLOGIES BETWEEN SLO AND PNEUMOLYSIN :
A comparison of the nucleotide sequences of the slo and ply genes suggest that these genes have evolved from a common ancestral gene, but that their sequences have diverged considerably. Overall about 50% base sequence homology exists between the two genes. However, a much greater degree of homology has been detected between the two toxins at the predicted amino acid sequence level. These relationships are described in detail elsewhere (7). Here we summarise the main features of the structural homologies between SLO and pneumolysin.

The low molecular weight form of SLO is very similar in size to pneumolysin (Fig. 2). Thus, inactivation of toxin activity by oxidation cannot be due to the formation of intramolecular disulfide bridges. Sensitivity to oxidation could be due to the formation of intermolecular disulfide bridges between SLO (or pneumolysin) and other proteins secreted by the producing organism. This is consistent with the observation that sensitivity to oxidation decreases during purification of SLO or pneumolysin (1).

A best fit programme aligns the sequences of the low molecular weight form of SLO and pneumolysin at the single Cys residues (Fig. 2) and reveals that 42% of the residues are identical (7). Alignment on the basis of structural similarity between amino acids matches 65% of the residues (7). Identical and structurally similar residues are distributed throughout the whole lengths of SLO and pneumolysin. In addition the hydropathicity profiles of these molecules, aligned at the single Cys residues, are almost indistinguishable (7). Thus, SLO and pneumolysin are structurally very similar molecules, even though their genetic determinants have undergone a considerable degree of divergence. This suggests that function has served as a selective pressure for the conservation of an overall structural similarity, which is important for toxin activity.

Previous studies with thiol-blocking agents have suggested that cysteine plays an important role in SLO and pneumolysin activities (11). The single Cys residues in these SLO and pneumolysin is located within a 12 residue sequence which is identical in both molecules (Fig. 3). Indeed, this is the longest continuous region of identity between the two toxins.

```
     526                            542
      M A R E C T G L A W E W W R K V I

      K I R E C T G L A W E W W R T V Y
     424                            440
```

Figure 3 : Identical sequences encompassing the single Cys residues in SLO and pneumolysin.

The location of the Cys residues within this very strongly conserved sequence suggests that this region represents a functionally important structure.

The nucleotide sequence of a third thiol-activated toxin gene, the listeriolysin determinant (llo) from Listeria monocytogenes, is currently being determined by P. Cossart and colleagues in the Pasteur Institute, Paris. Their preliminary data has revealed that a sequence encoded by the 3' end of the llo gene shares a considerable degree of homology with the C-terminal regions of SLO and pneumolysin (P. Cossart, this volume). Thus, conservation of sequence homologies, at least at the C-terminal ends of thiol-activated toxins, appears to extend across genus, in addition to species, barriers. Since these organisms are taxonomically diverse, this argues strongly that function has served as a selective pressure to maintain conserved sequences and therefore that these sequences are likely to be functionally important.

The availability of the cloned and sequenced slo, ply and llo genes will now permit detailed structure-function studies to be focused on regions which sequence conservation suggests to be functionally important. As an initial step in such studies we have constructed a number of nonsense mutations in the slo gene by inserting a synthetic translation termination codon at defined sites within the gene (Fig. 2). Mutants which terminate translation immediately proximal to the "Cys conserved sequence" completely abolish toxin activity. A mutant which prevents translation of the five C-terminal residues of SLO reduces hemolytic activity 200 fold, indicating that the extreme C-terminal residues are important for activity (Fig. 2). It is not yet clear whether the reduction in activity in this mutant is due to the deletion of residues at an important "active site" or due to a more gross alteration in the structure of the molecule. More refined mutants, differing in single residues, will be required to analyse these regions in detail and such mutants are currently being constructed. To facilitate the production and purification of mutant gene products we have linked the slo and ply genes to strong E. coli promoters (see Mitchell, Walker, Saunders, Kehoe,Andrew and Boulnois, this volume).

In addition to defined mutants in the cloned and sequenced thiol-activated toxin genes, monoclonal antibodies which block toxin activity at particular steps would facilitate structure-function studies. An anti-SLO monoclonal antibody which blocks hemolytic activity, but not SLO binding to erythrocytes has recently been isolated (12). The truncated gene products of the defined nonsense mutants described in Fig. 2 should facilitate the mapping of the epitopes to which such monoclonal antibodies are directed. A combination of structurally defined mutants, gene fusions between different thiol-activated toxin genes and monoclonal antibodies which inhibit defined steps in cell lysis will provide powerful tools to analyse the detailed structure-function relationships in this important group of pore-forming toxins.

ACKNOWLEDGMENTS
Work in the authors laboratories which is summarised here is supported by grants from the UK MRC (grant number G8702676CB to MK and G8409870CB to GB)

REFERENCES

1. Alouf, J.E. (1980). Pharmacol. Ther 11 : 661-717.
2. Bhakdi, S., M. Roth, A. Szeigoleit and J. Tranum-Jensen (1984). Infect. Immun. 46 : 394-400.
3. Bhakdi, S. and J. Tranum-Jensen. (1985). Infect. Immun. 47 : 52-60.
4. Bhakdi, S. and J. Tranum-Jensen (1985). Microbial Pathogenesis 1 : 5-14.
5. Duncan, J.L. and R. Schlegel. (1975). J. Cell Biol. 67 : 160-173.
6. Kehoe, M. and K. Timmis (1984). Infect. Immun. 43 : 804-810.
7. Kehoe, M., J. Walker, L. Miller and G. Boulnois (submitted for publication).
8. Oliver, D. (1985). Ann. Rev. Microbiol. 39 : 615-648.
9. Sarvas, M. (1986). Curr. Top. Microbiol. Immunol. 125 : 103-125.
10. Walker, J.A., R.L. Allen, P. Falmagne, M. Johnson and G. Boulnois (1987) Infect. Immun. 55 : 1184-1189.
11. Geoffroy, C., A.M. Gilles and J.E. Alouf. (1981). Biochem. Biophys. Res. Commun. 99:781-788.
12. Hugo, F., J. Reichwein, M. Arvand, S. Kramer and S. Bhakdi (1986) Infect. Immun. 54, 641 - 645.

Fehrenbach et al. (Eds.), Bacterial Protein Toxins, Zbl. Bakt. Suppl. 17
© Gustav Fischer, Stuttgart, New York, 1988

Studies on Structure and Functions of Elongation Factor 2 in Relation to ADP Ribosylation Using its cDNA

K. Kohno[2], T. Nakanishi[2], F. Ohmura[1] and T. Uchida[1, 2]

[1]Institute for Molecular and Cellular Biology, Osaka University, 1–3 Yamada-oka, Suita, Osaka, 565 Japan
[2]National Institute for Basic Biology, Myodaiji-chou, Okazaki, Aichi 444, Japan

ABSTRACT

Polypeptide chain elongation factor 2 (EF-2) cDNA has been cloned from wild type hamster cell and also a mutant hamster cell line containing non-ADP-ribosylatable EF-2. The mutant conferring resistance to diphtheria toxin (DT) and Pseudomonas aeruginosa exotoxin A (PA) is a G-to-A transition in the first Nucleotide of condon 717 (Gly- Arg). Transfection of mouse L cells with a recombinant EF-2 cDNA differing from the wild-type only by this G-to-A transition confers resistance to PA. The degree of toxin resistant protein synthesis of stable transfectants are dependent on the ratio of non-ADP-ribosylatable EF-2 to wild type EF-2. Non-ADP-ribosylatable and functionable EF-2 molecule and its gene were studied and discussed.

KEYWORDS

EF-2, non-ADP ribosylation, toxin resistance, cDNA, transfection, amino acid substitution, mutation, hot spot.

INTRODUCTION

Eukaryotic polypeptide chain elongation factor 2 (EF-2), a single polypeptide chain of Mr. about 95K, is essential for protein synthesis in all eukaryotes. EF-2 catalyzes the GTP hydrolysis-dependent translocation of peptidyl-tRNA from the ribosome A site to the P site during peptide chain elongation (Weissbach 1976, Kaziro, 1978). Eukaryotic EF-2 has one unique amino acid named diphthamide which is a post translationally modified histidine residue (Van Ness, 1980, Bodley, 1984). EF-2 contains a diphthamide residue that can be specifically ADP-ribosylated and inactivated in the presence of NAD by fragment A of diphtheria toxin (DT) or by Pseudomonas aeruginosa exotoxin A (PA) (Pappenheimer, 1983, Honjo, 1968, Gill, 1969). A single molecule of fragment A of DT introduced into the cytoplasm is sufficient to kill the cell (Yamaizumi, 1978). The enzymatic activity of DT is essential for its lethal activity, because CRM197 lacking only the enzymatic activity by missence mutation has no toxicity to susceptible cells and animals (Uchida, 1972). The two toxins have the same enzymatic activity as NAD:EF-2-ADPribose transferase, but humans, monkeys and hamsters are sensitive to DT whereas mice and rats are insensitive to DT, but very sensitive to PA. To examine the relationships between the structure and the functions of EF-2, several approaches have been reported as follows:purification and properties of EF-2, and the isolation and characterization of DT-and PA-resistant cells. As the next step in these studies, we wish to isolate a cDNA clone encompassing hamster EF-2. Here we report isolation of the cDNA and comparative studies of sequence homology among EF-2 and several GTP binding proteins. Furthermore we cloned EF-2 cDNA from DT-and PA-resistant cells and identified its mutation conferring resistance to DT and PA by transient and long-term expression assay with recombinant EF-2 cDNA.

MATERIALS AND METHODS

Cells and Cell Culture: Chinese hamster ovary cells, CHO-K1 (Pro⁻), CHO Gat⁻ (auxotroph for glycine, adenosine, and thymidine)cells and Mouse L cells deficient in thymidine kinase activity were used. CHO-K1 cells and L cells were routinely maintained in alpha MEM without nucleosides, and CHO Gat⁻ cells were maintain in alpha MEM with nucleosides, supplemented with 8% fetal calf serum (FCS). KEE1, KE1, KN2, and KN7 cells were isolated previously as DT-and PA-resistant cells from CHO-K1 cells (Kohno, 1985), and GE1 cells were also established as toxin-resistant cells from Gat⁻ cells (Kohno, 1987).

Cloning and Sequencing: Two mixtures of 16 tetradecamer oligodeoxyribonucleotides (5'-TCₐTGₜACₐTCₐAA and 5'-TCₐTGᵨACₐTCₐAA-3') constructed from the amino acid sequence of a peptide (Phe-Asp-Val-His-Asp) released by tryptic digestion of rat EF-2 specifically ADP ribosylated by DT(Robinson, 1974) were used to screan a rat liver cDNA library. Positive clones were isolated to obtain a full-sized hamster cDNA, two hamster cDNA library from CHO K1 cells and KEE1 cells were constructed following the Okayama and Berg method (Okayama, 1983). Using a vector pcD that permits the expression of cDNA in mammalian cells.

Northern Blot analysis: Total RNA was isolated from exponentially growing cells by their homogenization with 4M guanidinium thiocyanate, followed by ultra-centrifugation through a 5.7 M CsCl cushion. Poly(A)⁺RNA was purified once by oligo(dT)-cellulose chromatography (P-L Biochemicals, Type 7). Samples (RNA) were subjected to electrophoresis in 1% agarose formaldehyde gel, transferred to a nitrocellulose filter (Schleicher & Schull, BA85) (32), and hybridized with appropriate probes labelled by nick translation (10^8 cpm/ug) or with a multiprime DNA labelling system (10^9 cpm/ug)(Amersham). Prehybridization (3.5 hr at 42 C) and hybridization (15-20 hr at 42 C) were carried out as described previously (Kohno, 1986). Positive clones were isolated as described elsewhere (Kohno, 1987).

Transient Expression Assay: Plasmid DNA containing EF-2 cDNA transfected to mouse L cells. After transfection and subsequent incubation for 48 hr, the medium was replaced by F 12 containing 10% fetal calf serum and 2 uCi/ml of [³H]leucine. The cultures were incubated for 2 hr, and then the incorporation of [³H]leucine into the acid-insoluble fraction was measured.

Southern Blot Analysis: High molecular weight hamster genomic DNAs from wild-type and DT-resistant CHO cells were isolated. DNAs were separated on agarose gel and transferred to a Zeta-Probe blotting membrane (Bio-Rad). Probes were labelled by a multiprime DNA labelling system (Amersham, 1-2 x 10^9 cpm/ug), and blots were hybridized at 65 C for 22 hr in 10 x Denhardt's solution, 5 x SSC, 50mM sodium phosphate (pH 7), 1% SDS, and 500 ug/ml denatured herring sperm DNA. The filter was washed twice with 3 x SSC, 0.5% SDS at room temperature for 10 min, and then washed with 0.1 x SSC, 0.1% sodium pyrophosphate, and 1% SDS at 65 C for 5 min. Two-Dimensional Gel Analysis:Cell extracts were prepared and as described previously without dialysis (Kohno, 1985).

RESULTS AND DISCUSSION

Isolation of Hamster EF-2 cDNA: About 50,000 transformants were screened from a rat liver cDNA library. One of five positive clones contained DNA sequences complementary to a part of rat EF-2 mRNA and encoding the 15 amino acids containing ADP ribosylation site, the peptide produced by trypsin digestion of EF-2 (Robinson, 1974). To examine the length of EF-2 mRNA derived from rat and hamster cells using the fragment of the rat cDNA as a probe. The length of the EF-2 mRNA was approximately 3 Kbp in each case, which is sufficient to encode a protein of about 100 kDa. Restriction fragment DNA fo the rat EF-2 cDNA was used for screen a CHO cDNA library to isolate a hamster EF-2 cDNA. Twenty-five positive clones were isolated from about 70,000 transformants, and all showed similar restriction maps. The largest insert, found in clone, pHEW1, was sequenced. Analysis of the complete nucleotide sequence of the cloned cDNA showed that it contained one long open reading frame coding for 858 amino acid residuesfollowed by a TAG termination codon and that the other frames were interrupted by multitermination codons (Kohno, 1987). Partial sequence is shown in Fig 1. The cDNA insert is pHEW1 contains a 77-bp 5'-untranslated region, a 2574-bp coding sequence, and a 282-bp 3'-untranslated region. The translational initiation site was assigned to the first methionine codon ATG at position 1-3. The 3'-untranslated region is characterized by an additional pdy(A)$^+$ tail signal, 5'-AATAAA-3', located 12 nucleotides upstream from the poly(A)$^+$ tail.

Protein Primary Structure of Hamster EF-2: The primary structure of hamster EF-2 deduced from the cDNA pHEW1 nucleotide sequence is partially shown in Fig 1. Hamster EF-2 contains 857 amino acids (excluding the initiation methionine) and the calculated Mr. is 95,192 without modification. Nineteen residues of the amino-terminal region and 1 residue of the carboxyl-terminal region of rat EF-2 have been identified by Takamatsu (1985). A 15-amino acid peptide produced trypic digestion of ADP ribosylated rat and bovine EF-2 has been sequenced (Robinson, 1974, Brown, 1979). All these sequences are found in hamster EF-2. Van Ness et al (1980) showed that amino acid specifically ADP-ribosylated by DT is

```
 -77 TCCGCCGCAGCCGCAGCCATCGTCGGCGCCCCTCGCTCTTCTCCTGTGCCCGTGAGAATCCGTCGCCATCCGCCACT   -1

   1 ATG GTG AAC TTC ACG GTA GAC CAG ATC CGT GCC ATT ATG GAC AAG AAA GCC AAC ATC CGG AAC ATG TCA GTC ATC GCT CAC GTG GAC CAC   90
   1 Met Val Asn Phe Thr Val Asp Gln Ile Arg Ala Ile Met Asp Lys Lys Ala Asn Ile Arg Asn Met Ser Val Ile Ala His Val Asp His   30

  91 GGC AAG TCC ACA CTG ACG GAC TCC CTG GTG TGC AAG GCG GGT ATC ATC GCC TCT GCA AGA GCC GGT GAG ACA CGC TTC ACA GAC ACC CGC  180
  31 Gly Lys Ser Thr Leu Thr Asp Ser Leu Val Cys Lys Ala Gly Ile Ile Ala Ser Ala Arg Ala Gly Glu Thr Arg Phe Thr Asp Thr Arg   60

 181 AAG GAC GAA CAG GAG CGC TGC ATC ACT ATC AAG TCC ACG GCC ATC TCC CTC TTC TAT GAG CTC TCT GAG AAT GAC CTG AAC TTC ATC AAG  270
  61 Lys Asp Glu Gln Glu Arg Cys Ile Thr Ile Lys Ser Thr Ala Ile Ser Leu Phe Tyr Glu Leu Ser Glu Asn Asp Leu Asn Phe Ile Lys   90

 271 CAG AGC AAG GAT GGA TCT GGC TTT CTC ATC AAC CTC ATC GAC TCT CCA GGC CAT GTG GAT TTC TCC TCA GAG GTG ACA GCT GCA CTT CGT  360
  91 Gln Ser Lys Asp Gly Ser Gly Phe Leu Ile Asn Leu Ile Asp Ser Pro Gly His Val Asp Phe Ser Ser Glu Val Thr Ala Ala Leu Arg  120

 361 GTC ACC GAT GGA GCT CTT GTG GTG GTG GAC TGT GTG TCT GGT GTG TGC GTG CAG ACT GAG ACC GTG CTG CGG CAG GCC ATT GCC GAG CGC  450
 121 Val Thr Asp Gly Ala Leu Val Val Val Asp Cys Val Ser Gly Val Cys Val Gln Thr Glu Thr Val Leu Arg Gln Ala Ile Ala Glu Arg  150

 451 ATC AAG CCT GTC CTG ATG ATG AAT AAG ATG GAC CGT GCC CTG CTT GAG CTG CAG CTG GAG CCT GAG GAA CTA TAC CAG ACC TTC CAG CGC  540
 151 Ile Lys Pro Val Leu Met Met Asn Lys Met Asp Arg Ala Leu Leu Glu Leu Gln Leu Glu Pro Glu Glu Leu Tyr Gln Thr Phe Gln Arg  180

 541 ATT GTG GAG AAT GTC AAC GTC ATC ATT // CAG TAC CTG AAT GAA ATC AAG GAC AGT GTG GTG GCT GGC TTC CAG TGG GCC ACT AAG GAG GGC 2070
 181 Ile Val Glu Asn Val Asn Val Ile Ile // Gln Tyr Leu Asn Glu Ile Lys Asp Ser Val Val Ala Gly Phe Gln Trp Ala Thr Lys Glu Gly  690

2071 GCT CTC TGT GAG GAG AAC ATG CGT GGT GTG CGC TTC GAT GTC CAT GAT GTG ACC CTA CAT GCT GAT GCC ATC CAC CGA GGA GGT GGT CAG 2160
 691 Ala Leu Cys Glu Glu Asn Met Arg Gly Val Arg Phe Asp Val His Asp Val Thr Leu His Ala Asp Ala Ile His Arg Gly Gly Gly Gln  720

2161 ATC ATT CCC ACA GCT CGT CGT TGT CTG TAT GCC AGT GTG TTG ACT GCA CAG CCC CGC CTC ATG GAG CCT ATC TAC CTG GTG GAG ATT CAG 2250
 721 Ile Ile Pro Thr Ala Arg Arg Cys Leu Tyr Ala Ser Val Leu Thr Ala Gln Pro Arg Leu Met Glu Pro Ile Tyr Leu Val Glu Ile Gln  750

2251 TGT CCT GAA CAG GTC GTG GGT GGC ATC TAC GGT GTC CTG AAC AGG AAG CGT GGC CAT GTG TTT GAA GAG TCC CAG GTG GCT GGC ACC CCC 2340
 751 Cys Pro Glu Gln Val Val Gly Gly Ile Tyr Gly Val Leu Asn Arg Lys Arg Gly His Val Phe Glu Glu Ser Gln Val Ala Gly Thr Pro  780

2341 ATG TTT GTA GTC AAG GCC TAT CTT CCA GTC AAC GAG TCC TTT GGT TTT ACA GCT GAC CTG CGC TCC AAC ACT GGT GGC CAA GCT TTC CCC 2430
 781 Met Phe Val Val Lys Ala Tyr Leu Pro Val Asn Glu Ser Phe Gly Phe Thr Ala Asp Leu Arg Ser Asn Thr Gly Gly Gln Ala Phe Pro  810

2431 CAG TGT GTG TTC GAC CAC TGG CAG ATT CTG CCC GGG GAC CCG TTC GAC AAC AGC AGC CGT CCC AGC CAA GTG GTG GCT GAG ACC CGC AAG 2520
 811 Gln Cys Val Phe Asp His Trp Gln Ile Leu Pro Gly Asp Pro Phe Asp Asn Ser Ser Arg Pro Ser Gln Val Val Ala Glu Thr Arg Lys  840

2521 CGC AAA GGT CTA AAG GAG GGC ATC CCA GCA CTG GAC AAC TTC CTG GAC AAA CTG TAG GCAGGCTTGCACAGCCACACACTGCACAGTGCCCACCCATCAG 2620
 841 Arg Lys Gly Leu Lys Glu Gly Ile Pro Ala Leu Asp Asn Phe Leu Asp Lys Leu                                                   858

2621 AAGACACCTTGAGACTGTCCCCATAATGCTGCTCTGGAGGTGGCTGGGGCCACCCTGCCATTGAGCACTAACACTTGATGCCGACTCTATTTATTTCGGAATTTCCGAGGCAGTGGAGT 2739

2740 CGCCCTCTGCAGGCTGGACTGGCTGGCGGGCCATGGGGTGGGCAGGACACAGCTCTTTATCATTTTCAGAGGGAAAAATGCTCAGATATCAAACATCTAAATAAATGCATTCAGAGG 2856
```

Fig.1. Nucleotide sequence and deduced amino acid sequence of the cDNA insert in pHEW1 encoding hamster EF-2 cDNA(Kohno, 1986). The undelined amino acids(positions 2-20, 702-717, and 858) are the ones that completely matched those of rat EF-2 identified by peptide analysis of purified EF-2.

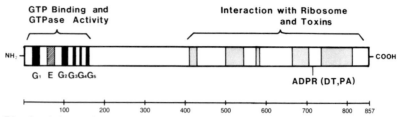

Fig.2. Schematic representation of the structure of EF-2(Kohno, 1986). The hatched box G & E indicate the homologous regions with GTP binding proteins or with only elongation factors. The shaded boxes correspond to the homologous regions between EF-2 and EF-G.

2-[3-carboxyamido-3-(trimethyl-ammonio)propyl] histidine, designated diphthamide, which is an unusual amino acid modified posttranslationally. The sequence analysis provides direct evidence that the modified amino acid is a histidine(715). Functional domain of EF-2: Functional domain of EF-2 was studied by sequence homology among EF-2 and several GTP binding proteins. As shown is Fig 2, five regions in the amino-terminal position of EF-2, corresponding to about 160 amino acids excluding the region E is considered to contain the domains essential for GTP binding and GTP ase activity. The carboxyl-terminal half of EF-2 contains several regions that have 34-75% homology with bacterial EFG, thus the carboxyl-terminal half is considered to contain the domain involved in the interaction of EF-2 with the ribosome and toxins.

Cloning and Expression of Toxin-resistant EF-2 cDNA: To obtain cDNA of non-ADP ribosylatable EF-2, a cDNA library derived from a DT-resistant CHO-K1 cell line (KEE1)(Kohno, 1985) was also prepared in the expression vector. Two clones, pD46 and pD51, were obtained from screening of about 70,000 transformants by fragment of rat EF-2 cDNA as probe. To know whether the two clones contained the first initiation codon ATG, 5' region of about 460bp was sequenced. The inserts started from nucleotide position number +50 in pD46, and +65 in pD51 in the coding regions of EF-2 cDNA. To examine whether these clones express the resistance to DT and PA, we constructed plasmid in which two clones (downstream of 513bp 3'terminal) were recombined with 5'region of EF-2-cDNA (upstream of 513bp) of wild type pHEW1to made full-length cDNA. When these recombinants, termed pWD46 and pWD51, were transferred into L cells by the calcium-phosphate method, cells transferred with pWD51 DNA showed protein synthesis in the presence of PA, while those with pWD46 did not (Table 1). This shows that pD51 contains the nucleotide sequence conferring resistance to PA in the EF-2 cDNA, which is limited to the downstream region from 513bp. Next we examined the sequences of the 520bp

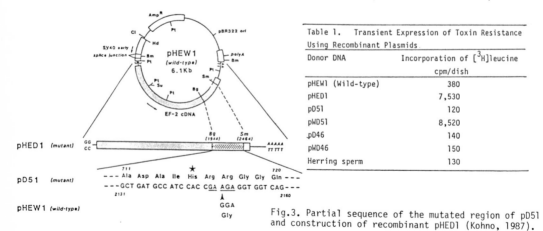

Table 1. Transient Expression of Toxin Resistance Using Recombinant Plasmids.

Donor DNA	Incorporation of $[^3H]$leucine
	cpm/dish
pHEW1 (Wild-type)	380
pHED1	7,530
pD51	120
pWD51	8,520
pD46	140
pWD46	150
Herring sperm	130

Fig.3. Partial sequence of the mutated region of pD51 and construction of recombinant pHED1 (Kohno, 1987).

fragments between the Bgl II and Sma I restriction sites, which contain the coding region of diphthamide. The sequence of the fragment from pD51 was compared with that of wild type EF-2 cDNA. G-to-A transition in the first nucleotide of codon 717 of pD51 was found, while the transition was not seen in pD46. The G-to-A transition in pD51 resulted in substition of Arg for Gly at a position two amino acid residues to the carboxyl-terminal side of the histidine residue, which is posttranslationally modified to diphthamide in wild-type EF-2 (Fig 3). To determine whether this point mutation was responsible for the resistance of the mutation to DT and PA, plasmid pHED1 was constructed by substituting the Bgl II-Sma I fragment from pD51 for the corresponding fragment in the cloned wild-type cDNA in pHEW1 (Fig 3). The plasmid pHED1 contained a full-length EF-2 cDNA that differs at only one base composed to the wild-type hamster sequence in pHEW1. L cells were transfected with either pHED1 or pHEW1 by the calcium phosphate method and protein synthesis of the transfected cells in the presence of PA was determined. Cells with pHED1 showed PA-resistant incorporation of [3H] leucine, while a little incorporation was detected in cells transfected with pHEW1 (Table 1). [3H] leucine incorporation by cells transfected with pHED1 or pHEW1 was dependent on the DNA concentration. Slightly higher PA-resistant [3H]-leucine incorporation was seen in cells transfected with pHEW1 than in cells treated with herring sperm DNA as a negative control. This was due to increased production of wild-type EF-2, because cells transfected with pHEW1 could produce both endogenous native mouse EF-2 and exogenous wild-type hamster EF-2. But, this slight resistance was temporary and later all the cells were killed by toxin. Similar expression of resistance to DT was also observed in human cultured cells transfected with pHED1. These results show that pHED1 encodes EF-2 cDNA which is resistance to both DT and PA. On the other hand, L cells transfected with pWD46 did not show any protein synthesis in the presence of PA. As mentioned above cells transfected with pHEW1 showed slight incorporation of [3H] leucine at early time after exposure to PA, however, pD46 contains a nucleotide sequence that causes loss of the function of wild-type EF-2 as a translocase. Thus we compared the nucleotide sequence of pD46 with that of wild type pHEW1. Only one base substitution in the coding region of pD46 was detected. This point mutation is a C-to-T transition in the second nucleotide of codon 207, and caused amino acid substitution of leucine for proline. We reported previously that ADP-ribosylatable EF-2 was not detected in KEE1 cells by two demential gel electrophoresis following the cell extracts treated with [32P] NAD and fragment A of DT (Kohno, 1985). This amino acid substitution may result in nonfunctionable and non-ADP-ribosylatable EF-2 or very rapid degradation of EF-2 in cell. Relationships between ratio of non-ADP-ribosylated EF-2 to wild-type EF-2 and the degree of toxin-resistant protein synthesis of stable transfectants: When mouse L cells transfected with pHED1 were incubated for 20 days in the presence of 50 ug/ml PA, resistant colonies appeared. There are various sizes of colonies in the plates. One the other hand, in cells transfected with pHEW1, no colonies were formed in the presence of toxin. Seven PA-resistant colonies from L cells transfected with pHED1 were selected at random for further analysis. Cellular protein synthesis of each toxin resistant cell line treated with various concentrations of PA for 24 was studied. Protein synthesis of wild type L cells was completely blocked by 0.01 ug/ml PA whereas LpD56 and LpD59 cells showed about 65% of the protein synthsis observed in the absence of PA. Similar resistance to toxin was seen at wide range dose of PA. Similar results were obtained with other transfectants, even when they showed different degrees of resistance to PA. Fig 4A shows that results of Northern blot analysis of these transfectants and of wild type CHO cells and L cells. Hamster EF-2 mRNA can be distinguished from mouse EF-2 mRNA under highly stringent conditions. Transfectant Lp53, which expressed the mutant EF-2 cDNA in pHED1, produced about twice as much hamster EF-2 mRNA as that produced by wild-type hamster cells (Fig 4A). It was expected that if a sufficient amount of mRNA for non-ADP-ribosylatable EF-2 were transcribed, protein synthesis of transfectants would not be decreased by toxin. However, protein synthesis in the presence of toxin was only about 65% of that in the absence of toxin (Fig 4A). Similar results were obtained in analyses of six other transfectants. In these transfectants, incorporation of [^{3}H] leucine in the presence of PA depended on the ratio of their productions of toxin-resistant hamster EF-2 mRNA to that of total EF-2 mRNA. We confirmed that the proportion of non-ADP-ribosylatable EF-2 reflected the estimated ratios of mutant to total EF-2 mRNA. ADP-ribosylated EF-2 can be separated from non-ADP-ribosylated EF-2 by two-dimensional gel electrophoresis (Kaneda, 1984, Kohno, 1985). As shown in Fig 4B, after treatment with DT fragment A, all the EF-2 in control L cells can be ADP-ribosylated, with an acidic shift of its isoelectric point. By contrast, after treatment with DT fragment A, EF-2 in the transfectants is separated into two spots corresponding to recipient mouse EF-2 (ADP-ribosylatable) and mutant hamster EF-2 (non-ADP-ribosylatable)(Fig 4B). The intensities of the spots were measured by microdensitometry. The ratios of non-ADP-ribosylatable to total EF-2 were 51, 40, and 31% for LpD53, LpD10, and LpD11, respectively, which agree fairly well with the percentages of mutant EF-2 mRNA and leucine incorporations in the presence of toxin. This fact suggests that ADP-ribosylated EF-2 molecules temporarily bind to ribosomes and thus compete with non-ADP-ribosylated EF-2 molecules.

Presence of a "Hot Spot" for Conferring Resistance to toxins: The results of Southern blot hybridization analysis with whole insert cDNA of pHEW1 as a probe under stringent conditions indicated that EF-2 gene in CHO cells is a single copy gene and that there are two functional copies of the gene per cell. The mutation of KEE1 cells in codon 717 results in a local change in the DNA sequence from GAGGA to GAAGA, creating an MboII restriction site. Wild-type EF-2 cDNA completely digested with MboII generates a 874-bp MboII fragment, whereas mutated EF-2 cDNA gives two fragments of 707 and 167 bp. Twelve cDNA clones from the cDNA library prepared from KEE1 cells were selected at random and their cDNAs were completely digested with MboII. Seven cDNA clones showed the same G-to-A transition mutation but the other five cDNAs did not (data not shown). This is consistent with KEE1 cells bearing two different mutations as mentioned before. The results of RNA blot hybridization analysis of the CHO-K1 and KEE1 cells. Judging from the intensities of the spots corresponding to EF-2 mRNA, KEE1 cells produced as much EF-2 mRNA as wild-type CHO-K1 cells. These results show that

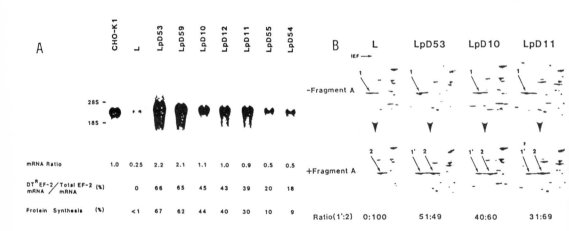

Fig. 4. Expression of toxin-resistant EF-2 derived from pHED1
A, Northern blot analysis. B, ADP-ribosylatable and non-ADP-ribosylatable EF-2 were analysed by two dimentional gel electrophoresis(Kohno, 1987).

each allele in the EF-2 gene locus of KEE1 is transcribed and further indicate that EMS treatment caused G-to-A transition at nucleotide 2149 of one allele with no change at this position in the other allele. To determine whether a G-to-A transition in codon 717 is present in other independently isolated toxin-resistant mutants, we examined these mutants for the presence of a novel restriction fragment of the EF-2 gene produced by the transition. Probing of total genomic DNA from CHO-K1 cells completely digested with MboII with a 160-bp HinfI fragment from genomic EF-2 generates a single fragment of 1297 bp. The mutant allele gives rise to two fragments of 1042 and 255 bp. We previously isolated and characterized several DT-resistant CHO cell lines that are EF-2 structural gene mutants: KE1, KN2, KN7, and KEE1 from CHO-K1 cells (Kohno, 1985) and GE1 from CHO Gat⁻ cells. KE1 and GE1 were selected after EMS mutagenesis, whereas KN2 and KN7 were selected after N-methyl-N'-nitro-N-nitrosoguanidine treatment. Wild-type CHO-K1 and CHO Gat⁻ gave a single band of about 1300 bp, but all the mutants gave a new 255-bp band derived from the mutated allele and the normal 1297 bp. All four independently isolated CHO DT-resistant cells showed the same RFLP. Consequently, the site presented here is a hot spot for causing resistance of hamster EF-2 molecules to DT. Why could we not find the mutation of the His-715 residue? One would predict that the replacement of His-715 by another amino acid in EF-2 would result in toxin resistance, since another residue might not be ADP-ribosylated by toxins since it would not be modified post-translationally. But, when expression assay in our system using mutant EF-2 cDNA (His-715- Lys) prepared by site-directed mutagenesis was tested, toxin resistant protein synthesis of the cells transfected with the mutant cDNA was less than that of cells transfected with wild type cDNA. This result suggests that products of the mutant have no function as translocase during the polypeptide elongation step, and that non ADP ribosylatable and functionable EF-2 are very restricted. This cDNA can be used for co-transformation of a given gene as selectable marker. We almost determined whole sequence of genomic DNA of EF-2 obtained from CHO cells. EF-2 protein occupies about 0.3% of total cellular proteins. The gene is highly and non-tissue specifically expressed in cell. This promoter is good for production of useful proteins.

REFERENCES

Bodley, J.W., P.C.Dunlop, and B.G.Van Ness (1984). Diphthamide in elongation factor 2:ADP-ribosylation, purification,properties. Methods Enzymol, 106, 378-387.

Brown, B.A., and J.W.Bodley (1979). Primary structure at the site in beef and wheat elongation factor 2 of ADP-ribosylation by diphtheria toxin. FEBS Lett. 103, 253-255.

Gill, D.M., A.M.Pappenheimer Jr., R.Brown, and J.T.Kurnick (1969). Studies on the mode of action of diphtheria toxin. J. Exp. Med., 129, 1-21.

Honjo, T., Y.Nishizuka, O.Hayaishi, and I.Kato (1968). Diphtheria toxin-dependent adenosine diphosphate ribosylation of aminoacyl transferase II and inhibition of protein synthesis. J. Biol. Chem., 243, 3553-3555.

Igelwski, B.H., and D.Kabat (1975). NAD-dependent inhibition of Protein synthesis by Pseudomonas aeruginosa toxin. Proc. Natl. Acad. Sci. U.S.A., 72, 2284-2288.

Kaziro, Y. (1978). The role of guanosine 5'-triphosphate in polypeptide chain elongation. Biochem. Biophys. Acta., 505, 95-127.

Kohno, K., T.Uchida, E.Mekada and Y.Okada (1985). Characterization of diphtheria toxin resistant mutants lacking receptor function or containing non-ribosylatable elongation factor 2. Somat. Cell and Mol. Genet., 11, 421-431.

Kohno, K., T.Uchida, H.Ohkubo, S.Nakanishi, T.Nakanishi, T.Fukui, E.Ohtsuka, M.Ikehara and Y.Okada (1986). Amino acid sequence of mammalian elongation factor 2 predicted from the cDNA sequence: Homology with GTP-binding proteins. Proc. Natl. Acad. Sci. U.S.A., 83, 4978-4982.

Kohno, K., and T.Uchida (1987). Highly frequent single amino acid substitution in mammalian elongation factor 2 results in expression of resistance to EF-2-ADP-ribosylating toxins. J. Biol. Chem., (in press).

Moehring, T.J., and J.M.Moehring (1977). Selection and characterization of cells resistant to diphtheria toxin and pseudomonas exotoxin A: Presumptive translation Mutants. Cell, 11, 447-454.

Moehring, T.J., and J.M.Moehring (1979). Characterization of the diphtheria toxin-distance system in Chinese hamster ovary cells. Somat. Cell Genet., 5, 453-468.

Okayama, H., and P.Berg (1983) A cDNA cloning vector that Permits expression of cDNA inserts in mammalian cells. Mol. Cell. Biol., 3, 280-289.

Pappenheimer, A.M.Jr., P.C.Dunlop, K.W.Adolph, and J.W.Bodley (1983). Occurrence of Diphthamide in Archaebacteria. J. Bacteriol., 153, 1342-1347.

Robinson, E.A., O.Henriksen, and E.S.Maxwell (1974). Elongation factor 2. J. Biol. Chem., 249, 5088-5093.

Uchida,T., A.M.Pappenheimer,Jr., and A.A.Harper (1972). Reconstitution of diphtheria toxin from two nontoxic cross reacting mutant toxins. Science, 175, 901-903.

Van Ness, B.G., J.B.Howard, and J.W.Bodley (1980). ADP-ribosylation of elongation factor 2 by diphtheria toxin. J. Biol. Chem., 255, 10710-10716.

Weissbach, H., and S.Ochoa (1976). Soluble factors required for eukaryotic protein synthesis. Rev. Biochem. 45, 191-216.

Yamaizumi, M., E.Mekada, T.Uchida, and Y.Okada (1978). One molecule of diphtheria toxin fragment A introduced into a cell. Cell, 15, 245-250.

Fehrenbach et al. (Eds.), Bacterial Protein Toxins, Zbl. Bakt. Suppl. 17
© Gustav Fischer, Stuttgart, New York, 1988

Genetics of Hemolysins in Aeromonas Hydrophila

T. Chakraborty, V. Husslein, B. Huhle, H. Bergbauer, T. Jarchau, H. Hof[1]
and W. Goebel

Institut für Genetik und Mikrobiologie der Universität Würzburg, Röntgenring 11,
D-8700 Würzburg
[1]Institut für Hygiene und Mikrobiologie der Universität Würzburg, Josef-Schneider-Str. 2,
D-8700 Würzburg

ABSTRACT

The cloning and identification of two cytotoxic hemolysins (other
than the phospholipase) from the gram-negative bacterium Aeromonas
hydrophila is presented. The partial nucleotide sequence of one of
these cytotoxins, aerolysin is presented together with its
regulatory region.   This region contains several prominent
sequences which are probably involved in the regulation of this
gene.   The role of aerolysin in Aeromonas infections is
demonstrated by testing isogenic pairs of aerolysin-producing and
aerolysin-deficient strains in a mouse toxicity model. Finally,
the absence of aerolysin sequences in some Aeromonas isolates has
led to the identification of a genetically unrelated cytotoxic
hemolysin in this species.

KEYWORDS

Aeromonas hydrophila, cytotoxic hemolysins, aerolysin, nucleotide
sequence, mouse toxicity

Aeromonas spp. are ubiquitous inhabitants of fresh water
environments throughout the world. Recent attention has focussed
on A. hydrophila and A. sobria because of their repeated isolation
from contaminated food and water samples and their association
with human disease (Daily,1981; Gracey, 1982; Janda,1984).   The
clinical picture of Aeromonas infections range from severe watery
diarrhea, soft wound infections to septicemia and meningitis
(Freij,1984). Many isolates of this species produce exotoxins
including enterotoxin, cytotoxic haemolysins,phospholipase and
proteases (Ljungh,1983).   The role of these toxins in Aeromonas
infections however remain unclear.
In order to understand the role of the haemolysins in Aeromonas
infections we have used recombinant DNA techniques to clone and

identify these toxins. We report here on the detection and isolation of two cytotoxic haemolysins in Aeromonas hydrophila and describe the genetics and role of one of these toxins, aerolysin, in Aeromonas associated infections.

The cytotoxic haemolysin, aerolysin, has been implicated as an important virulence factor in Aeromonas-associated infections (Daily, 1981). It is a single polypeptide that is synthesised as a 54kD preprotoxin containing a typical signal sequence at the amino-terminus (Howard, 1985). The signal is removed cotranslationally, and the resulting protein is released from the bacteria as an inactive protoxin. Subsequent processing at the carboxy-terminus of the protein is accomplished by the action of one of the proteases secreted in situ by the bacteria, or by reaction with other proteases such as trypsin. Processing of the protoxin results in an increase of at least one thousand fold in activity (Howard, 1985). The protein is thought to exert its mode of action by binding to the target cell membrane with subsequent aggregation and pore formation (Howard, 1982). However, an internal target of the toxin has also be suggested (Thelestam, 1981).

We have previously reported the cloning of the aerolysin determinant from a clinical isolate (AH2) of Aeromonas hydrophila. The cloned gene was found to exhibit both haemolytic and cytotoxic activities . Genetic mapping of the cloned fragment using transposon mutagenesis with Tn 1000 and deletion analysis with restriction endonucleases led to the delineation of the structural gene aerA. Furthurmore, flanking regions which modulate the activity (aerB) and expression (aerC) of the aerolysin gene were mapped (Chakraborty, 1986).

Using antibody raised against purified aerolysin we have shown that the toxin is present in the periplasm in its protoxin form in Escherichia coli. In contrast, aerolysin is found in its mature form in the supernatant fluids of Aeromonas hydrophila. Thus, although the protein is recognised as extracytoplasmic in E. coli, it accumulates in the periplasm rather than outside.

DNA SEQUENCE FEATURES OF THE AEROLYSIN GENE

Using the data obtained previously for the location of the aerolysin gene, we have sequenced regions corresponding to the aerC and aerA regions. From the sequence the longest reading frame is 492 amino acids long which would correspond to a protein of 54.2kD. There are no other reading frames long enough to encode a protein as large as aerolysin. The direction of the reading frame obtained corresponds to the one previously determined by aerolysin-β galactosidase fusions. The translation product of the first 69 bp has all the features of a typical 23 amino acid signal peptide. It contains positively charged amino acids immediately following the initiator methionine, a central hydrophobic core, followed by more polar amino acids and an alanine adjacent to the scissile bond. The first amino acid of proaerolysin is therefore the alanine at position 24 and this corresponds well to the previously published amino acid sequence of the N-terminal end of aerolysin (Buckley, 1981). Apart from the signal peptide the sequence is remarkably hydrophilic, which is somewhat surprising for a membrane pore-forming protein. However, the nucleotide sequence of another pore forming toxin, alpha toxin of S. aureus also indicates that this is a very hydrophilic protein (Grant, 1984). The pore forming outer membrane proteins also lack hydrophobic sequences (Mizuno, 1983). A common feature of these proteins appears to be the aggregation within the membrane leading to channel formation. In this respect , a small region of homology between aerolysin and alpha toxin has been noted by T. Buckley(pers.comm).

The inactive protoxin is converted to mature toxin by the proteoly tic removal of about 25 amino acids from the carboxy-terminus. This would place the site of activation between amino acids 447 and 449 assuming trypsin induced activation of the protoxin. We note that the G + C content of aerolysin is 59%, suggesting that the gene is endogenous to this bacterial species.

Insertions within the region preceding aerA have previously been shown to affect the the expression of aerolysin. The nucleotide sequence of this region is unusual in two respects. Firstly, the A + T content of this region is 61% contrasting with an A + T content of 41% for coding regions within the sequence.Secondly, there are no extended reading frames for 269 nucleotides upstream of the aerolysin gene implicating this region as a regulatory region. A core sequence of ATAAAA is repeated 8 times within this region in both orientations, two other copies of this sequence are present within the first 90 amino acids of the aerolysin gene.

In order to map transcriptional start sites within the aerC region we used S1 analysis of RNA extracted from both A.hydrophila AH 2 and E. coli recombinants habouring the aerolysin determinant.These experiments revealed the presence of two transcripts,transcribing in opposite orientations, within the aerC region. The 5'terminus of the aerolysin transcript was found to be 70 bp upstream of the aerA initiator codon. Within the untranslated region of this transcript the sequence AAAAATAA is present twice in the same orientation with a third direct repeat of this sequence located 14 bp after the start of the gene. At the spatial regions of the -10 and -35 regions of the transcript there appears to be only poor homology at the -10 region (CTGATAT) and good consensus at the -35 region (TTGAGTC) for bacterial promotors (McClure,1985). A possible ribosome binding site is located 4bp from the initiator methionine and is depicted in Fig.1 . The 5'end of the second transcript is located 197 bp away from the start of the aerolysin gene transcript . This transcript contains a 6.4kD open reading frame that would be read from the opposite DNA strand. There appears to be poor homology to the consensus sequences at -10 (AGAGAAT) and -35 (TATTTACTTAA) regions although the -35 region bears some resemblance to similar regions of the P'ʀ promotor of phage lambda and the ctxA gene of Vibrio cholera(Mekalanos,1983). Directly preceeding the -35 region of this promotor is an extended region of hyphenated dyad symmetry ,suggesting it may have a role in regulation of this promotor. Intriguingly, a 12 bp sequence GAATAAACCGGG present in the untranslated region of this transcript occurs as a direct repeat 540 bp away within the coding region of the aerolysin gene. This putative polypeptide encoded for by this transcript has an overall acidic nature.

The partial sequence encompassing the 5'end of the non-coding region of the aerolysin cloned from a fish isolate has been reported(Howard, 1986). A comparison of the two sequences reveals the following features: Firstly, there is very strong homology, 87% at the nucleotide level, within the coding region of the aerolysin gene of both isolates despite being isolated from geographically distant regions and unrelated hosts. Secondly, the A + T richness and the length of the aerC region has been conserved between the two isolates ; however ,none of the sequence features described above are detectable in the aerC-equivalent region of the fish isolate. Furthurmore, the overall nucleotide similarity between the two sequences is 47% and there are no extended regions of homology.

Taken together, the results suggest a complex regulatory function for the aerC region. The presence of several prominent repeated sequences, their juxtaposition to the promotors, the length and inherent nature of this A + T rich sequence suggest that the aerolysin gene may be regulated both negatively and positively.

```
  1   CCATGCGCCTGAGCCGCTGCCGCCAGGACGACTGACCCGCCAGCGGAAAATCCCCCCATC   60

 61   CCGGCCCATAGTTAAGGCTCCTCCTGCACTTGACCATGGGCCGCCACATGAAACCCGCCA   120

121   TCCTTCTTCTCCTCTCTCTGCCCTTTTGTATCCAGGCTGCCGGAGCGCGAACTCTGGCTG   180

181   GTGGAACTGGAACACAACGACGGCCTGCGCCTGCAGTTTCAGGGAGCCGAACTCGAACTG   240

241   GGCAGCGCCCGGCTGGAGGGCATTCGGCAGTTATCTGATTTGAGGCCCGGTATGCGTCTG   300

301   GCCATCTGAGCCGTGATGCGTGGCCGAGCCAAATTGGTCTTGCCCCCCAGGCACGGCCGT   360

361   CGGATGCCTGGCGGCGGGCGCAGGCACCCCTGATCCGCACAAGGCGCCGGGACGCTCTCG   420

                                            SD
421   ATGGCGGGGCTGGGGGAGGTGGCGTTTGATCATCATACCCGCTGGCTCAACGGGGGGCCC   480

481   GGTGACATGCAACCCGGACGCGAGCTGGTGCTGACCCGGGATGAAGCAGGGAGCCTGCAG   540

                                      <  11      10 >
541   GAGATCCTGGTCGTCAATCCGGAAGATGAAATCACGGAATAAAACCGGGAAATATCTATT   600
                                                            ***
                         <  9
601   CTCTGTCTTATCCAATAAGTCAGGATATTTAAGAATATATAAAATTGTTAGACTTTTATT   660
***   Pc·      ***

661   TCATTTAAAGAGGACCGCTTATAAGTATTTAGTCATTAAAGTGATAGCTCTAATTCAAAC   720

                            8 >                 7 >
721   GTTTTCGTCATATTGAGATCATGAAATTAAATATTCCTGCTTGAGTCTAAATAACCTCGG   780
                                              ***     Pa
                       <  6  5 >
781   CTGATATGGTGGTCTGGCGTGCTGCTTGTTAATAAAAATAACCCTCTCATTCGTGTCGTT   840
*****

        4 > SD                      3 >
841   CTCCAAAAATAAGGGGTTGCTATGAAAGCACTCAAAATAACAGGCTTGTCATTAATCATT   900
  1                   MetLysAlaLeuLysIleThrGlyLeuSerLeuIleIle      13

901   TCCGCCACGCTGGCCGCCCAGACCAATGCTGCAGAGCCCATCTATCCTGACCAGCTGCGG   960
 14   SerAlaThrLeuAlaAlaGlnThrAsnAlaAlaGluProIleTyrProAspGlnLeuArg   33

961   CTGTTCTCTCTTGGGGAAGATGTCTGCGGTACTGATTATCGTCCAATTAACCGGGAAGAA   1020
 34   LeuPheSerLeuGlyGluAspValCysGlyThrAspTyrArgProIleAsnArgGluGlu   53

1021  GCACAGAGTGTCCGGAATAATATTGTGGCCATGATGGGGCAGTGGCAAATCAGTGGGTTG   1080
 54   AlaGlnSerValArgAsnAsnIleValAlaMetMetGlyGlnTrpGlnIleSerGlyLeu   73
```

Fig 1. Sequence of the aerC region of the aerolysin gene and the amino terminal sequence of the protein. The numbers denote the presence of the core sequence ATAAAA and its respective orientation is indicated. The promotors Pa and Pc indicated are for the aerolysin gene and the putative 6.4kD polypeptide respectively. The -10 and -35 regions of the promotor are indicated with *** and the putative ribosome binding site with the letters SD.

THE ROLE OF AEROLYSIN IN AEROMONAS-ASSOCIATED INFECTIONS

The pathogenic potential of aerolysin was evaluated by constructing isogenic mutants of AH2 carrying specific deletions within the aer determinant on the chromosome. This was achieved by introducing deleted derivatives of the aer determinant, cloned onto a pMB1 -based mobilizable vector, into A. hydrophila AH 2. Such vectors are unable to replicate stably in AH 2 and are rapidly lost by segregation. In order to detect mutants, a kanamycin resistance gene from the transposon Tn 903, was used as a selectable marker with the cloned DNA sequence. The plasmid pHPC3-702 carries a 1.4kb KpnI fragment encoding resistance to kanamycin in place of the 1.8kb fragment from the aer determinant on plasmid pHPC3-700. E. coli recombinants haboring pHPC3-702 are completely devoid of both hemolytic and cytotoxic activities. This plasmid was mobilized into a spontaneously derived nalixidic acid derivative of AH 2 (AB 3). Subsequent in vivo recombination and segregation of the plasmid produced genetic recombinants that had the resident aerA aerB region replaced by the substitution mutation carried on pHPC3-702 (Fig.2.). One such recombinant was used in subsequent studies. DNA hybridization was used to confirm the genetic structure of AB 3 aer-5. Immunoblots performed with specific antisera directed against aerolysin showed that it was absent in both cell lysates and supernatant fluids of AB3 aer-5.

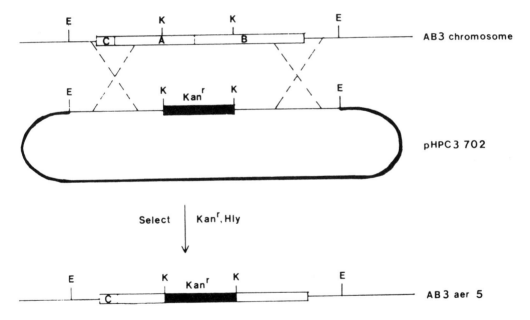

Fig 2. Construction of the aerolysin-deficient strain AB3 aer-5.A double cross-over event occuring between flanking homologous regions lead to replacement of the normal aerA aerB region by the kan[r] deletion-substitution. The 1.8kb KpnI fragment of Aeromonas DNA has been replaced by a 1.4kb KpnI fragment resistance to kanamycin.Thickened lines represent vector pSUP205 DNA sequences while open boxes depict A. hydrophila sequences. E = EcoRI; K = KpnI.

DETECTION OF THE AEROLYSIN GENE IN AEROMONAS SPP.

A gene probe comprising of a 1039bp fragment from the aerA gene was used to detect the presence of the aerolysin gene in clinical and environmental isolates of A. hydrophila. All strains tested were both hemolytic on human blood agar plates and showed cytotoxicity to Chinese Hamster Ovary and HeLa tissue culture cell lines. All 20 clinical isolates were found to have sequences homologous to the DNA probe. However, only 26 of 29 environmental isolates showed homology to the DNA probe. This suggested the presence of a second cytotoxic haemolysin in this species.

MOLECULAR CLONING OF A SECOND CYTOTOXIC HAEMOLYSIN FROM A.HYDROPHILA

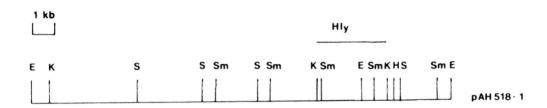

Fig. 3. A partial restriction endonuclease map of the Aeromonas DNA insert in plasmid pAH518-1. The region encoding the cytotoxic hemolysin is shown. E = EcoRI; H = HindIII; K = KpnI; S = SalI; Sm = SmaI.

A gene bank from a strain devoid of aerolysin sequences was constructed and screened for the presence of a cytotoxin. Eleven cosmid clones were obtained that showed cytotoxicity to Chinese Hamster Ovary cells. All clones were also found to possess haemolytic activity. Digestion with restriction endonucleases showed fragments common to all cosmid clones. One such recombinant, designated pAH 518 was used in furthur studies. A partial map of a subclone pAH 518-1 harbouring two contigous EcoRI fragments is shown in Fig.3 . The region coding for the haemolytic activity was determined by deleting pAH518-1 with restriction endonucleases and the minimal fragment still encoding haemolytic activity is located on a 2.1 KpnI fragment depicted in Fig.3 . E. coli recombinants harboring this recombinant also exhibit cytotoxicity in the CHO tissue culture assay. A polypeptide of 58kD is common to all recombinants expressing hemolytic and cytotoxic activity. No cross reacting polypeptides were detected in an immunoblot assay using specific antisera to aerolysin. As expected, recombinants harboring the second hemolysin do not hybridize to the aerolysin gene probe. A cytotoxic activity not neutralizable by specific antiserum to aerolysin has recently been reported in Aeromonas spp.(Notermans, 1986). The cloning of a second cytotoxic factor should now allow

We next determined the 50% lethal dose (LD_{50}) of both the parental strain and its isogenic aerolysin-deficient mutant. The results are depicted in Table 1. Intraperitoneal injection of mice with the parental strain AB3 showed a LD_{50} of around 5×10^7 cells while the aerolysin-strain had a LD_{50} of more than 8×10^8 cells. To exclude the possibility that unlinked mutations affecting toxicity had been introduced during the construction of AB 3 aer-5, we reintroduced the wild type aer determinant into this strain. A double cross-over event leading to integration of the wild type ·aerA aerB genes was detected by plating on blood agar plates and scoring for hemolytic colonies. Several stable transconjugants were obtained, and one such transconjugant (AB3 aer-5 rev-1) was checked for its genetic structure using DNA hybridization and for aerolysin production in hemolysin and cytotoxin assays. As can be seen from Table 1, full toxicity was regained with the strain AB 3aer-5 rev-1 which had regained a LD_{50} of 5×10^7 cells.

All deaths of mice were recorded 30h post inoculation; the majority of mice succumbed 18h after i.p. injection. Pure cultures of AB 3 could be isolated form individually homogenized livers and spleens of dead mice. High concentrations of bacteria were also detected in the blood samples of these mice. No loss of antibiotic markers could be detected upon plating onto selective/non-selective plates. These results clearly demonstrate the association of toxin with lethality in mice extends previous results obtained with wild type isolates producing varying levels of aerolysin (Daily,1981). The systemic infection obtained with the mouse model is rapid, reflecting well the rapid course of wound infections and septicemia seen with human infections.

Table 1. Mortality of mice after peritoneal injection of AB3, AB3 aer-5 and AB3 aer-5 rev-1.

Strain	No. of cells injected	No. of mice dead/ No. tested
AB3 [a]	8×10^8	5/5
	6×10^8	9/9
	4×10^8	5/5
	2×10^8	5/5
	1×10^8	3/5
	5×10^7	1/5
AB3-5 [b]	8×10^8	0/5
	6×10^8	1/9
	4×10^8	0/5
	2×10^8	0/5
	1×10^8	0/5
	5×10^7	0/5
AB3-5 rev1 [c]	8×10^8	5/5
	6×10^8	5/5
	4×10^8	5/5
	2×10^8	5/5
	1×10^8	3/5
	5×10^7	2/5

clarification on the presence and role of this toxin in Aeromonas infections.

REFERENCES

Buckley, J.T., L.N. Halasa K.D. Lund and S. Macintyre (1981). Purification and some propertìes of the hemolytic toxin aerolysin. Can. J. Biochem. 59,430-435.

Chakraborty,T., B. Huhle, H. Bergbauer and W. Goebel (1986). Cloning, expression and mapping of the Aeromonas hydrophila aerolysin gene determinant in Escherichia coli K-12. J. Bacteriol. 167, 368-374.

Daily,O.P., S.W. Joseph, J.C. Coolbaugh and colleagues (1981). Association of Aeromonas sobria with human infection. J. Clin. Microbiol. 13, 769-777.

Freij,B.J. (1984). Aeromonas: biology of the organism and diseases of children. Pediatr. Infec. Dis. 3, 164-175.

Gracey,M., V. Burke and J. Robinsin (1982). Aeromonas associated gastroenteritis. Lancet ii. 1304-1306.

Grant, G.S. and M. Kehoe (1984). Primary sequence of the alpha toxin gene from Staphylococcus aureus Wood 46. Infec. Immun. 46, 615-618.

Howard, S.P. and J.T. Buckley (1982). Membrane glycoprotein receptor and hole forming properties of a cytolytic protein toxin. Biochemistry.21, 1662-1667.

Howard S.P., and J.T. Buckley (1985). Activation of the hole forming toxin aerolysin by extracellular processing. J. Bacteriol. 163, 336-340.

Howard, S.P. and J.T. Buckley (1986). Molecular cloning and expression in Escherichia coli of the structural gene for the hemolytic toxin aerolysin from Aeromonas hydrophila. Mol. Gen. Genet. 204, 289-295.

Janda, J.M., E. J. Bottone, C. V. Sinner and D. Calcaterra (1983). Phenotypic markers associated with gastrointestinal Aeromonas hydrophila isolates from symptomatic children. J. Clin. Microbiol. 17, 588-591.

McClure, W.R. (1985). Mechanism and control of transcription initiation in procaryotes. Ann. Rev. Biochem. 54, 171-204.

Mekalanos, J.J., D.J. Swartz, G.D.N. Pearson and colleagues (1983). Cholera toxin genes: Nucleotide sequence, deletion analysis and vaccine development. Nature. 306, 551-557.

Mizuno,.T., M.-Y. Chou, and M. Inouye (1983). A comparative study on the genes for the three porins of Escherichia coli outer membrane. J. Biol. Chem. 258, 6932-6940.

Notermans, S.H.W., A. Havelaar, W. Jansen and colleagues (1986). Production of "Asao Toxin" by Aeromonas strains isolated from feces and drinking water. J. Clin. Microbiol. 23, 1140-42.

Thelestam, M., and Ljungh A. (1981). Membrane demaging and cytotoxic effects on human fibroblasts of alpha- and beta-hemolysin from Aeromonas hydrophila. Infec. Immun. 34, 949-954.

Fehrenbach et al. (Eds.), Bacterial Protein Toxins, Zbl. Bakt. Suppl. 17
© Gustav Fischer, Stuttgart, New York, 1988

Epitope Mapping of the S1 Subunit of Pertussis Toxin

A. Bartoloni, M. Bigio, R. Rossi and R. Rappuoli[1]
A. Robinson, L. A. E. Ashworth and L. I. Irons[2]
D. Burns and C. Manclark[3]
H. Sato[4]

[1]Sclavo Research Center, Via Fiorentina 1, 53100 Siena, Italy
[2]Vaccine Research and Production Laboratory, Porton Down, Salisbury, Wilts, SP4 OJG, England
[3]Division of Bacterial Products, Center for Drugs and Biologics, Food and Drug Administration, Bethesda, MA 20892, U.S.A.
[4]Department of Applied Immunology, National Institute of Health 10–35, 2-Chome, Kamiosaki Shinagawa-ku, Tokyo, Japan

Monoclonal antibodies against the S1 subunit of pertussis toxin have been shown to be able to protect mice from the intracerebral challenge with virulent B. pertussis, and CHO cells from the toxic effect of pertussis toxin (Sato et al., 1984). This observation raised the possibility that the S1 subunit could be used as a vaccine against whooping cough. Following the cloning and sequencing of the pertussis toxin operon (Nicosia et al., 1986; Locht and Keith, 1986), the S1 subunit was expressed in large amounts as a fusion protein in E. coli (Nicosia et al., 1987). The S1 fusion protein showed the same NAD-ribosyl transferase activity of pertussis toxin, suggesting that the natural and recombinant S1 subunits had a similar folding.

The recombinant S1 subunit was used to immunize mice, rabbits and goat and, although we obtained high titer antibodies which recognized the native pertussis toxin as well as the recombinant molecule, little protection was observed either in vitro (CHO cells assay) or in vivo (intracerebral challenge of mice). In order to solve this apparent discrepancy (the observation that monoclonal antibodies against the subunit S1 are able to neutralize the activity of the toxin, while polyclonal antibodies against the same subunit are not able to do so), we decided to map the epitopes recognized by the protective monoclonal antibodies.

We have expressed in E. coli the S1 subunit of pertussis toxin, the corresponding subunits from B. parapertussis and B. bronchiseptica (which have 11 and 4 aminoacid substitutions respectively, Arico' and Rappuoli, 1987) and several 5' and 3' deletions of the S1 subunit. Following partial purification, the recombinant molecules have been used in a Western blot assay for reaction with a panel of anti-S1 monoclonal antibodies obtained from different laboratories. Preliminary data show that these reagents will allow fine mapping of the epitopes of the subunit S1; in fact, some of the monoclonal antibodies recognize only part of the constructions and many of the do not recognize the full length molecules of B. parapertussis and/or B. bronchiseptica which differ by only a few aminoacid substitutions.

References

Arico', B., and R. Rappuoli (1987). Bordetella parapertussis and Bordetella bronchiseptica contain transcriptionally silent pertussis toxin genes. J. Bacteriol., 169, 2847-2853.

Locht, C., and J.M. Keith (1986). Pertussis toxin gene: nucleotide sequence and genetic organization. Science, 232, 1258-1264.

Nicosia, A., M. Perugini, C. Franzini, M.C. Casagli, M.G. Borri, G. Antoni, M. Almoni, P. Neri, G. Ratti, and R. Rappuoli (1986) Cloning and sequencing of the pertussis toxin genes: operon structure and gene duplication. Proc. Natl. Acad. Sci. USA, 83, 4631-4635.

Nicosia, A., and R. Rappuoli (1987). Promoter of the pertussis toxin operon and production of pertussis toxin. J. Bacteriol., 169, 2843-2846.

Sato, Y., M. Kimura, and H. Fukimi (1984). Development of a pertussis component vaccines. Infect. Immun., 46, 422-428.

Fehrenbach et al. (Eds.), Bacterial Protein Toxins, Zbl. Bakt. Suppl. 17
© Gustav Fischer, Stuttgart, New York, 1988

Specificity and Synergism of Bacillus Thuringiensis israelensis Toxins on Mosquito Larvae

C. Bourgouin, A. Delecluse and G. Rapoport

Unité de Biochimie Microbienne, Institut Pasteur, Rue du Docteur Roux, 28, F-75724 Paris Cedex 15

Bacillus thuringiensis israelensis (Bti) during sporulation produces crystalline inclusions toxic to larvae of Diptera such as mosquito and blackfly that are vectors of tropical diseases (malaria, onchocerciasis). The crystals are made of three main polypeptides with molecular weight of 28 kDa, 68 kDa and 130 kDa. The crystal genes have been located on a 72 MDa plasmid by curing experiments. In addition to the toxicity to dipteran larvae, the solubilized crystal is haemolytic for erythrocytes. Whereas the haemolytic activity has been attributed to the 28 kDa protein, the larvicidal protein was not clearly identified. Some authors proposed a synergistic action between at least two of the 3 main proteins of the crystal (Wu and Chang, 1985). One way to resolve this issue was to clone the crystal protein genes. We cloned the 28 kDa and the 130 kDa protein genes (Bourgouin and others, 1986) from the 72 MDa plasmid of Bti 4Q2-72. The 28 kDa protein gene was similar to the gene cloned by others and it was shown that the gene product is responsible for the haemolytic activity. Recombinant clone RX8 containing the 130 kDa protein gene was highly active against both Culex pipiens and Aedes aegypti larvae. The region encoding the 130 kDa was similar to the gene cloned by Sekar and Carlton (1985) but as well as the 130 kDa gene, plasmid pRX8 also contains the 2 ORFs (ORF1, ORF2) previously cloned and sequenced by Thorne and others (1986).

In order to determine the role of the 130 kDa gene and the ORF1 and ORF2 in the mosquitocidal activity, we subcloned the 130 kDa gene and the ORF1-ORF2 in the plasmids pRX8-2 and pRX8-3, respectively (fig). The recombinant clones RX8-2

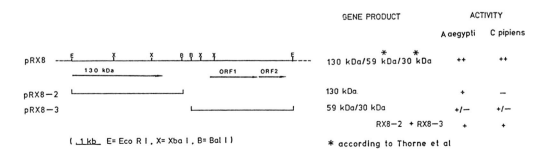

and RX8-3 were assayed for toxicity on both A. aegypti and C. pipiens larvae. Clone RX8-2 was specifically toxic to A. aegypti larvae, with a weaker activity than clone RX8, and not active on C. pipiens larvae. Weak toxicity of RX8-3 was detected both on A. aegypti or on C. pipiens larvae. However, when cultures of RX8-2 and RX8-3 were mixed, the activity on C. pipiens larvae was restored.

These results indicate that, first the 130 kDa protein is specifically active against A. aegypti larvae, and secondly that the activity of the mixed clones on larvae of C. pipiens is due to a synergistic action between the 130 kDa and products of ORF1 and ORF2. Experiments are in progress to characterize the products of the two ORFs and to determine if both are involved in the synergism described here. We do not know whether such a synergistic effect occurs in vivo. We showed that the purified 130 kDa protein fraction was active against A. aegypti larvae and also against C. pipiens larvae. The discrepancy between this result and those obtained with the cloned 130 kDa protein could be explained by two hypothesese : a) the 130 kDa fraction used contained undetectable amounts of ORF1-ORF2 products which act in synergism, or b) as observed, this fraction contained two molecular species of 130 kDa protein, and one could be specifically active on A. aegypti larvae and the other one on C. pipiens larvae.

Bourgouin, C., A. Klier, and G. Rapoport (1986). Characterization of the genes encoding the haemolytic toxin and the mosquitocidal delta-endotoxin of Bacillus thuringiensis israelensis. Mol. Gen. Genet., 205, 390-397.

Sekar, V., and B. C. Carlton (1985). Molecular cloning of the delta-endotoxin gene of Bacillus thuringiensis var. israelensis. Gene, 33, 151-158.

Thorne, L., F. Garduno, T. Thompson, D. Decker, M. Zounes, M. Wild, A. M. Walfield, and T. J. Pollock (1986). Structural similarity between the Lepidoptera -and Diptera- specific insecticidal endotoxin genes of Bacillus thuringiensis subsp. "kurstaki" and "israelensis". J. Bacteriol., 166, 801-811.

Wu, D., and F. N. Chang (1985). Synergism in mosquitocidal activity of 26 and 65 kDa protein from Bacillus thuringiensis subsp. israelensis crystal. FEBS Lett., 190, 232-236.

Fehrenbach et al. (Eds.), Bacterial Protein Toxins, Zbl. Bakt. Suppl. 17
© Gustav Fischer, Stuttgart, New York, 1988

Molecular Cloning of the Adenylate Cyclase Toxin of Bordetella Pertussis

R. M. Brownlie, J. G. Coote and R. Patron

Department of Microbiology, University of Glasgow, Glasgow G12 6QH, U. K.

ABSTRACT

A recombinant plasmid, pRMB1, was identified which restored adenylate cyclase
(AC) and haemolytic activities to a Tn5-insertion mutant of B. pertussis,
BP348. However, B. pertussis AC activity was not expressed in E. coli
harbouring pRMB1. A 10 kb BamH1 fragment from pRMB1 was subcloned into the
expression vectors pIC20H and pGLW11. Expression of the B. pertussis AC only
occurred when the BamH1 fragment was inserted in the correct orientation with
respect to the promoters contained in the vectors. Although expression of AC
depended on a promoter from the vector, the AC was translated from its own
start codon. However, AC activity in E. coli harbouring recombinant plasmids
was about 100-fold less than that in B. pertussis.

KEYWORDS

Adenylate cyclase, molecular cloning, Bordetella pertussis, expression,
haemolysin.

INTRODUCTION

Bordetella pertussis produces an adenylate cyclase (AC) which differs from
that of other prokaryotes in being largely extra-cytoplasmic and activated by
the eukaryotic regulatory protein calmodulin. This AC is now recognized as a
toxin from its ability to enter and intoxicate a variety of mammalian cells by
elevation of their cAMP levels. It has been suggested that AC may assist
survival of the pathogen in the host by interfering with phagocyte function
(Confer and Eaton, 1982). Here we describe the cloning of the AC genes and
their expression in E. coli.

RESULTS AND DISCUSSION

A gene library of B. pertussis was constructed in the broad-host-range vector
pLAFR1. Recombinant plasmids were transferred by conjugation to a Tn5-
insertion mutant of B. pertussis, BP348 (Weiss and others, 1983). A plasmid,
designated pRMB1, was identified which restored both the haemolytic and AC
activities to strain BP348. However, AC activity was not detected in

cytoplasmic fractions of E. coli DH1 harbouring pRMB1 (Table 1).
In Southern blot analysis, a hybridization probe to pRMB1 hybridized to the
same BamH1 fragments of both B. pertussis and B. parapertussis chromosomal
DNA, but not to any chromosomal fragments from three strains of the related
B. avium.
A 10 kb BamH1 fragment from pRMB1 was subcloned into the expression vector
pIC20H (which contains a lacZ promoter) to give a plasmid designated pRMB3, and
into the expression vector pGLW11 (which contains a tac promoter) in different
orientations to give plasmids designated pRMB6 and pRMB7. These plasmids were
transferred by transformation into E. coli CAA8306 (cya). AC activity was
detected in cytoplasmic fractions of E. coli CAA8306 when harbouring pRMB3 or
pRMB6 but not when harbouring pIC20H or pRMB7 (Table 1). This activity was
enhanced when calmodulin was present in the reaction mixture. It would appear
that the AC structural gene was transcribed from the lacZ promoter in the case
of pRMB3 and from the tac promoter in the case of pRMB6. As expression from the
tac promoter of pGLW11 requires a start codon, the 10 kb BamH1 fragment must
contain the start codon of the AC structural gene. Specific AC activity in
E. coli CAA8306 harbouring either pRMB3 or pRMB6 was about 100-fold less than
that obtained from B. pertussis cytoplasmic fractions and this may be due to
inefficient translation of the B. pertussis DNA in E. coli. Further work is
required to determined whether the AC enzymic activity, expressed in E. coli,
also has "toxic" activity and is able to elevate cAMP levels in neutrophils.

Table 1 Expression of adenylate cyclase activity in E. coli
strains harbouring cloned B. pertussis DNA.

Strain	Adenylate cyclase activity (pmol cAMP min^{-1} mg^{-1} protein)	
	Calmodulin absent	Calmodulin present[1]
E. coli DH1 pRMB1	<1[2]	<1
E. coli CAA8306 pIC20H	<1	<1
E. coli CAA8306 pRMB3	5.1	31.3
E. coli CAA8306 pRMB6	5.2	25.6
E. coli CAA8306 pRMB7	<1	<1

Supernates of sonicated cells were assayed for AC activity. 1, Bovine liver
catalase (Sigma; 1mg ml^{-1} final conc.) was used as a source of calmodulin.
2, Limit of detection.

ACKNOWLEDGEMENTS

We are grateful to Dr. A. Weiss and Dr. B. Kiely for kindly providing strains.
This work was supported by a grant from the Medical Research Council.

REFERENCES

Confer, D.L. and Eaton, J.W. (1982). Phagocyte impotence caused by invasive
bacterial adenylate cyclase. Science, 217, 948-950.
Weiss, A.A., Hewlett, E.L., Myers, G.A. and Falkow, S. (1983). Tn5-induced
mutations affecting virulence factors of Bordetella pertussis. Infection and
Immunity, 42, 33-41.

Fehrenbach et al. (Eds.), Bacterial Protein Toxins, Zbl. Bakt. Suppl. 17
© Gustav Fischer, Stuttgart, New York, 1988

The Gamma-Haemolysin Determinant of Staphylococcus aureus Comprises Two Linked Cistrons

J. C. Cooney, J. P. Arbuthnott and T. J. Foster

Department of Microbiology, Moyne Institute, Trinity College, Dublin 2, Ireland

ABSTRACT

The determinant coding for the γ-haemolysin of S. aureus has been cloned. It comprises of two linked cistrons, hlgA and hlgB, which code for 32 kDa and 36 kDa polypeptides components of γ-toxin, respectively.

KEYWORDS

Gamma-haemolysin, gamma-toxin, molecular cloning, Tn5 mutagenesis, complementation, minicells, Western blotting.

INTRODUCTION

Gamma-haemolysin (γ-toxin) of S. aureus requires the synergistic action of two polypeptides (Guyonnet et al., 1968; Taylor and Bernheimer 1974). The role of γ-toxin in the pathogenesis of S. aureus infections is not known. Elevated anti-γ-toxin titres were detected in sera of osteomyelitis patients (Taylor and Plommet, 1973) showing that the toxin is expressed during chronic infections. The unusual haemolytic pattern of Toxic Shock Syndrome-associated S. aureus isolated is due to the expression of γ-toxin by strains that lack the capacity to synthesize α- or β-toxins (Clyne et al., 1987).
    The hlg determinant from strain Smith 5R has been cloned (Mulvey and Arbuthnott, 1986). Here we report genetic analysis of the cloned hlg determinant by Tn5 mutagenesis. Two cistrons have been identified and characterized by in vitro complementation tests, and their gene products, have been identified.

RESULTS

An 3kb HindIII fragment was cloned from λhlg into pBR322, but was weakly haemolytic. A 6kb fragment was then subcloned into the expression vector pKK233-2 to form pJC09. Zones of haemolysis were readily detectable around E. coli (pJC09) colonies after incubation for 16 h.
    Several Tn5 insertions which lacked haemolytic activity were isolated and mapped (Fig 1). Lysates of E. coli cells carrying the mutant plasmids were loaded into wells in agarose incorporating rabbit erythrocytes. Enhanced haemolysis was

observed between several of the extracts. This *in vitro* complementation defined
two cistrons (hlgA and hlgB) (Fig 1), which are separated by about 300bp.
Southern hybridization analysis of genomic DNA with hlgA and hlgB probes confirmed
that hlgA and hlgB are linked in the *S. aureus* chromosome.

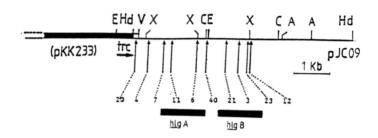

Fig 1:   Map of pJCO9
The vertical lines indicate the positions of Tn5 insertions,
the bars labelled hlgA and hlgB are the deduced locations
of the two cistrons. Restriction sites are abbreviated as
follows: A, Accl; C, Clal; E, EcoRl; Hd, HindIII; V,
EcoRv; X, Xbal.

Western immunoblotting and minicel experiments showed that hlgA encodes a polypeptide of 32 kDa while hlgB specifies a 36 kDa protein which correspond to the
polypeptide components of purified γ-toxin (M. Clyne, personal communication).
This was confirmed by the *in vitro* complementation that also occured (i) between
extracts of *E. coli* carring pJCO9 hlgA::Tn5 and the purified 36 kDa peptide and
(ii) between *E. coli* pJCO9 hlgB::Tn5 extracts and the purified 32 kDa protein.

ACKNOWLEDGEMENTS

We are grateful to Marguerite Clyne for generously supplying purified γ-toxin
and antiserum.

REFERENCES

Clyne, M., J.C.S. de Azavedo and J.P. Arbuthnott, 1987. Production of gamma
   hemolysin by Toxic Shock Syndrome associated strains of *Staphylococcus aureus*
   (Manuscript in preparation).

Guyonnet, F., M. Plommet and C. Bouillane 1968. Purification de l'hemolysine
   gamma de *Staphylococcus aureus*. C.R. Acad. Sci. 267: 1180-1182.

Taylor, A.G. and A.W. Bernheimer 1974. Further characteristics of Staphylococcal
   gamma haemolysin. Infect. Immun. 10: 54-59.

Taylor, A.G. and M. Plommet 1973. anti gamma-haemolysin as a diagnostic test in
   staphylococcal osteomyelitis. J. Clin. Path. 26: 409-412.

Fehrenbach et al. (Eds.), Bacterial Protein Toxins, Zbl. Bakt. Suppl. 17
© Gustav Fischer, Stuttgart, New York, 1988

Genetic Regulation of the Exported Virulence Protein (YOPs) of Yersinia

G. Cornelis, J.-C. Vanooteghem, M.-P. Sory, T. Michiels, T. Biot and C. Sluiters

Unité de Microbiologie, Université de Louvain UCL 54.90 B-1200 Bruxelles

ABSTRACT

The product of *virF* acts as a diffusible positive regulator of the virulence functions of *Yersiniae*. It activates transcription of plasmid genes encoding excreted proteins (*yop* genes) at 37°C. Its own transcription appears to be thermodependent. It acts on yop genes from *Y.pseudotuberculosis* as well as on genes from *Y.enterocolitica*.
The region encoding *virF* governs in *E. coli* the synthesis of two polypeptides of 19 and 21 kDa. It is not yet clear whether the product of *virF* is one of these polypeptides.

KEYWORDS

Yop, *Yersinia*, virulence, regulon.

INTRODUCTION

Virulent *Y.enterocolitica* strains restrict their growth at 37°C, in rich medium deprived of calcium. This property, called calcium dependency, correlates with pathogenicity. It is conditioned by a 70kb plasmid called pYV. A 20 kb region of this plasmid, containing at least four genes called *virA, B, C* and *F* conditions the requirement for calcium at 37°C (Cornelis *et al.*1986). In growth restriction conditions, *Y.enterocolitica* releases several pYV encoded proteins (POMPs). The genes encoding these proteins (*yop* genes) are scattered over pYV, outside the calcium region. Transcription of these *yop* genes increases by factors of 3.5 (*yop*84) to 200 (*yop*51) when temperature is shifted from 25 to 37°C. Mutations in *virF* severely affects transcription of *yop*51 (Cornelis *et al.*1987). The aim of the present work was to characterize *virF*.

RESULTS

1. The mutation in plasmid pGC1152-9 defining *virF* consists of an insertion of Tn*813* into *Eco*R1 fragment 8 of pYV. This mutation suppresses the calcium requirement for growth at 37°C and prevents the production of POMPs. *Bam*H1 restriction fragment

6 of pYV was cloned onto the mobilizable vector pSUP202. *Y.enterocolitica* W22703(pGC1152-9)(pSUP202-B6) was found to restrict its growth and to release the POMPs at 37°C in absence of calcium. Hence, mutations in *virF* can be complemented in trans.

2. In order to estimate the role of *virA*, *B*, *C* and *F* on transcription of the yops, we cloned the gene *yop*51 onto a mobilizable derivative of ∾pACYC184. We subsequently tackled *yop*51 with transposon Tn2507 containing the *cat* gene without its promotor. This construct, called pTM243, was introduced in W22703 carrying a wild-type pYV plasmid or *virA*, *B*, *C* and *F* mutants. The cat gene of pTM243 was efficiently transcribed at 37°C but not at 25°C, in the presence of pYV. Mutations in *virA*, *B* and *C* reduced transcription while *virF* completely abolished transcription.

3. Sub-clones of fragment B6 were tested for their ability to complement pGC1152-9. Among the clones tested, only one, called pGC630, spanning coordinates 31-35.6 kb of pYV did complement. In particular, *Eco*R1 fragment 8, spanning 32.8-34 kb did not complement.

4. In *E.coli* minicells, plasmid pGC630 directed the synthesis of two polypeptides of MW 19 and 21 kDa. *Eco*R1 fragment 8 encodes the 21 kDa polypeptide.

5. *Y.enterocolitica* W22703(pTM243) does not transcribe *cat*. However, there is clear thermodependant transcription of *cat* in W22703(pTM243) (p630). Hence, *virF* acts independently of other pYV genes.

6. Transcription of *virF* was analyzed by Northern blot, using *Eco*R1 fragment 8 as a probe. Strong transcripts of approximately 1500 and 1150 nucleotides were detected in cultures of *Y.enterocolitica* W22703(pYV) shifted for 2 hours at 37°C. Transcripts were much less abundant in cultures maintained at 25°C.

7. In order to check whether *virF* from *Y.enterocolitica* could activate transcription of a *yop* gene from *Y.pseudotuberculosis*, we introduced the gene *yop*26 from *Y. pseudotuberculosis* into *Y.enterocolitica* W22703(pGC1256), a mutant affected in the corresponding *yop*25 gene. The recombinant *Y.enterocolitica* clearly produced the 26 Kda protein of *Y.pseudotuberculosis*.

REFERENCES

Cornelis G., Sory M.-P., Laroche Y., and Derclaye I. (1986). Genetic analysis of the plasmid region controlling virulence in *Yersinia enterocolitica* 0:9 by mini-mu insertions and *lac* gene fusions. Microbial Pathogenesis, 1, 349-359.
Cornelis G., Vanooteghem J.-C., and Sluiters C. (1987). Transcription of the yop regulon from *Y. enterocolitica* requires trans acting pYV and chromosomal genes.Microbial Pathogenesis, 2, 367-379.

Fehrenbach et al. (Eds.), Bacterial Protein Toxins, Zbl. Bakt. Suppl. 17
© Gustav Fischer, Stuttgart, New York, 1988

Regulation of Pertussis Toxin Expression

R. Gross, A. Nicosia, B. Aricò and R. Rappuoli
Sclavo Research Centre, Via Fiorentina 1, 53100 Siena, Italy

Pertussis toxin is expressed by virulent B. pertussis (phase I), but not by avirulent B. pertussis (phase III) strains and by phase I B. parapertussis and B. bronchiseptica. It has been proposed that a transactivating factor (Vir), present in phase I but not in phase III B. pertussis strains, is necessary for the expression of pertussis toxin and other virulence factors. Cloning of the pertussis toxin genes from B. pertussis (Nicosia, 1986) has allowed us to investigate the regulation of their expression at the molecular level. Recently it has been shown that the expression of the pertussis toxin operon is regulated on the transcriptional level (Nicosia, 1987).

For the present study we have constructed a promotor probe vector for Bordetella and we use this vector to investigate the regulation of pertussis toxin expression. By deletion analysis of the 5' untranslated region of the pertussis toxin operon we demonstrate that a sequence upstream of the promotor up to the –170 region is necessary for the expression and that this region is inactive in phase III organisms. We also transferred the various constructions into phase I B. parapertussis and B. bronchiseptica and we show that these species are able to activate the pertussis toxin promotor as efficiently as B. pertussis. Both species contain the complete toxin operon, but do not transcribe it (Aricò, 1987a). It has been speculated that the reason for this is the accumulation of mutations in the promotor region of these species. Therefore we cloned the 5' untranslated region upstream of the promotor from B. bronchiseptica in front of the promotor from B. pertussis. We show that this construction is indeed inactive. Recently it has been shown that the B. pertussis strain 18323 contains several common mutations with B. parapertussis and B. bronchiseptica in the promotor region (Aricò, 1987b)). This strain has been shown to produce much less pertussis toxin than other B. pertussis isolates, probably due to these mutations in the regulatory region of the pertussis toxin operon.

REFERENCES

Aricò, B., Rappuoli, R. (1987). <u>Bordetella parapertussis</u> and <u>Bordetella bronchiseptica</u> contain transcriptionally silent pertussis toxin genes. <u>J. Bacteriol.</u>, <u>169</u>.

Aricò, B., Gross, R., Smida, J., Rappuoli, R. (1987). Evolutionary relationships in the Genus <u>Bordetella</u>. Submitted.

Nicosia, A., Perugini, M., Franzini, C., Casagli, M.C., Bossi, M.G., Antoni, G., Almoni, M., Neri, P., Ratti, G. and Rappuoli, R. (1986). Cloning and sequencing of the pertussis toxin genes: operon structure and gene duplication. <u>Proc. Natl. Acad. Sci.</u>, <u>83</u>, pp. 4631–4635.

Nicosia, A., Rappuoli, R. (1987). Promoter of the pertussis toxin operon and production of pertussis toxin. <u>J. Bacteriol.</u>, <u>169</u>.

Fehrenbach et al. (Eds.), Bacterial Protein Toxins, Zbl. Bakt. Suppl. 17
© Gustav Fischer, Stuttgart, New York, 1988

Cloning and Expression in Escherichia coli of the α-Toxin Determinant from Clostridium perfringens

D. Leslie[1], N. Fairweather[2], C. Dougan[2] and M. Kehoe[1]

[1]Department of Microbiology, Medical School, University of Newcastle upon Tyne,
 Framlington Place, Newcastle upon Tyne, NE2 4HH, U.K.
[2]Wellcome Biotechnology Ltd., Langley Court, Beckenham, Kent, BR3 3BS, U.K.

Clostridium perfringens has been reported to produce as many as seventeen different toxins, which are designated by the letters of the Greek alphabet (1). The species is divided into five toxigenic types according to the ability of strains to produce particular combinations of the four major toxins, namely the α, β, ϵ, and ι-toxins (2). The large number of different toxins which can be produced by each strain makes it difficult to assess the contribution of individual toxins to virulence or to purify individual toxins in sufficient quantities for studies on their structure or mechanisms of action. Most studies to date have utilised partially purified toxin preparations or crude anti-toxin sera (3). To overcome these problems we have initiated a genetic analysis of C. perfringens toxins by cloning toxin determinants in E. coli.

Like other workers (4), we initially encountered difficulties in expressing cloned C. perfringens genes in E. coli. To avoid potential problems of promoter recognition, we cloned Eco RI generated fragments of C. perfringens Type A DNA in front of a strong E. coli promoter (into the cat gene of pACYC184). E. coli harbouring one of the resulting recombinants, called pDAZ 01, expressed a C. perfringens haemolysin at easily detectable levels. This haemolysin possesses properties which identify it as the C. perfringens α- toxin. It causes a hot-cold haemolysis of human and sheep erythrocytes and produces a lethicinase activity on egg yolk plates. Both of these activities are inhibited by anti-alpha toxin serum. The material released from the periplasm of E. coli / pACYC184 by osmotic shock contains low levels of phospholipase C activity detectable by in vitro assays employing p-Nitrophenylphoshorylcholine as substrate. This activity is increased 4-5 fold in strains harbouring pDAZ 01. The recombinant phospholipase C activity, but not the control level, is completely inhibited by anti-alpha toxin serum. In addition, the anti-alpha serum reacts with a M_r 43,000 polypeptide in immunoblots of total cell protein from E. coli/pDAZ 01, whereas this polypeptide is not expressed by the control, E. coli/pACYC184 strain. The DNA sequences cloned in pDAZ01 hybridize under high stringency conditions to DNA isolated from type A   C. perfringens.

The data summarised above indicates that the C. perfringens α-toxin determinant has been cloned and is expressed in E. coli. The cloned gene will facilitate studies on the structural relationships between the α-toxin and phospholipase C s produced by other pathogenic bacteria, and studies on the role of κ-toxin in virulence.

REFERENCES

1. Smith, L.Ds. (1979) Reviews of Infectious Diseases 1 (2) 254-262.
2. McDonel J.L. (1986) In Pharmacology of Bacterial Toxins pp. 477-517 Eds Dornor, F. and Drews, J.
3. Möllby, R., Nord, C.E. and Wadstrom, T. (1973) Toxicon 11 : 139-147.
4. Garnier, T. and Cole S.T. (1986) J. Bact. 168(3) 1189-1196.

Fehrenbach et al. (Eds.), Bacterial Protein Toxins, Zbl. Bakt. Suppl. 17
© Gustav Fischer, Stuttgart, New York, 1988

Cloning of the Genetic Determinant of the Group B Streptococcal Hemolysin in E. Coli

R. Lütticken, O. Schneewind, A. Schmidt and E. Mühlenbrock

Institut für Hygiene, Universität Köln, Goldenfelsstr. 21, D-5000 Köln 41

ABSTRACT

Chromosomal DNA from a CAMP factor-negative *Streptococcus agalactiae* strain was used to clone the determinant of the group B streptococcal hemolysin in *E. coli.*. Plasmid pUC8 was used as vector. One *E. coli* colony carried a recomibant plasmid pCO707, which confers hemolytic activity to several *E. coli* hosts. Hemolytic activity of the respective strains was consistently on blood agar plates and in broth medium containing starch. By transposon mutagenesis the genetic determinant for hemolysis could be located to a DNA fragment of about 800 base pairs.

KEYWORDS

Hemolysin, group B streptococcus, *Streptococcus agalactiae* , genetics.

Several attempts to purify the hemolysin from *Streptococcus agalactiae* (group B streptococcus = GBS) have been reported on, in order elucidate the chemical nature and mode of action of this potential virulence factor (Dal and Monteil, 1983, 1984; Ferrieri, 1982; Marchlewicz and Duncan, 1980, 1981; Tsaihong and Wennerstrom, 1983). In none of these studies purifaction of free hemolysin to homogeneity could be achieved; this is largely due to the fact that the group B streptococcal hemolysin (GBS Hly) can only be detected in culture supernatants when a carrier molecule is present, like serum albumin, starch or other macromolecules. Moreover, the GBS Hly seems to be non-immunogenic. Nevertheless its sensitivity to proteolytic enzymes points to its proteinaceous nature. Thus, it resembles streptolysin S from *S. pyogenes* in many respects.

To obtain a deeper insight in this interesting cytolysin, we performed a study on its genetic basis. For this purpose chromosomal DNA from the ß-hemolyzing GBS strain 74-360 (CAMP factor-negative) was cloned into *E. coli* MC1000 (Casabadan and Cohen, 1980) using pUC8 (Vieira and Messing, 1982) as plasmid vector and employing standard recombinant DNA techniques.

One *E. coli* clone obtained, clearly shows ß-hemolysis on blood agar plates and in blood broth containing starch. The recombinant plasmid identified in this clone, pCO707, carries a 3.9 kilobases (kb) insert of streptococcal DNA (Fig. 1). This insert was further characterized physically and functionally by restriction enzymes and by transposon mutagenesis with Tn5 (McKinnon, Bacchetti, and Graham, 1982). The results of these experiments (depicted in Fig. 1) localized the GBS hemolysin determinant (GBS hly) on a DNA fragment of about 0.8 kb. Plasmid pCO707 also confers the Hly+ phenotype to two other *E. coli* hosts, JM103 and DH5 respectively. In none of the *E. coli* transformants pigment production was observed although this trait apparently is genetically linked with the Hly determinant in the orignial streptococcal host (Wennerstrom, Tsaihong, and Crawford, 1985).

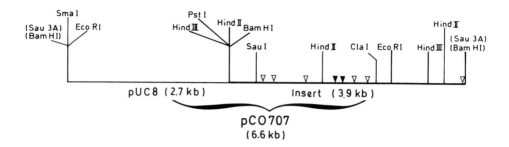

Fig. 1: Linear restriction enzyme map of the recombinant plasmid pCO707 specifying hemolysis. This plasmid of about 6.6 kb size carries a 3.9 kb insert of group B streptococcal DNA ligated to the vector pUC8. By transposon mutagenesis with Tn5 the group B streptococcal hemolysin determinant could be tentatively loacted on the insert: insertion at locations marked by the closed triangles abolish hemolysis; other insertions (open triangles) did not affect hemolysis.

Subcloning experiments are now being performed to eventually define the hemolysin determinant of GBS.

ACKNOWLEDGEMENTS

This work was supported by grant Lu 212/4 from the Deutsche Forschungsgemeinschaft. We are grateful to Dr. Patricia Ferrieri, Minneapolis, MN, for providing the GBS strain 74-360 and to Dr. J. Kreft, Würzburg for constant advice. The technial help of Miss B. Rauschenberger is greatly appreciated.

REFERENCES

Casabadan, M.J. and S.N. Cohen (1980). Analysis of gene control signals by DNA fusion and cloning in Escherichia coli. *J. Mol. Biol., 138,* 179-207.

Dal, M.C. and H. Monteil (1984). Hemolysin from Streptococcus agalactiae. In: Alouf, J.E., F.J. Fehrenbach, J.H. Freer, and J. Jeljaszewicz (Eds.), *Bacterial Protein Toxins.* Academic Press, London, pp. 363-364.

Dal, M.-C., and H. Monteil (1983). Hemolysin produced by group B Streptococcus agalactiae. *FEMS Microbiol. Lett., 16,* 89-94.

Ferrieri, P. (1982). Characterization of a hemolysin isolated from group B Streptococci. In: Holm, S. E., and P. Christensen (Eds.), *Basic Concepts of Streptococci and Streptococcal Diseases.* Reedbooks, Chertsey, Surrey, pp. 142-143.

Marchlewicz, B.A., and J.L. Duncan (1981). Lysis of erythrocytes by a hemolysin produced by a group B Streptococcus sp. *Infect. Immun., 34,* 787-794.

Marchlewicz, B.A., and J.L. Duncan (1980). Properties of a hemolysin produced by group B streptococci. *Infect. Immun., 30,* 805-813.

McKinnon, R.D., S. Bacchetti, and F.L. Graham (1982). Tn5 mutagenesis of the transforming genes of human adenovirus type 5. *Gene, 19,* 33-42.

Tsaihong, J.C., and D.E. Wennerstrom (1983). Effect of carrier molecules on production and properties of extracellular hemolysin produced by Streptococcus agalactiae. *Current Microbiol., 9,* 333-338.

Vieira, J., and J. Messing (1982). The pUC plasmids, an M13mp7-derived system for insertion mutagenesis and sequencing with synthetic universal primers. *Gene, 19,* 259-268.

Wennerstrom, D.E., J.C. Tsaihong, and J.T. Crawford (1985). Evaluation of the role of hemolysin and pigment in pathogenesis of early onset group B streptococcal infection. In: Kimura, Y., S. Kotami, and Y. Shiokawa (Eds.), *Recent Advances in Streptococci and Streptococcal Diseases.* Reedbooks, Bracknell, Berkshire, pp. 155-156.

Fehrenbach et al. (Eds.), Bacterial Protein Toxins, Zbl. Bakt. Suppl. 17
© Gustav Fischer, Stuttgart, New York, 1988

Identification of a Chromosomal Locus Crucial for the Virulence of Listeria monocytogenes: The Listeriolysin O Gene Region

J. Mengaud[1], J. Chenevert[1], Ch. Geoffroy[2], J.-L. Gaillard[3], B. Gicquel-Sanzey[1] and P. Cossart[1]

[1]Unité de Génie Microbiologique, [2]Unité des Antigènes Bactériens, Institut Pasteur, Rue du Docteur-Roux, 28, F-75724 Paris Cédex 15
[3]Laboratoire de Microbiologie, Faculté de Médecine Necker-Enfants Malades, F-75730 Paris Cédex 15

ABSTRACT

In culture supernatants of a Tn 1545-induced non hemolytic mutant of *Listeria monocytogenes,* by immunoblotting with an anti-serum raised against purified listeriolysin O,we have detected the presence of a truncated protein of 52000D (the secreted listeriolysin O is 60000D).The region of insertion of the transposon has been cloned and sequenced.The transposon had inserted in an open reading frame.The homologies detected between this ORF, streptolysin 0 and pneumolysin demonstrate that the transposon had indeed inserted in the listeriolysin O gene. As the non hemolytic mutant was non virulent, our work demonstrates that a genetic determinant essential for virulence is the Listeriolysin O gene or its adjacent region.

KEYWORDS

Listeria monocytogenes, hemolysin, listeriolysin O, Tn 1545, virulence.

Listeria monocytogenes is a facultative intracellular bacterium responsible for severe infections in human and animals.Its virulence is generally attributed to its capacity to survive and replicate inside the macrophages (Mackaness,1962). Recent data indicate that penetration into the host is also a crucial step of the infectious process (Gaillard and others,1987). However, the factors responsible for this virulence are still to be identified.

Among various factors incriminated as responsible for the virulence, the hemolysin(s) secreted by *L.monocytogenes* is (are) suspected on the basis of two types of data: i) all clinical isolates of *L.monocytogenes* are hemolytic. Non hemolytic species belonging to the genus *Listeria* are avirulent when tested in the murine model (Rocourt and other, 1983). ii) a non hemolytic (Hly -) mutant obtained by insertion of a single copy of the conjugative transposon Tn 1545 in the chromosome was avirulent (Gaillard and others,1986).The exact nature of the hemolytic factors(s) was unclear. But recently, the purification of a hemolytic factor from culture supernatant of *L.monocytogenes* has been achieved (Geffroy and others,1987).The secreted listeriolysin O is a 60 KD protein belonging to the group of SH-activated cytotoxins (Smyth and others, 1978).

We have used a rabbit antiserum raised against this highly purified protein to detect, by immunoblotting the presence of listeriolysin O in the culture supernatant of the Tn1545-induced Hly-mutant. It contained a shorter polypeptide of 52 KD which reacted with the antiserum.This result indicated that Tn 1545 had inserted in the structural gene of listeriolysin O gene.

Taking advantage of a resistance gene carried by the transposon, we cloned the region where Tn1545 had inserted (Mengaud and others, submitted). A 400 base-pair DNA fragment containing the Listeria-Tn1545 junction was then sequenced : the transposon had inserted in an open reading frame. The deduced protein sequence was highly homologous to streptolysin O (M.Kehoe, personal communication) and pneumolysin (Walker and others, as shown in Fig 1).

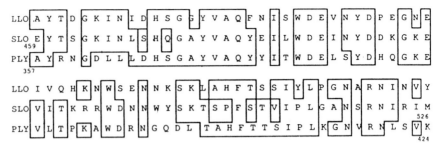

Figure 1 : Comparison of the deduced aminoacid sequence of listeriolysin O (LLO) with streptolysin O (SLO) and pneumolysin (PLY). Boxes denote common residues. Numbers refer to aminoacid positions in the protein sequence, in the case of SLO and PLY.

These homologies lie in the carboxyterminal end of pneumolysin and streptolysin O : for these two proteins, this region corresponds to the region of highest homology. In addition, it is the region where the unique cystein, thought to be essential for activity, is located. The homologies detected confirm the insertion of the transposon in the Listeriolysin O gene.

This work demonstrates that the nonhemolytic avirulent mutant previously described (Caillard and others, 1986) results from the insertion of Tn1545 within the structural gene of listeriolysin O gene and reveals that a genetic determinant essential for the virulence of *Listeria monocytogenes* is the listeriolysin O gene or its adjacent regions.Our results confirm the relationships between SH-activated cytotoxins. But it should be noted that the hemolytic activity of listeriolysin is optimal at pH 5 and undetectable at pH 7, which is not the case for streptolysin and pneumolysin.These differences are probably an indication that these cytotoxins have different roles in different types of pathogenicity.

REFERENCES

1. Gaillard J.L., Berche P., Mounier J., Richard S., and P. Sansonetti. 1987, Penetration of *L.monocytogenes* into the host: a crucial step of the infections process.Ann. Inst. Pasteur/Microbiol., 138, 241-284.
2. Gaillard J.L., Berche P. and Sansonetti P., 1986, Transposon mutagenesis as a tool to study the role of hemolysin in the virulence of Listeria monocytogenes. Infection and Immun., 52, 50-55.
3. Geffroy C., Gaillard J.L., Alouf J. and Berche P., 1987, Purification, characterisation and toxicity of sulfhydryl activated hemolysin (Listeriolysin O) form *Listeria monocytogenes,* Infection and Immun., 55,1641-1646.
4. Mackaness, G.B., 1962, Cellular resistance to infection. J. Exp. Med., 116, 381-406.
5. Mengaud J., Chenevert J., Geoffroy C., Gaillard J.L. and Cossart P. Identification of the structural gene encoding the SH-activated hemolysin of L.monocytogenes: Listeriolysin O is homologous to streptolysin and pneumolysin .Infection and Immun.,(in press).
6. Rocourt J., Alonso J.M. and Seelinger H.P.R., 1983, Virulence comparée des cinq groupes génomiques de *Listeria monocytogenes (sensu lato),* Ann. Microbiol. (Inst.Pasteur) 134A, 354-364.
7. Smyth C.J. and Duncan J.L., 1978, Thiol-activated (oxygen-labile) cytolysins p. 2-129-183. in J. Jeljaszewicz and T. Wadstrom (eds), Bacterial toxins and cell membranes. Academic Press, Inc., New-York.
8. Walker J.A., Allen R.L., Falmagne P.,Johnson M.K. and Boulnois G.,1987, Molecular cloning, characterisation and complete nucleotide sequence of the gene for Pneumolysin, the sulfhydryl-activated toxin of *Streptococcus pneumoniae*, Infection and Immun.,55, 1184-1189.

Fehrenbach et al. (Eds.), Bacterial Protein Toxins, Zbl. Bakt. Suppl. 17
© Gustav Fischer, Stuttgart, New York, 1988

Expression of the Pneumolysin Gene in E. Coli: Purification of Recombinant Pneumolysin and Some Biological Properties

T. Mitchell[1], J. Walker[1], K. Saunders[1], M. Kehoe[2], P. Andrew[1] and G. Boulnois[1]

[1]Department of Microbiology, Medical Sciences Building, University of Leicester, Leicester, LE1 7RH, U.K.
[2]Department of Microbiology, Medical School, Newcastle University, Newcastle, U.K.

ABSTRACT

The pneumolysin gene has been expressed in E. coli and the recombinant toxin purified. The gene is expressed faithfully in E. coli and the recombinant toxin is neutralised by anti SLO, inhibited by cholesterol and inhibits the respiratory burst of human PMNLs.

KEY WORDS

Thiol-activated toxins, Pneumolysin, Purification, recombinant protein, polymorphonuclear leukocytes.

Pneumolysin, the thiol-activated toxin of Streptococcus pneumoniae, is one of a family of immunologically related, hydrophobic, cytolytic agents, produced by diverse Gram-positive bacterial pathogens. All of these toxins are irreversibly inactivated by cholesterol (Smyth and Duncan, 1978).

In the case of SLO, the thiol-activated toxin of Streptococcus pyogenes, toxin molecules recognise and bind to cholesterol in target membranes and following lateral diffusion in the membrane, oligomerise to give rise to transmembrane channels that lead to cellular lysis (Bhakdi and Tranum-Jensen, 1986). At concentrations that have no effect on cell viability, pneumolysin inhibits respiratory burst and bactericidal activity in both polymorphonuclear leukocytes (PMNLs) and monocytes. In addition, pneumolysin inhibits chemotaxis and random migration of PMNLs (Paton and Ferrante, 1983). The mode of action of pneumolysin on these cell types is unknown.

In an attempt to probe the structure and function of pneumolysin, we recently reported the molecular cloning and complete nucleotide sequence of the pneumolysin gene in E. coli (Walker and others, 1987). Here we report preliminary findings on the expression of the pneumolysin gene in E. coli, purification of the recombinant product and some of its biological characteristics.

We have previously reported the complete nucleotide sequence of the pneumolysin gene and some 3kb of flanking sequences (Walker and others, 1987). Using this information several fragments of DNA carrying the entire pneumolysin gene with varying amounts of 5' and 3' flanking DNA were cloned in pUC18 or pUC19 such that the pneumolysin gene was expressed with or against the lac promoter. One such plasmid pJW208 expressed $2x10^4$ HU/ml of culture and this expression was stable.

An extract of an overnight culture of MC1061(pJW208) was prepared by sonication and cell debris removed by centrifugation. This extract was applied onto a hydrophobic interaction column and protein eluted with a decreasing salt gradient. Then haemolytic fractions were subjected first to ion exchange chromatography and finally molecular exclusion chromatography. Haemolytic fractions from the final chromatography were analysed by SDS-PAGE which demonstrated that this material was composed of a single polypeptide. The pure material chromatographed as a single peak on a second molecular exclusion column and subsequent N-terminal amino acid sequencing (see below) also confirmed purity. The recombinant pneumolysin had a specific activity of 8×10^6 haemolytic units (HU)/mg protein. The yield from 1 litre of overnight culture was 0.5mg with a 10% recovery.

The nucleotide sequence of the pneumolysin gene revealed the presence of two inframe ATG translation initiation codons, only one of which would yield a polypeptide with the correct N-terminal amino acid sequence (Walker and others, 1987). To ensure that expression of the pneumolysin gene in E. coli involved selection of the correct ATG start the N-terminal amino acid sequence of the purified recombinant protein was determined. The sequence was NH_2-Ala-Asn-Lys-Ala-Val-Asn-Asp-Phe and is identical to native pneumolysin (Walker and others, 1987).

The haemolytic activity of the purified recombinant pneumolysin was inhibited by cholesterol and neutralised by antisera raised against SLO. When the purified recombinant pneumolysin was used to immunise rabbits, the resulting antisera neutralised both recombinant and native pneumolysin. Pre-immune sera had no neutralising activity.

Purified recombinant pneumolysin inhibited the respiratory burst of human PMNLs as judged by H_2O_2 production by phorbol myristate acetate (PMA)-treated cells. For example, 0.1, 0.25, and 2.5 HU of recombinant pneumolysin per 10^6 PMNLs reduced H_2O_2 production by 21%, 51% and 71% respectively. These levels of pneumolysin had no effect on PMNL viability.

The scene is now set for a detailed analysis of pneumolysin structure and function via modification of the DNA sequence of the gene.

REFERENCES

Bhakdi, S., and J. Tranum-Jensen (1986) Membrane damage by pore-forming bacterial cytolysins. Microbial Pathogenesis, 1, 5-14.

Paton, J.C., and A. Ferrante (1983) Inhibition of human polymorphonuclear leukocyte respiratory burst, bactericidal activity, and migration by pneumolysin. Infect. Immun, 41, 1212-1216.

Smyth, C.J., and J.L. Duncan (1978) Thiol-activated (oxygen-labile) cytolysins. In: J. Jeljaszewicz and T. Wadstrom (Eds.) Bacterial Toxins and Cell Membranes. Academic Press Inc., New York, pp.129-183.

Walker, J.A., R.L. Allen, P. Falmagne, M.K. Johnson, and G.J. Boulnois (1987) Molecular cloning, characterization, and complete nucleotide sequence of the gene for pneumolysin, the sulfhydryl-activated toxin of Streptococcus pneumoniae. Infect.Immun, 55, 1184-1189.

Fehrenbach et al. (Eds.), Bacterial Protein Toxins, Zbl. Bakt. Suppl. 17
© Gustav Fischer, Stuttgart, New York, 1988

Nucleotide Homology of the Genes Encoding Staphylococcal Enterotoxins SEB and SEC 1, 2 and 3

S. Notermans, K. Wernars and C. J. Heuvelman

National Institute of Public Health and Environmental Hygiene, P. O. Box 1, 3720 BA Bilthoven, The Netherlands

The amino acids 15 through 29 of staphylococcal enterotoxin B (SEB) and staphylococcal enterotoxin C_1 (SEC_1) are identical. A DNA-probe, based on the nucleotide sequence of the SEB molecule and coding for the amino acids 15 through 29 was synthesized and tested for hybridization with the DNA of Staphyloccoccus aureus strains producing SEB, SEC_1, SEC_2 and SEC_3 and other enterotoxins. Hybridization reactions were only observed with strains producing SEB and SEC_1. No hybridization occurred with strains producing SEC_2 and SEC_3 or other toxins. These results show the existence of more than one type of SEC.

A number of staphylococcal enterotoxins (SE) has been differentiated by serological techniques and are classified by the letter designation SEA through SEE. Three subtypes of SEC, numbered 1, 2 and 3 have been described (Borja and Bergdoll, 1977; Reiser and others, 1984). The immunological differences between these subtypes are small and complete neutralization occurs with heterologous antibodies (Reiser and others, 1984).
The complete amino acid sequence of SEB and SEC_1 has been determined (Huang and Bergdoll, 1970; Schmidt and Spero, 1983) showing extensive homology between the amino acid sequence of both toxins. Therefore, such a homology could exist with the subtypes SEC_2 and SEC_3. Recently the nucleotide sequence of the SEB gene from S.aureus has been determined (Jones and Khan, 1986). The amino acid sequence 15 through 29 of the SEB molecule is identical to that of SEC_1. We used a 42-mer synthetic DNA-probe coding for this region of the SEB molecule to determine if this synthetic DNA-probe reacts with DNA of both SEB and SEC 1, 2 and 3, and other SE-producing strains of S.aureus.

The S.aureus strains used included reference strains (FRI 196E, S6, 14458, FRI 137, FRI 361, FRI 913, FRI 1151M, FRI 326E, FRI 1183 and SET 23 producing SEA, SEA/SEB, SEB, SEC_1, SEC_2, SEC_3, SED, SEE, TSST-1 and TSST-1 resp.) and wild type strains. The DNA-probe synthesized (5'-AGTAAATTCACTGGTTTGATGGAAAATATGAAA-GTTTTGTAT-3') was labeled according tot Maxam and Gilbert (1980) with γ-^{32}P-ATP. A colony-hybridization procedure was used for testing homology between the DNA-probe and the DNA of S.aureus. The colonies were lysed on a Gene Screen Plus membrane (du Pont) by a combination of NaOH treatment and steaming as described by Maas (1983). Using a hybridization mixture (without formamide) essentially containing 1.0 M NaCl, the optimum hybridization temperature was 41^6C.

The synthetic 42-mer DNA-probe reacted with all 20 SEB-producing S.aureus strains and with 8 out of 31 strains producing SEC (see Table 1). Among the latter only those producing SEC_1 were detected with this probe.

TABLE 1 Hybridization Reaction of a Synthetic 42-mer DNA-probe, Encoding for the Amino Acids 15 through 29 of SEB, with Different Strains of S.aureus

Toxin produced	Number of strains tested	Number of strains with hybridization signals
SEA	4	0
SEB	20	20
SEC	31	8 *
SED	4	0
SEE	1	0
TSST-1	4	0
Negative	8	0

* SEC_1 = positive, SEC_{2+3} = negative

Strains producing other toxins and toxin-negative strains did not show any reaction. Our DNA-probe had a nucleotide sequence similar to that published by Jones and Khan (1986) and encoded for the amino acids 15 through 29 of the SEB molecule as produced by strain S6. This part of the amino acid sequence is identical to that of SEC_1, produced by strain FRI 137. Staphylococcal enterotoxins are differentiated according to their immunological activity. Enterotoxins SEC_1, SEC_2 and SEC_3 can be distinguished from each other by their different patterns in iso-electric focussing. Furthermore SEC_3 has serine as the N-terminal residue, whereas the SEC_1 and SEC_2 have glutamic acid for their N-terminal residue (Schmidt and Spero, 1983; Reiser and others, 1984). Our results demonstrate that, although SEC_1 is serologically and chemically similar to SEC_2 and SEC_3, clear differences exist in the nucleotide sequence encoding for these toxins.

Borja, C.R., and M.S.Bergdoll (1967). Purification and partial characterization of enterotoxin C produced by Staphylococcus aureus strain 137. Biochemistry, 6, 1467-1473.

Huang, I.Y., and M.S.Bergdoll (1970). The primary structure of staphylococcal enterotoxin B. J.Biol.Chem., 245, 3518-3525.

Jones, C.L., and S.A.Khan (1986). Nucleotide sequence of the enterotoxin B gene from Staphylococcus aureus. J.Bacteriol., 166, 29-33.

Maas, R. (1983). An improved colony hybridization method with significantly increased sensitivity for detection of single genes. Plasmid, 10, 296-298.

Maxam, A.M., and W.Gilbert (1980). Sequencing end-labeled DNA with base-specific chemical cleavages. Methods Enzymol., 65, 499.

Reiser, R.F., R.N.Robbins, A.L.Noleto, S.P.Khoe, and M.S.Bergdoll (1984). Identification, purification, and some physicochemical properties of staphylococcal enterotoxin C_3. Infect.Immun., 45, 625-630.

Schmidt, J.J., and L.Spero (1983). The complete amino acid sequence of staphylococcal enterotoxin C_1. J.Biol.Chem., 258, 6300-6305.

Fehrenbach et al. (Eds.), Bacterial Protein Toxins, Zbl. Bakt. Suppl. 17
© Gustav Fischer, Stuttgart, New York, 1988

DNA Sequence Analysis of Staphylococcal Epidermolytic Toxins

P. W. O'Toole and T. J. Foster

Department of Microbiology, Moyne Institute, Trinity College, Dublin 2, Ireland

ABSTRACT

The complete nucleotide sequence of the eta gene of Staphylococcus aureus has been determined. The DNA sequence and the deduced amino acid sequence of ETA were compared with those of ETB. Three major regions of homology were observed. Analysis of a deletion mutant indicated that the promoter and regulatory signals responding to the accessory gene regulator (agr) of S. aureus were retained in the 250 nucleotides upstream from the coding sequence.

KEYWORDS

Epidermolytic toxin A, Staphylococcus aureus, DNA sequence analysis, regulation of expression.

INTRODUCTION

Strains of S. aureus associated with the Staphylococcal Scalded Skin Syndrome synthesize either or both of the epidermolytic toxins, ETA and ETB (Bailey, de Azavedo, and Arbuthnott, 1980). These antigenically distinct proteins cause splitting of the granular skin layer of neonates in certain mammalian species. We have previously cloned the eta and etb genes in bacteriophage and plasmid vectors in E. coli (O'Toole and Foster, 1986a, 1986b). The eta gene was expressed from its own promoter in E. coli, whereas expression of etb was dependent on the trc promoter of the vector plasmid. The DNA sequence of the eta gene has been determined, allowing the coding sequence and the deduced primary structure of ETA to be compared with the corresponding sequences of ETB (Lee and others, 1987).

RESULTS

The coding sequence for eta was identified by computer-search for residue identity with an oligonucleotide back-translated from the published 23 amino-terminal amino acids of ETA (Johnson, Metzger and Spero, 1979). The primary translation product of the open reading frame had a 38 residue signal sequence, which gave a protein of molecular weight 26,950 after secretion. This agrees with the published size of ETA determined electrophoretically (Johnson and co-workers,

1975). A presumptive promoter (TTGTTT-16-TATAAT) and potential ribosome binding site (GGATG) were identified by fidelity with consensus sequences and spacing (McLaughlin, Murray and Rabinowitz, 1981; Rosenberg and Court, 1979).

The DNA sequence of etb has recently been determined (Lee and colleagues, 1987). The coding sequences of eta and etb have 440/840 residue identities (52% homology), reasonably spread throughout the lengths of the genes. It is likely that they have a common evolutionary origin. In addition, a sequence of 29 nucleotides containing dyad symmetry which is located upstream from the eta coding sequence has 28 residues identical to a sequence spanning the putative eth promoter. The presumptive promoter of etb is quite dissimilar to the consensus E. coli promoter, perhaps explaining its failure to function in the Gram negative host.

The aligned amino acid sequences of ETA and ETB have 40% residue identity, including 3 regions of locally elevated homology (67% in one case). The hydrophathy plots of the toxins indicate that the conserved regions are predominantly hydrophilic sequences. Overall, the hydropathy plots are very similar, suggesting that the secondary and tertiary structures are also conserved, possibly to retain a conformation necessary for interaction with the appropriate substrate or receptor in the epidermis.

One deletion created during DNA sequence analysis retained the structural gene and 256 residues upstream from the initiation condon. This fragment, when introduced into S. aureus on a shuttle plasmid, directed expression of eta under control of agr (Recsei and colleagues, 1986). This shows that the promoter and regulatory signals which respond to agr are within the 256 residues retained by this deleted fragment.

REFERENCES

Bailey, C.J., J.C. de Azavedo, and J.P. Arbuthnott (1980). a comparative study of two serotypes of epidermolytic toxin from Staphylococcus aureus. Biochim. Biophys Acta **624**, 111-120.

Johnson, A.D., J.F. Metzger, and L. Spero (1975). Production, purification and chemical characterization of Staphylococcus aureus exfoliative toxin. Infect. Immun., 12, 1206-1210.

Johnson, A.D., L. Spero, J.S. Cades, and B.T. de Cicco (1979). Purification and characterization of different types of exfoliative toxin from Staphylococcus aureus. Infect. Immun., 24, 679-684.

Lee, C.Y., J. Schmidt, A.D. Johnson-Winegar, L. Spero, and J.J. Inadolo (1987). Sequence determination and comparison of the exfoliative toxin A and B genes from Staphylococcus aureus. J. Bacteriol., (in press).

McLaughlin, J.R., C.L. Murray, and J.C. Rabinowitz (1981). Unique features in the ribosome binding site sequence of the gram-positive Staphylococcus aureus. J. Biol. Chem. 256, 11283-11291.

O'Toole, P.W., and T.J. Foster (1986a). Molecular cloning and expression of the epidermolytic toxin A gene of Staphylococcus aureus. Microb. Pathogen., 1, 583-594.

O'Toole and T.J. Foster (1986b). Epidermolytic toxin serotype B of Staphylococcus aureus is plasmid-encoded. FEMS Microbiol. Letts., 36, 311-314.

Rosenberg, M., and D. Court 1979. Regulatory signals involved in promotion and termination of RNA transcription. Annu. Rev. Genet., 13, 318-354.

Fehrenbach et al. (Eds.), Bacterial Protein Toxins, Zbl. Bakt. Suppl. 17
© Gustav Fischer, Stuttgart, New York, 1988

Genetically Engineered Diphtheria Toxin Mutants as Immunogenic Carriers for Heterologous Antigens

A. Phalipon[1], V. Cabiaux[2] and M. Kaczorek[1]

[1]Institut Pasteur, U. A. G. G., 28, rue du Dr Roux, F-75015 Paris Cédex 15
[2]Université libre de Bruxelles, Laboratoire des Macromolécules aux Interfaces, B-1050 Bruxelles

ABSTRACT

Tripartite fusion proteins comprising a mutant diphtheria toxin CRM228 (DT), the hepatitis B surface antigen (HBsAg) from hepatitis B virus and β-galactosidase (βgal) were obtained by expression of hybrid genes in E.coli. These soluble fusion proteins, purified in one step by chromatography affinity to βgal were shown to induce synthesis of anti-HBs antibodies and anti-diphtheria toxin antibodies in guinea pigs (A. Phalipon and M. Kaczorek, 1987). In order to analyze immunogenicity of DT-HBs without any fused βgal part, an expression vector was constructed which allows separation of the protein of interest and the βgal part. For this purpose, a synthetic oligonucleotide (coll) was introduced between tox228 and lacZ genes, which codes for a peptide sequence specifically recognized by collagenase. Mild proteolysis with collagenase is specific for the coll peptide resulting in separation of DT-HBs and βgal portions. Isolation of the fused proteins DT-HBs by a second affinity chromatography step will provide a material pure enough to carry out immunization and to analyze immunogenicity of DT-HBs alone.

KEYWORDS

Recombinant DNA, expression vector, affinity chromatography, collagenase, vaccines.

RESULTS

Genetic engineering offers a novel approach to the preparation of immunogenic proteins of predetermined antigenicity, i.e. the construction of hybrid genes carrying inserts encoding specific antigens. DT is particularly amenable to such an approach since a number of nontoxic still immunogenic DT mutants are available. We have previously cloned and sequenced tox228 encoding a non toxic mutant DT CRM228 carrying two amino-acid exchanges one each in the A and B chain (Kaczorek and co-workers, 1983).
By expression in E.coli, we have prepared soluble DT-βgal fusion proteins which induce protective antibodies to wild type DT.

Next, we have constructed tripartite fusion proteins by insertion of a 42 amino-acids determinant of HBsAg into the NH$_2$-end of fragment B of DT-β gal hybrids. Immunization experiments showed that the soluble purified proteins were capable to elicit antibodies recognizing respectively wild type DT and 22 nm HBsAg particles. However, antibodies were not protective against diphtheria toxin, which indicates that at least one major DT epitope involved in toxin neutralization is located at the site of HBsAg insertion in fragment B (Phalipon and Kaczorek, 1987).
In order to study the immunogenicity of the DT-HBs proteins without the βgal portion, we constructed a vector pTHPCOLL which allows expression and purification of a new hybrid protein : DT-HBs-Coll-β gal. In this protein, the sequence coll (Gly-Pro-Val) encoded three times by a 42 bp synthetic oligonucleotide, is specifically recognized by collagenase from Achromobacter iophagus (1). Controlled digestion of DT-HBs-Coll-βgal protein, purified by affinity chromatography to βgal, leds to proteolysis by collagenase specifically into the coll peptide. This result demonstrates that the coll peptide is accessible to collagenase within the conformational structure of the fusion protein. Moreover, in the same conditions, the DT-HBs proteins are not proteolysed by collagenase. Hence, introduction of the coll sequence between DT-HBs and βgal allows purification of the DT-HBs protein after collagenolysis followed by a second affinity chromatography step.

CONCLUSION

Until a host/vector system will be available in Corynebacterium diphtheriae, obtention of genetically engineered diphtheria toxins will proceed in E.coli. The production and the purification of such hybrid toxins is greatly enhanced by βgal fusions which stabilize and allow an one step purification of the hybrid protein. The pTHPCOLL vector, we describe here, directs synthesis of such a fusion protein from which, moreover, the DT-HBs portion can be purified after a specific proteolysis with a collagenase. This will provide us sufficient quantities of DT-HBs fusion protein to analyze its immunogenicity in animals.
This work suggests that the modification of highly immunogenic DT by insertion of heterologous antigenic sequences is a promising approach towards novel vaccines.

REFERENCES

Kaczorek, M., Delpeyroux, F., Chenciner, N., Streek, R.E., Murphy, J.R., Boquet, P. and Tiollais, P. (1983). Nucleotide sequence and expression of the diphtheria tox228 gene in E.coli. Science 221, 855-858.
Phalipon, A. and Kaczorek, M. (1987). Genetically engineered diphtheria toxin fusion proteins carrying the hepatitis B surface antigen. Gene, in press.

(1)Achromobacter collagenase was a gift of B. KEIL (Institut Pasteur, Paris).

Fehrenbach et al. (Eds.), Bacterial Protein Toxins, Zbl. Bakt. Suppl. 17
© Gustav Fischer, Stuttgart, New York, 1988

Characterization of the Serratia. marcesens Hemolysin Determinant

K. Poole, E. Schiebel and V. Braun

Mikrobiologie II, Auf der Morgenstelle 28, Universität Tübingen, D-7400 Tübingen

ABSTRACT

The nucleotide sequence of a 7.5 kilobase pair fragment of DNA comprising the hemolysin determinant of Serratia marcesens was determined. Two large open reading frames were identified, designated shlA and shlB, capable of encoding proteins with predicted molecular weights of 165,046 and 61,836, respectively. Overexpression of the genes in Escherichia coli permitted the identification and subcellular localization of the gene products, both of which were found in the cell envelope. The molecular weights of the proteins as deduced from SDS-polyacrylamide gel electrophoresis was in agreement with that predicted from the nucleotide sequence. Based on detergent solubility and sucrose density gradient centrifugation the shlB gene product was localized more specifically to the outer membrane. Expression and localization of the shlA gene product, the presumed hemolysin, was independent of the shlB gene product, although hemolytic activity absolutely required both gene products.

KEYWORDS

Serratia marcesens, hemolysin determinant, nucleotide sequence, shlAB, subcellular localization, hemolytic activity.

INTRODUCTION

Serratia marcesens is increasingly recognized as an important opportunistic pathogen. Clinical isolates are often hemolytic on blood agar. The ability of hemolytic bacteria to induce the release of inflammatory mediators (Scheffer and others, 1985), with a possible attendant increase in vascular permeability, edema and granulocyte accumulation, suggests that hemolysin production may be an important component of the pathogenicity of this organism. Unlike the E. coli hemolysin, which is secreted into the culture medium (Springer and Goebel, 1980), the S. marcesens hemolysin remains cell-associated, and Serratia colonies ellicit only narrow zones of hemolysis on blood agar (Braun and others, 1985). In contrast to the E. coli hemolysin, too, the S. marcesens hemolysin exhibits no requirement for calcium ions for activity and hemolysis by S. marcesens requires that the cells be actively metabolizing (Braun and others, 1985). Preliminary data also suggests that the number of genes and the size of gene products involved in the hemolytic phenotype in S. marcesens differs from that in E. coli (Braun and others, 1987).

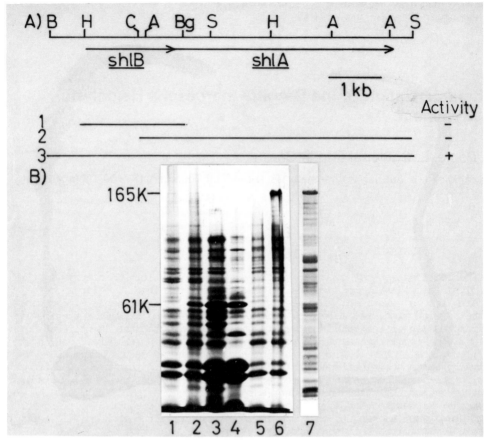

Fig. 1: A) Physical map of the Serratia marcesens hemolysin
determinant. The location and orientation of the genes is
indicated. DNA inserts in plasmids transformed into E. coli,
as well as the presence (+) or absence (-) of hemolytic activity
in transformants harbouring these plasmids, is also shown.
A, AvaI, B, BamHI, Bg, BglII, C, ClaI, H, HpaI, S, SalI.
B) Expression and localization of the S. marcesens hemolysin
determinant gene products in E. coli. Whole cell protein extracts
(lanes 1,2,5,6), cell envelopes (lanes 3,7) and outer membranes
(lane 4) were prepared from strains harbouring recombinant
plasmids carrying no insert, lanes 1 and 5 , the shlB gene
(insert 1 above), lanes 2-4 and the shlA gene (insert 2 above),
lanes 6 and 7. Strains harbouring the shlB gene express a
protein of 61 kD mol. wt. (lane 2) which is localized in the
outer membrane (lane 4). Similarly, the presence of the shlA
gene correlates with the production of a protein of 165 kD
mol. wt. (lane 6) present in the cell envelope (lane 7).

Braun, V., H.Günter, B.Neuss, and C.Tautz (1985). Hemolytic activity of
   Serratia marcesens. Arch.Microbiol., 141, 371-376.
Braun, V., B.Neuss, Y.Ruan, E.Schiebel, H.Schöffler, and G.Jander (1987).
   Identification of the Serratia marcesens hemolysin determinant by cloning
   into Escherichia coli. J.Bacteriol., 169, 2113-2120.
Scheffer, J., W.König, J.Hacker, and W.Goebel (1985). Bacterial adherence and
   hemolysin production from Escherichia coli induces histamine and leukotriene
   release from various cells. Infect.Immun., 50, 271-278.
Springer, W., and W. Goebel (1980). Synthesis and secretion of hemolysin by
   Escherichia coli. J.Bacteriol., 144, 53-59.

Fehrenbach et al. (Eds.), Bacterial Protein Toxins, Zbl. Bakt. Suppl. 17
© Gustav Fischer, Stuttgart, New York, 1988

Use of Oligodeoxynucleotide as a Probe for Exfoliative Toxin A Gene Detection

S. Rifai[1], V. Barbançon[1], Y. Piémont[1] and P. Falmagne[2]

[1]Laboratoire de Toxinologie Bactérienne, Institut de Bactériologie 3, rue Koeberlé,
 F-67000 Strasbourg
[2]Laboratoire de Chimie Biologique de la Faculté des Sciences, Université d'Etat, 21, Avenue
Maistriau, B-7000 Mons

ABSTRACT

An oligodeoxynucleotide was synthetized after purification of exfoliative toxin
type A (ETA) from Staphylococcus aureus. This oligonucleotide hybridize
specifically with purified chromosomal DNA of ETA productive strain. Use of
this labeled probe allowed detection of ETA gene.

KEYWORDS

Staphylococcus aureus, exfoliative toxin type A, oligodeoxynucleotide, specific
hybridization, ETA gene detection.

We have determined the peptidic sequence of the staphylococcal exfoliative
toxin type A (ETA) purified in our laboratory (Piémont and Monteil, 1983). The
sequence of the first twenty-five aminoacids from the NH_2-terminus of the
protein was compared to that previously described by Johnson and co-workers
(1977). This comparison allowed the observation of a good correlation between
the two sequences, but some differences were noticed. From the peptidic
sequence of these aminoacids we deduced the nucleic acid sequence to construct
a synthetic oligodeoxynucleotide (74-mere) (Gene Assembler, Pharmacia) We used
the codons the more frequently encountered in E.coli (Grantham and co-workers,
1980). This oligodeoxynucleotide was labeled at its 5' end using $[\gamma^{32}P]$ATP; the
^{32}P-labeled oligonucleotide was used for ETA gene detection.

This oligonucleotide hybridize specifically with the purified chromosomal DNA
of ETA productive S.aureus strains and no such hybridization was observed with
unproductive ETA strains nor with ETB productive strains. Several restriction
patterns obtained after simple and multiple digestions of DNA from an ETA
strain allowed a hybridization of the probe with a 3.4 kb Hind III fragment.

Moreover the same result was noticed when the probe was hybridized to
chromosomal DNA extracted from an ETA + ETB productive S.aureus strain. Hence

we supposed that the ETA gene was located over the same chromosomal fragment in both strains.
Amount of total purified DNA as low as 500 ng was detected by our labeled probe. Likewise 30 ng of a 3.4 kb Hind III fragment recovered from an agarose gel can be detected by hybridization.

We showed that this probe could be used for the identification of ETA productive S.aureus strains. After isolation of S.aureus in our laboratory, the probe revealed wether the gene of ETA toxin was present or not.

Finally this oligonucleotide will be useful for the screening of a genomic bank to the purpose of ETA cloning.

REFERENCES

Grantham, R., C.Gautier, M.Gouy, R.Mercier, and A.Pave (1980). Codon catalog usage and the genome hypothesis. Nucleic Acid Res., 8, 49-62.
Johnson, A.D., L.Spero, J.S.Cades, and B.T. de Cicco (1979). Purification and characterization of different types of exfoliative toxin from Staphylococcus aureus. Infect. Immun., 24, 679-684.
Piémont, Y., and H.Monteil (1983). New approach in the separation of two exfoliative toxins from Staphylococcus aureus. FEMS Microbiol. Letters, 17, 191-195.

Fehrenbach et al. (Eds.), Bacterial Protein Toxins, Zbl. Bakt. Suppl. 17
© Gustav Fischer, Stuttgart, New York, 1988

Cloning of Several δ-Endotoxin Genes from B. thuringiensis Strains Active against Spodoptera Littoralis

V. Sanchis[1], D. Lereclus[1, 2], J. Ribier[1], G. Menou[1], D. Martouret[2] and M.-M. Lecadet[1]

[1]Unité de Biochimie Microbienne, Institut Pasteur, 28, Rue du Dr. Roux, F-75724 Paris Cédex 15
[2]Station de Recherches de lutte biologique, INRA, La Minière, F-78280 Guyancourt

It is currently suggested that multiple and different δ-endotoxin genes acting independantly or synergistically could contribute to determine the host range specificity in Lepidopteran active strains of B. thuringiensis. As deduced from DNA hybridization experiments and from crystal protein analysis, this is apparently the case for strains aizawai 7-29 and entomocidus 601, strains which have been characterized for their efficiency against the cotton leaf worm Spodoptera littoralis.
From strain aizawai 7-29 a plasmid copy of the δ-endotoxin gene, contained on a 18 kb BamHI fragment, was previously cloned in E. coli (pBT 45-1) (Klier and others, 1985). This gene is located on a 45 Md plasmid (pBT45) which, transferred into B. cereus 569, directed the synthesis of crystalline inclusions which were poorly toxic against S. littoralis, but that were preferentially active against Pieris brassicae, as defined by the LC50 ratio towards the two insect species.
Fig. 1 shows the structural organization of the pBT45 plasmid, as determined by electron microscope examination, restriction map analysis and hybridization

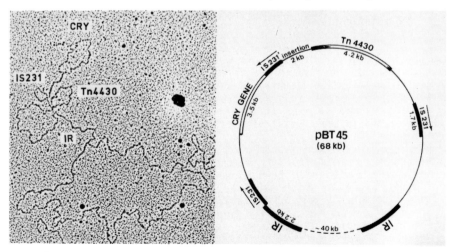

Fig. 1 : Electron micrograph of the self-annealed pBT45 molecule. Model for the structural organization of the plasmid.

experiments. It appears that the crystal gene is associated with the transposable elements Tn4430 and IS231. The model proposed in Fig. 1 strongly suggests that these elements are parts of a composite transposon delimited by two inverted repeated sequences (IR). This structure is similar to that of the resident pBT42 plasmid in the berliner 1715 strain. However pBT45 contains two DNA inserts (2 kb each) inside and at the end of two IS231 elements. The δ-endotoxin gene carried on plasmid pBT45 is structurally identical to the plasmid gene from the berliner strain (Wabiko and others, 1986), as is a second δ-entodoxin gene contained on a 14 kb BamHI fragment cloned from total aizawai 7-29 DNA. This second gene (pHTA1) expressed in E. coli led to the synthesis of genuine crystals that were also preferentially active against P. brassicae larvae. It appears therefore that this type of crystal gene and its surrounding sequences are duplicated in strain aizawai 7-29. A third gene (pHTA4), contained on a 6 kb BglII fragment, was cloned from total DNA of aizawai 7-29 (Fig. 2). This third gene displayed a quite

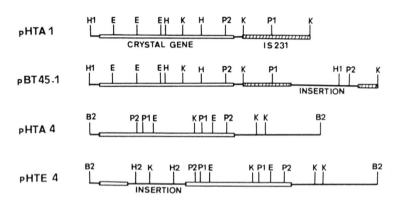

Fig. 2 : Physical map of the different cloned δ-endotoxin genes from strains aizawai 7-29 and entomocidus 601. Abbreviations are : B2 = BglII, E = EcoRI, H = HindIII, H1 = HpaI, H2 = HincII, K = KpnI, P1 = PstI, P2 = PvuII.

different physical map and directed, in E. coli, the synthesis of a 130-140 Kda protein which was not significantly active against the two insect species cited above. A similar gene (pHTE4), contained on a 7.5 kb BglII fragment, and isolated from total DNA of the entomocidus 601 strain also did not induce any larvicidal activity against either insect. It must be noted that a 1.5 kb DNA sequence apparently unrelated to the crystal gene is inserted in the gene originating from strain entomocidus 601.

As a consequence of the multiplicity of the δ-endotoxin genes in strain aizawai 7-29, several gene copies have been cloned, apparently belonging to different structural types ; one of which (pHTA4), also present in the entomocidus 601 strain, had not previously been characterized. Finally, we recently cloned a DNA fragment whose product is specifically toxic against S. littoralis. Studies are now in progress to characterize this new recombinant clone.

Klier, A., Lereclus, D., Ribier, J., Bourgouin, C., Menou, G., Lecadet, M-M., and Rapoport, G. (1985). In : J. A. Hoch, P. Setlow (Eds.), Molecular Biology of Microbial Differentiation, Amer. Soc. Microbiol., Washington.
Wabiko, H., Raymond, D. L., and Bulla, L. A. Jr (1986). DNA, 5, 305-314.

Fehrenbach et al. (Eds.), Bacterial Protein Toxins, Zbl. Bakt. Suppl. 17
© Gustav Fischer, Stuttgart, New York, 1988

Molecular Cloning of Clostridium perfringens Alpha Toxin

R. W. Titball, S. E. C. Hunter, B. C. Morris, A. D. Shuttleworth and T. Rubidge

CDE Porton Down Salisbury, Wilts, UK SP4 OJQ

ABSTRACT

The gene encoding phospholipase C (alpha toxin) in C. perfringens type A has been
isolated and cloned into E. coli using a plasmid vector. The toxin encoding DNA
codes for both the structural gene and the gene promoter. The cloned gene product has been purified and is identical with native C. perfringens alpha toxin
with respect to molecular weight, iso-electric point, immunogenicity, toxicity
and thermal stability. The E. coli cloned gene has been used to examine the DNA
of a variety of phospholipase C synthesising bacteria for comparability with the
C. perfringens alpha toxin gene.

KEYWORDS

Clostridium perfringens alpha toxin, alpha toxin cloning, phospholipase C cloning.

INTRODUCTION

Clostridium perfringens is the etiological agent of a wide variety of diseases of
man and animals (Stephen and Pietrowski, 1981) and the pathogenic potential of
this bacterium can be largely ascribed to the wide variety of toxins produced by
the bacterium. (McDonel, 1986).

Of the toxins produced, phospholipase C (alpha toxin) has received the most
attention. Many workers have elucidated some biophysical properties of the
purified protein, however, little is known of the genetic basis of toxin production, or the relationship of the structure of the molecule to its toxicity and
antigenicity.

We have set out to examine these areas in detail with a long term view towards
using genes encoding toxoids to induce protection against alpha toxin.

RESULTS AND DISCUSSION

A library of Hind III restriction endonuclease digestion fragments of
C. perfringens NCTC 8237 chromosomal DNA has been constructed in E. coli using
the plasmid vector pUC18. of 2,000 clones screened two synthesised phospholipase C.

Analysis of the recombinant plasmids from these clones has revealed that a 3.1 kb DNA insert encoded the gene for phospholipase C (alpha toxin). Expression was not affected by the orientation of the DNA insert in the vector plasmid, nor by the addition of IPTG to the growth medium, indicating that the DNA insert encodes both the structural and regulatory domains of the gene.

Restriction endonuclease digestion analysis of the DNA insert indicated that generally only enzymes with A-T rich recognition sequences cut the DNA. This result is in accordance with the G-C content of 24-27 moles% for C. perfringens chromosomal DNA (Breed, 1975).

The phospholipase C synthesised within E. coli containing the recombinant plasmid accumulated within the periplasmic space. This result is typical of that observed for a protein possessing an N-terminal signal sequence, directing export of the protein across a cell membrane (Scott and Silhavy, 1982).

The E. coli -cloned alpha toxin was biochemically and immunologically similar to the native C. perfringens alpha toxin: the molecular weight of 44,300 determined for both proteins is comparable with many previous reported values for the native toxin determined by SDS-PAGE (McDonel, 1986). Both proteins reacted with a single line of identity in a double diffusion test system against polyvalent anti-C. perfringens A serum, suggesting that many or all epitopes are shared.

Many workers have reported that C. perfringens alpha toxin appears as a number of forms after electrofocusing (IEF) (Mollby, 1978). We found that both the C. perfringens toxin and the E. coli cloned toxin appeared as two major forms after IEF (pI 5.48 and 5.6).

Using dot blot and Southern blot techniques a sequence complimentary to the alpha toxin encoding DNA was detected in C. perfringens types A,B,C and D capable of synthesising phospholipase C and in a strain of C. perfringens type B which failed to synthesise detectable phospholipase C in vitro. The sequence was not detected in C. novyi, C. sordellii or a selection of other phospholipase C synthesising bacteria.

REFERENCES

Breed, R S (1975). Bergeys Manual of Determinative Bacteriology. Williams and Wilkins, Baltimore, Maryland.

McDonel, J L (1986). Toxins of Clostridium perfringens Types A,B,C,D and E. In: F Dorner and J Drews (Eds), Pharmacology of Bacterial Toxins, Pergamon Press, Oxford, pp 477-506.

Mollby, R (1978). Bacterial Phospholipases. In: J Jeljaszewicz and T Wadstrom (Eds), Bacterial Toxins and Cell Membranes. Academic Press, New York, pp 367-424.

Scott, D E and T J Silhavy (1982). Molecular components of the signal sequence that function in the initiation of protein export. J. Cell. Biol, 95, 689-696.

Stephen, J and R A Pietrowski (1981). Bacterial Toxins. Nelson and Sons, Surrey.

Toxin-Lipid Interaction

Fehrenbach et al. (Eds.), Bacterial Protein Toxins, Zbl. Bakt. Suppl. 17
© Gustav Fischer, Stuttgart, New York, 1988

Secondary and Tertiary Structure of Membrane Proteins

J. P. Rosenbusch

Biozentrum, University of Basel, Klingelbergstr. 70, CH-4056 Basel

ABSTRACT

The structure of porin from E. coli outer membranes is compared
with those of the reaction center of Ps. viridis and of bacteriorhodopsin from H. halobium. The contributions of various
forces affecting their folding within the bilayer are considered. It is widely accepted that hydrophobicity and α-helical
configuration play significant roles in membrane protein structures. Nevertheless, it seems also clear that in membrane proteins facilitating transport of ions (and other polar solutes),
hydrophobicity and related parameters are unlikely to be the
only forces involved. Local and global charge neutralization,
as well as saturation of the entire hydrogen bonding potential
in the membrane domain of proteins by extensive hydrogen bonding networks may accomodate domains within membrane boundaries
that, judged merely from the distribution of hydrophobic residues in their primary sequence, would not be assigned to the
membrane domain. Though only qualitative at present, the considerations reported here may help in providing a better understanding of structures for which hydrophobicity parameters may
be incompatible with the functions of any particular protein.

KEYWORDS

Hydrogen-bonding networks, ion pairs, porin, reaction centers,
bacteriorhodopsin, ion channels.

Membrane-integral protein domains are typically considered as
hydrophobic moieties, arranged in α-helical configuration. This
notion was derived from the proton pumping bacteriorhodopsin,
the first membrane protein to reveal its structure at a near-
molecular (7 Å) resolution (Henderson & Unwin, 1975). The emerging structural concepts (Engelman and co-workers, 1980) received decisive support from the first high resolution (3 Å)
structure determination of a reaction center, a transmembrane
electron-translocating protein of photosynthetic bacteria
(Deisenhofer and co-workers, 1985). In view of its function,

the structure of its membrane domain indeed appears eminently plausible: within membrane boundaries, eleven α-helices containing only hydrophobic residues surround, and thus insulate, a chain of pigments involved in consecutive redox reactions. Many other transmembrane proteins, and bacteriorhodopsin belongs to this group also, facilitate the transport of polar solutes or ions. Such proteins may be expected a priori to contain polar groups and ionizable residues. Porin appears to be a typical example of such a protein, as it forms voltage-dependent water-filled channels across E. coli outer membranes (for a review, see Nikaido & Vaara, 1985). It is a very hydrophilic protein, and its secondary structure consists exclusively of β-pleated sheets (Rosenbusch, 1974; Kleffel and co-workers, 1985). Its reconstitution in phospholipid bilayers revealed that its membrane-spanning channels exist reversibly in close and open configurations (Schindler & Rosenbusch, 1978). Each trimer contains three such channels (Schindler & Rosenbusch, 1981; Engel and co-workers, 1985). Three-dimensional reconstruction of two-dimensional lipid-containing porin crystals by electronmicroscopy allowed visualizing the three pores per trimer (Dorset and co-workers, 1983; Engel and co-workers, 1985). Three-dimensional crystals (Garavito & Rosenbusch, 1980) have been analyzed by X-ray crystallography (Garavito and co-workers, 1983; Garavito & Rosenbusch, 1985) and yield resolution to beyond 3 Å. Though progress in obtaining its high resolution structure is slow, detailed electron density maps may soon be available.

The protein sequence of porin (Chen and co-workers, 1982) has revealed that polar and ionizable residues are spread over the entire sequence: there is a single segment of eleven residues devoid of charges, all other such segments being shorter. Segments without any polar residues are ≤6 residues long. Labelling the protein from the hydrophobic membrane core (Page & Rosenbusch, 1986) and using a photoactivatable, carbene-generating reagent (Brunner & Semenza, 1981) confirms the notion, obtained from the structural studies, that the bulk mass of the protein exists within membrane boundaries. Reactions of nucleophilic groups, such as arg, lys, and carboxyl groups with reagents of various sizes and partition coefficients reveal a sizeable number of such ionizable groups to be buried within the membrane, and inaccessible from within the channels (Schindler & Rosenbusch, 1981; Page & Rosenbusch, 1986). Considerations of topology, sequence and structure predictions support the spectroscopically determined figure which indicates that two-thirds of the backbone exist in β-configuration (Kleffel and co-workers, 1985; Vogel & Jähnig, 1986). Taken together, these data clearly suggest that independent of any details of structure prediction, porin cannot span the membrane without polar and ionizable groups occuring within the membrane core (Paul & Rosenbusch, 1985).

Though this finding is at variance with the notion that hydrophobic segments arranged in α-helical configuration constitute the only membrane-spanning domains, the properties of porin may contribute to an understanding of the mechanism of transport of ions across the membrane barrier; one illuminating example

being the voltage-gated sodium channel protein. Much interest
has been focused on this protein that catalyzes sodium flux
across axonal membranes upon an action potential (Hodgkin &
Huxley, 1952). In the past few years, the primary structure of
several such proteins from different sources have been elucidated by Numa's group (Noda and co-workers, 1984; 1986). Noteworthy in the present context is that the structure predictions
based on notions such as hydrophobicity and α-helicity (Kyte &
Doolittle, 1982) and on related criteria (Finer-Moore & Stroud,
1984; Guy, 1984) led to proposals of the structure that could
either not be subject to voltage-control, or would transgress
the very rules that were used to devise them.

The basic criteria may thus need reexamination. The hydrophobic
effect clearly is an important aspect. It is theoretically
well-founded (Tanford, 1980) and generally accepted that water-
soluble proteins assume globular shapes in aqueous solutions,
thus minimizing the contact area between their hydrophobic core
and the aqueous bulk phase. This is illustrated in a model
experiment (Fig. 1a) which shows the shape that a droplet of a
nonpolar substance assumes if it is deposited into an aqueous
bulk phase. It also seems intuitively obvious that a droplet of
(stained) water, introduced into an aqueous bulk phase, lacks
the cohesive forces necessary for its assuming an organized
structure, thus rapidly diffusing (Fig. 1b) and fading. A completely hydrophilic macromolecule has, of course, constraints
of its own and is likely to assume a random coil configuration
(e.g. polysaccharides).

In the model experiments shown in panels c and d, the environment of a membrane protein is simulated by an organic solvent
of low dielectric constant. If a hydrophobic droplet is added
to the organic solvent, it also disperses rapidly (Fig. 1c),
corresponding to the situation of polar substances in aqueous
bulk phases. This may be taken to mimic, with a grain of salt,
the currently favored notion of hydrophobic domains located
within the membrane core. On the contrary, if a polar solvent
is injected into the organic phase (Fig. 1d), it assumes a
stable globular shape, thus minimizing the surface area (hydrophobic effect) and maximizing hydrogen-bonding within the droplet. Should this cartoon undo currently accepted concepts?
Surely, this model experiment is a gross oversimplification.
Thus, a membrane protein, unlike a soluble protein, is exposed
to two bulk solvents rather than one, and the effects of the
aqueous phase on the extramembranous protein domains are obviously neglected in the model experiment. (Incidentally, the
fact that two bulk phases exist, may be one of the main reasons why membrane protein crystallization is not trivial).
Thus, the membrane domain of the photosynthetic reaction center
protein contains only hydrophobic residues within the membrane,
and in this respect, it is comparable to the situation of Fig.
1c. However, its very substantial extramembranes domains exhibit a high order and may position, very precisely, the points
of exit and entry of the transmembrane polypeptides on both
sides of the membrane. Together with the stabilizing antiparallel α-helical dipoles (Wada, 1976; Edmonds, 1983), these
factors may cause the structure to be highly ordered also with-

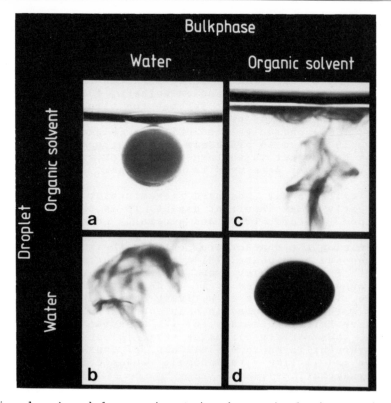

<u>Fig. 1</u> – A model experiment is shown simulating various
forces that may contribute to the shape that membrane
proteins may assume. Panel <u>a</u> illustrates the classical
hydrophobic effect (Tanford, 1980). A stained droplet of
organic solvent has been deposited just below the sol-
vent-air interface. The globular shape is due to the
minimization of the interface between water and the organic solvent. Due to matching the density of the organic
solvents used to that of water, the drop remains in its
original position. The photograph was taken 10 s after
deposition of a 5 µl droplet using an Eppendorf pipette.
Appropriate staining of droplets was performed for the
purpose of vizualisation. The experimental conditions in
<u>b</u>-<u>d</u> are analogous. Panel <u>b</u> shows the rapid diffusion of a
stained water droplet in an aqueous bulk phase. In panel
<u>c</u>, an organic solvent droplet has been introduced into
the same organic bulk solvent. In panel <u>d</u>, a stained
water droplet was introduced into the organic bulk solvent. In panel <u>b</u> and <u>c</u>, the contents of the droplets dis-
persed freely. With macromolecules, such as proteins, the
backbone would limit this dispersion, leading, presumably, to a random coil configuration. In panel <u>d</u>, the
aqueous droplet remains globular because of the minimization of its surface (hydrophobic effect), but also due
to the extensive hydrogen bonding network among the constituent water molecules within the droplet. It may thus
represent a model for porin which may expose polar groups
also on its <u>inter</u>molecular contact areas within the membrane.

in the crystal which appears to exhibit only very few amphi-
phile binding sites within the membrane domain (R. Huber, personal communication).

But what forces govern the structure of bacteriorhodopsin which
has most of its bulk mass within membrane boundaries and which
exhibits an apparently very hydrophobic surface (Engelman &
Zacchai, 1980) in the contact areas with the membrane? Are the
helical dipole moments and the few charged residues supposedly
within the membrane domain enough to stabilize this protein?
This is a particularly intruiging question because bacteriorhodopsin is unusually stable, with an irreversible thermal
denaturation occuring at 100°C (Jackson & Sturtevant, 1978).
Finally, bacteriorhodopsin monomers are likely to exhibit extensive interactions in the plane of the membrane, as this
protein is arranged in the purple patches of H. halobium as
lattices with an order that allows structural resolution to
reach 3.5 Å (Glaeser and co-workers, 1986).

Porin is, in the overall disposition in the membrane, similar
to bacteriorhodopsin. The bulk of its mass is located within
the membrane domain, with only small parts bulging out of
either side (for a review, see Rosenbusch, 1987). It forms two-
dimensional arrays that exhibit order to a resolution <5 Å
(Büldt and co-workers, 1986, and Massalski and co-workers, unpublished). In its solubilized state as well as within the membrane, it is unusually stable in all respect that have been
tested (Rosenbusch, 1974; Rosenbusch & Müller, 1977; Schindler
& Rosenbusch, 1985) so that intramolecular and intermolecular
interactions must be very strong. Because of these properties,
and its unusual polarity and secondary structure (see above),
it may be useful to study its organization within the membrane
as a complementary paradigm if it can indeed be considered a
typical membrane protein. The outer membrane of Gram-negative
bacteria in which it resides is quite unusual, of course
(Nikaido & Vaara, 1985), but it seems nonetheless worthy to
note that the functional studies were performed in membranes
reconstituted to bilayers with regular phospholipids, and that
its functional properties in this environment, determined by
conductance measurements, were identical to those determined
with outer membranes (Schindler & Rosenbusch, 1981). The structural studies also involved reconstructions of electron microscopic data in three dimensions of two-dimensional crystalline
lattices consisting of protein-phospholipid membranes (Engel
and co-workers, 1985). The packing in the small hexagonal form
of two-dimensional lattices appeared indistinguishable from
that of a hexagonal three-dimensional crystal habit. Since its
overall dimensions are in good agreement with the size of its
trimeric configuration in detergent solutions, it seems likely
that its structure does not undergo irreversible structural
perturbations under any of the conditions tested. Several further arguments reinforcing the notion of its location have been
reported elsewhere (Rosenbusch, 1987).

Although some of its structural peculiarities may not apply to
other of membrane protein systems, it nevertheless appears that
the principles guiding its structure are likely to be applic-

able to other membrane proteins as well. Surely, the model experiments shown in Fig. 1 are gross oversimplifications. As
mentioned, a membrane protein, unlike soluble proteins, is
exposed to two bulk phases rather than one. Thus, the membrane
protein of the reaction center, which contains only hydrophobic
residues, may have a well-ordered domain because of its very
substantial extramembranes domains which, together with the
stabilizing antiparallel α-helical dipoles, may contribute
significantly to the highly ordered structure of the membrane
domain also in the crystal. In a first approximation, the
structure of bacteriorhodopson, which exhibits a supposedly
very hydrophobic surface towards the membrane (Engelman &
Zacchai, 1980) would rely only on dipoles of its helices and
the effects the few charged residues within the membrane domain
may have to afford the highly unusual stability of this protein, which is critical in view of its temperature-tolerance,
mentioned above.

Considering the properties of porin may again be relevant in
this context. As indicated above, it seemed inconceivable at
the outset that polar and ionizable groups were included within
the membrane domain. The evidence that there is no typical
membrane domain in this protein has been summarized above. It
is folded in β-structure and contains polar and ionizable
groups evenly distributed throughout its sequence. Inspite of
these facts, it spans not only the outer membrane of Gram-negative bacteria, but can be reconstituted into phospholipid bilayers in a fully functional state. In fact, it had already
been postulated in 1974 that saturation of the hydrogen bonding
potential of polar residues renders them as hydrophobic as
nonpolar moieties (Chothia, 1974). It has also been reported
that ionizable groups are stable if buried in a low dielectric
medium, if they are electrically neutral and form hydrogen
bonds with neighboring donor and acceptor groups (Rashin and
Honig, 1984). According to these considerations, segments that
appear hydrophilic based on their primary structure may be
accommodated within the membrane.

The requirements of intramembranous domains may now be recon-
sidered as follows:
i) Nonpolar, α-helical segments may span the membrane, as it
occurs in photosynthetic reaction centers. To what extent the
helical dipoles (Wada, 1976; Edmonds, 1985) and van der Waals
interactions account in this instance for the high degree of
order in membrane domains is not clear. It seems beyond doubt
that much of the order in this protein is contributed by the
highly ordered and large extramembranous domains with their
intense intermolecular contacts. Uniquely relying on hydrophobicity and related parameters may help in identifying transmembrane segments, but hardly at the exclusion of any other
domain.
ii) The saturation of the hydrogen bonding potential of peptide
bonds within the backbone is likely to occur frequently in
α-helical configurations. However, any other periodic array
that fully saturates hydrogen bonding intrasegmentally would be
expected to be equally favorable energetically (Eisenberg,
1984). This may include structures such as 3_{10}, π, and 2.2_7

helices and 2, ribbons. No evidence for such structures has been obtained in membrane proteins, but again, the experience is very limited. Intersegmental hydrogen bonding, as it occurs in β-pleated sheet or barrel structures could again neutralize hydrogen bonding potentials. Indeed, in porin, this seems to be the predominant secondary structure occuring.
iii) If it is accepted that hydrogen bonding within the backbone renders the peptide bond "apolar", the same principle may apply to polar and ionizable residues, as discussed above. This notion could explain the properties of porin, and maybe also of bacteriorhodopsin, by calling for an open mind in predicting the structure of membrane channel proteins. So far, this has often invoked breaking the very rules that were used in the structure predictions (Guy and Hucho, 1987).

In conclusion, the existence of extensive hydrogen bonding networks and of electrostatic interactions which preserve local and global electroneutrality may complement the hydrophobic effect in folding and in stabilizing the structure of membrane proteins, including their intermolecular contacts which are so critical for obtaining them in crystalline order in two and three dimensions.

REFERENCES

Brunner, J., and G. Semenza (1981). Biochemistry, 20, 7174-7182.
Chen, R., C. Krämer, W. Schmidmayer, U. Chen-Schmeisser and U. Henning (1982). Biochem.J., 203, 33-43.
Chothia, C. (1974). Nature, 248, 338-339.
Deisenhofer, J., O. Epp, K. Miki, R. Huber, and H. Michel (1985). Nature, 318, 618-624.
Dorset, D.L., A. Engel, M. Häner, A. Massalski, and J.P. Rosenbusch (1983). J.Mol.Biol., 165, 701-710.
Edmonds, D.T. (1985). Eur.Biophys.J., 13, 31-35. Eiselé, J.-L. (1987). Experientia, in press.
Eisenberg, D. (1984). Annu.Rev.Biochem., 53, 595-623.
Engel, A., A. Massalski, H. Schindler, D.L. Dorset, and J.P. Rosenbusch (1985). Nature, 317, 643-645.
Engelman, D.M., R. Henderson, A.D. McLachlan, and B.A. Wallace (1980). Proc.Natl.Acad.Sci.US, 77, 2023-2027.
Engelman, D.M., and G. Zacchai (1980). Proc.Natl.Acad.Sci.US, 77, 5894-5898.
Engelman, D., and T.A. Steitz (1981). Cell, 23, 411-422.
Finer-Moore, J., and R. Stroud (1984). Proc.Natl.Acad.Sci.US, 81, 155-159.
Guy, R. (1984). Biophys.J., 45, 249-261.
Guy, R., and F. Hucho (1987). Trends Neurosci., 10, 318-321.
Garavito, R.M., and J.P. Rosenbusch (1980). J.Cell Biol., 86, 327-329.
Garavito, R.M., J. Jenkins, J.N. Jansonius, R. Karlsson, and J.P. Rosenbusch (1983). J.Mol.Biol., 164, 313-327.
Garavito, R.M., and J.P. Rosenbusch (1985). Methods Enzymol., 125, 309-328.
Glaeser, R.M., J. Baldwin, J.A. Cerka, and R. Henderson (1986). Biohpys.J., 50, 913-920.

Hodgkin, A.L., and A.F. Huxley (1952). J.Physiol. London, 117, 500-549.

Huang, K.-I., H. Bayley, M.-J. Liao, E. London, and H.G. Khorana (1981). J.Biol.Chem., 256, 3802-3809.

Jackson, M.B., and J.M. Sturtevant (1978). Biochem., 17, 911-915.

Katre, N.V., J. Finer-Moore, R.M. Stroud, S.B. Hayward (1984). Biophys.J., 46, 195-204.

Kleffel, B., R.M. Garavito, W. Baumeister, and J.P. Rosenbusch (1985). EMBO Journal, 4, 1589-1592.

Kyte, J., and R.F. Doolittle (1982). J.Mol.Biol., 152, 105-132.

Nikaido, H., and M. Vaara (1985). Microbiol.Rev., 49, 1-32.

Noda, M., S. Shimizu, T. Tanabe, T. Takai, T. Kayano, T. Ikeda, H. Takahashi, H. Nakayama, Y. Kanaoka, N. Minamino, K. Kangawa, H. Matsuo, M.A. Raftery, T. Hirose, S. Inayama, H. Hayashida, T. Miyata, and S. Numa (1984). Nature, 312, 121-127.

Noda, M., M. Ikeda, T. Kayano, H. Suzuki, H. Takashima, M. Kurasaki, H. Takahashi, and S. Numa (1986). Nature, 320, 188-192.

Page, M.P.G., and J.P. Rosenbusch (1986). Biochem.J., 235, 651-661.

Parsegian, A. (1969). Nature, 272, 586-590.

Paul, C., and J.P. Rosenbusch (1985). EMBO Journal, 4, 1593-1597.

Rashin, A.A., and B. Honig (1984). J.Mol.Biol., 173, 515-521.

Rosenbusch, J.P. (1974). J.Biol.Chem., 249, 8019-8029.

Rosenbusch, J.P. (1985). Bulletin Inst.Pasteur, 83, 207-220.

Rosenbusch, J.P. (1987). In: Bacterial Outer Membranes as Model Systems. M. Inouye (Ed.), John Wiley and Sons, pp. 141-162.

Schindler, H., and J.P. Rosenbusch (1978). Proc.Natl.Acad.Sci. US, 75, 3751-3755.

Schindler, H., and J.P. Rosenbusch (1981). Proc.Natl.Acad.Sci. US, 78, 2302-2306.

Schindler, M., and J.P. Rosenbusch (1982). J.Cell Biol., 92, 742-746.

Schindler, M., and J.P. Rosenbusch (1984). FEBS Letters, 173, 85-89.

Tanford, C. (1980). The Hydrophobic Effect. J.Wiley and Sons, New York.

Vogel, H., and F. Jähnig (1986). J.Mol.Biol., 190, 191-199.

Wada, A. (1976). Adv.Biophys., 9, 1-63.

Fehrenbach et al. (Eds.), Bacterial Protein Toxins, Zbl. Bakt. Suppl. 17
© Gustav Fischer, Stuttgart, New York, 1988

The Interaction of Ganglioside Carbohydrate with the Surface of Phosphatidylcholine and Phosphatidyl-Ethanolamine Bilayer Membranes

H.-J. Galla and M. Ollmann

Institut für Biochemie der TH Darmstadt, Petersenstraße 22, D-6100 Darmstadt

ABSTRACT

Pyrene labeled gangliosides were used to study their distribution in phosphatidylcholine bilayer membranes by the excimer formation technique. Labeled disialogangliosides PyG_{D1a} and PyG_{D1b} exemplify a system with nearly ideal mixing even in the presence of Ca^{2+}. Monosialogangliosides exhibit a preference for fluid bilayer regions. We observed a passive exclusion of G_{M3}, G_{M2} and G_{M1} from phosphatidylcholine domains that are rigidified by the Ca^{2+}-ions. Our experiments exclude a specific ganglioside-Ca^{2+}-interaction.
In phosphatidylethanolamine bilayer membranes the lipid phase transition temperature of fully hydrated membranes was reduced by G_{D1a} due to a disturbance of the hydrogen bonds between PE-molecules. This could not be observed with G_{M1} or G_{T1b}. From the spectroscopic determination of the hydration-dehydration process of PE membranes we were able to get information on the ganglioside headgroup orientation. G_{D1a} is found to be bend back to the bilayer surface whereas the headgroups of G_{M1} and G_{T1b} protrude out of the membrane surface into the aqueous phase.

KEYWORDS

Gangliosides, excimers, mixing behaviour with phosphatidyl-cholines, hydration of phosphatidylethanolamines

INTRODUCTION

Gangliosides are particularly abundant in cerebral grey matter but are also present in extraneuronal tissue. Their function and interaction with other lipid components and membrane proteins is far from beeing understood. It has been supposed that gangliosides serve as Ca^{2+}-storage and regulate nerve cell membrane permeability (Rahmann and Hilbig, 1983; Probst and others, 1984). In extraneuronal tissue gangliosides are receptors for bacterial toxins, hormones or viruses. The monosialoganglioside G_{M1} is a specific receptor for choleratoxin (Goins and others, 1986; Spiegel, 1985). The di- and trisialogangliosides G_{D1b} and G_{T1b} are reported to mediate the binding and the translocation of the tetanustoxin into the target cell (Lazarovici and Yavin, 1985). The function of gangliosides in the immune response of a cell and in the binding of antibodies is probably dependent on the chemical structure of the gangliosides and also on the conformational state of their headgroup.

In this paper we investigated the interaction between gangliosides and phosphatidylcholines as well as phosphatidylethanolamines in reconstituted membranes. Disialogangliosides exhibit a prominent feature in both types of model membranes due to their ideal mixing with phosphatidylcholines and due to their capacity to form hydrogen bonds with phosphatidylethanolamines.

RESULTS AND THEIR DISCUSSION

Thermotropic behaviour of pyrene-labeled gangliosides in phosphatidylcholine bilayers

Pyrene-labeled gangliosides (fig.1) were incorporated into dipalmitoylphosphatidylcholine (DPPC) bilayer membranes in molar ratios between 1 and 8 mol % with respect to the lipid.

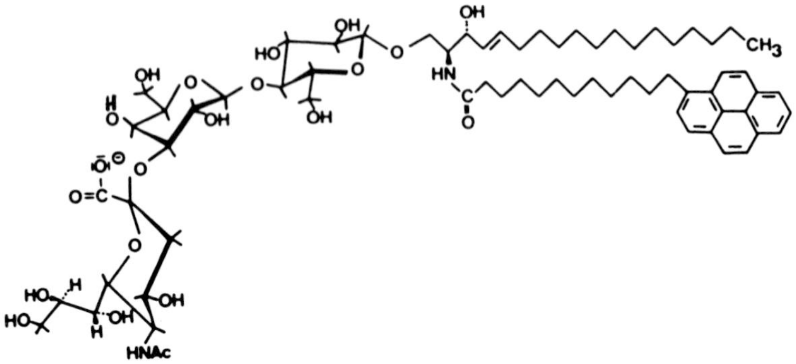

Fig. 1: Structure of pyrene-labeled monosialoganglioside PyG$_{M3}$ (N-12-(1-pyrene)dodecanoyl-lyso G$_{M3}$).

Pyrene derivatives are able to form excited dimers (excimers) if the sample is properly radiated (Galla and Hartmann, 1980). Typical fluorescence spectra clearly showing the monomer and the excimer band are given in fig. 2.

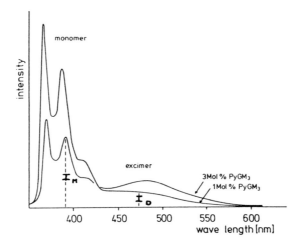

Fig. 2: Fluorescence spectra of PyG$_{M3}$ incorporated into dipalmitoylphosphatidylcholine bilayer membranes. Spectra for different ganglioside concentrations are taken at 45° C.
A broad excimer band around 470 nm appears beside the structured monomer band with increasing probe concentration.

From the intensity ratio I_D/I_M of the excimer to the monomer fluorescence emission it is possible to determine the coefficient of the lateral diffusion of the probe and it is possible to measure the thermotropic phase transition curve of the host lipid (Galla and Hartmann, 1980). Here we summarize the main results of our recent exhaustive study (Ollmann and others, 1987):

1) From the observed linear concentration dependence of the I_D/I_M-ratio with increasing pyrene-labeled ganglioside content we know that PyG$_{M1}$, PyG$_{M2}$, PyG$_{M3}$, PyG$_{D1a}$ and PyG$_{D1b}$ distribute homogeneously in fluid phosphatidylcholine bilayers. The lateral diffusion coefficient ($D_{diff} = 1,6 \times 10^{-7}$ cm^2/s) is comparable to the diffusion of the phosphatidylcholines themselves.

2) Ca^{2+}-ions up to 200 mM do not affect ganglioside diffusion significantly. Even in the presence of Ca^{2+} gangliosides do not tend to phase separate in fluid bilayer membranes.

3) The shape of the thermotropic phase transition curves obtained by the excimer technique yield information on the lateral distribution of pyrene probes between fluid and rigid domains within the bilayer membranes (Hresco and others, 1986). Fig. 3 summarizes some typical results. Fig. 3A is an example of a completely miscible probe with nonideal mixing behaviour. Pyrene labeled phosphatidylcholine was used as probe molecule. The height of the I_D/I_M – peak between 30 and 40° C is a measure of the probe's

preference for a fluid state. Below the phase transition temperature (T_m = 41°C) PyPC concentrates in fluid defects leading to a
local increase of the probe concentration and therefore to an
increased I_D/I_M ratio in comparison to the fluid phase, where the
probe is homogeneously distributed. Addition of Ca^{2+} induces a
drastic increase of the peak height.

Pyrene labeled gangliosides were used to determine the phase
transition of the DPPC host membrane in the absence and in the
presence of Ca^{2+} (fig. 3 B-D). In the absence of Ca^{2+} and with
PyG_{M3} as probe molecule the phase transition is indicated by a
plateau region of the I_D/I_M values between 35 and 40°C. With
PyG_{M1} this plateau disappears and with PyG_{D1a} the host lipid
phase transition is indicated by an increase in the I_D/I_M ratio.
The curves shown in fig. 3D are typical for a probe with ideal
mixing behaviour.

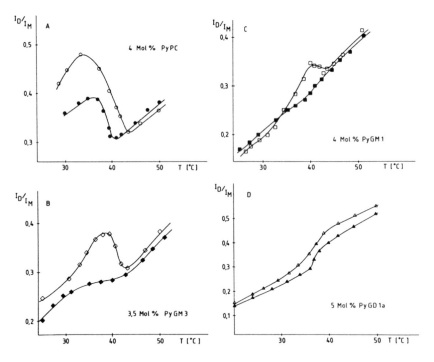

Fig. 3: Phase transition curves of DPPC measured
by the excimer formation technique using different
pyrene labeled lipids:
A) pyrene – labeled phosphatidylcholine (PyPC)
B) PyG_{M3} , C) PyG_{M1}, D) PyG_{D1a} .
Closed symbols are given in the absence and open
symbols in the presence of 200 mM Ca^{2+}.

Addition of Ca^{2+} triggers a tightening of the phosphatidylcholine
bilayer and induces a change in the lateral distribution of PyG_{M3}

and PyG_{M1} at the phase transition. The system passes into a nonideal distribution between fluid and rigid regions. Ca^{2+}-ions are able to recover the I_D/I_M peak. PyG_{D1a} however exhibits an almost ideal mixing behaviour. Even in the presence of 200 mM Ca^{2+} the peak could not be recovered. This clearly demonstrates that G_{D1a} performs a favourable interaction with phosphatidylcholine due to a best fit of the headgroup dipoles as was postulated by Maggio and others (1980).

We conclude, that the disialoganglioside is randomly distributed between fluid and rigidified parts of a membrane. Ca^{2+} is able to induce a ganglioside preference for the fluid phase with mono-sialo- but not with disialogangliosides. However, this effect is not caused by a specific Ca^{2+}-ganglioside interaction but by a tightening of the PC-membrane and a passive exclusion of the monosialogangliosides from the gel phase. These results together with the above mentioned diffusion data rule out a chelating effect of Ca^{2+} on gangliosides in PC-membranes.

Ganglioside-Phosphatidylethanolamine-interaction

Aqueous dispersions of phosphatidylethanolamines are known to form two types of solid lamellar phases depending on the mode of preparation (Seddon and others, 1983). The first type, a fully hydrated gel phase, forms rapidly by preparing the sample above the crystalline to liquid-crystalline phase transition temperature T_{m1}. This hydrated gel phase is metastabel with respect to a second, dehydrated crystalline phase. Dehydrated samples show a crystalline to liquid-crystalline phase transition at an elevated temperature T_{mh} (fig.4). The dehydrated phase can be generated either by dispersion of the lipid in the aqueous medium below T_{m1} or by incubating an initially hydrated sample at low temperature (4° C) for several days.

We investigated the effect of different gangliosides on the phase transition temperature of the hydrated PE-Phase (Fig. 5). Phase transition curves are measured by electron spin resonance using the temperature dependent partition of 2,2,6,6 tetramethylpiperi-dine-1-oxid (TEMPO) between the water and the lipid phase. The increase in the partition coefficient is a measure for the flui-disation of the membrane. Only G_{D1a} reduces the phase transition temperature of the host lipid by about 5° C. G_{M1} and G_{T1b} did not affect the PE-phase transition temperature. The negativ surface charge allone is therefore not responsible for this shift.

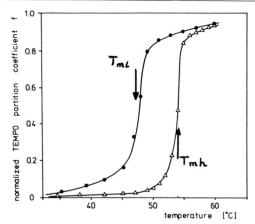

Fig. 4: Phase transition curves of fully hydrated and completely dehydrated dimyristoylphosphatidyl-ethanolamine (DMPE) bilayer membranes. The corresponding phase transition temperatures are T_{ml} = 48° C for the hydrated and T_{mh} = 54° C for the dehydrated phase. Transition curves are obtained by EPR-spectroscopy.

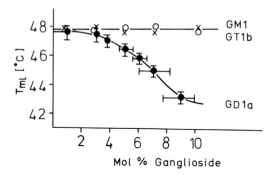

Fig. 5: The effect of gangliosides on the phase transition temperature of fully hydrated DMPE - membranes. G_{D1a} (●-●-●), G_{M1} (x-x-x) G_{T1b} (o-o-o).

Again obviously only the disialoganglioside strongly interacts with the lipids of the host membrane. We propose that the headgroup of G_{D1a} exhibits a conformation where the sialic acid residues are directed to the membrane surface and disturb the hydrogen bonds between the ammonium group and the phosphate group of neighboured PE-molecules. This hydrogen bond network stabilize the pure PE-layer. The carboxylic groups of the sialic acids function as hydrogen bond acceptors and may therefore invade into the surface region thus expanding the PE-layer. Consequently the phase transition temperature will be reduced. The fact that this is only induced by the disialoganglioside but not by monosialo- or trisialogangliosides gives raise to the assumption that only G_{D1a} assumes a conformation which allows the incorporation of the sialic acid residue into the PE-headgroup region. In comparison to the experiments with PC-membranes this is only possible if the oligosaccharide part of G_{D1a} is bend back to the membrane surface whereas with G_{M1} or G_{T1b} it protrudes out of the membrane into the aqueous space.

Additional information supporting the above hypothesis was ob- tained from the consideration of the stability of the hydrated phase. Pure DMPE converts from the hydrated to the dehydrated phase during incubation at 4°C. The choice of an appropriate time produces a situation, where part of the lipid is dehydrated and the rest remains hydrated. The corresponding phase transition curve exhibits two steps clearly demonstrating the coexistence of hydrated and dehydrated membrane regions. The midpoints of the two superimposed transitions are again T_{ml} and T_{mh}. The step

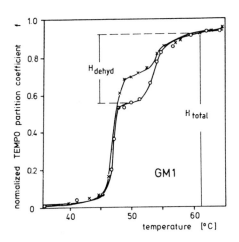

Fig. 6: Phase transition curves of hydrated DMPE/Ganglioside - samples, taken after incuba- tion at 4°C for 5 days: 1 mol % G_{M1} (o-o-o) and 2 mol % G_{M1} (x-x-x).

height, H_{dehyd}, with respect to the total height, H_{total}, is taken to quantify the amount of lipid in the dehydrated phase. In the presence of gangliosides the step height, H_{dehyd}, decreases with increasing ganglioside content. The effect, shown in fig. 6 for G_{M1}, depends on the ganglioside species.

The evaluation of the experiments is given in fig. 7. The fraction of lipid in the dehydated phase is given as function of ganglioside concentration for G_{M1}, G_{D1a} and G_{T1b}. From the extrapolation of the straight lines we obtain the concentration of ganglioside that is necessary to inhibit the dehydration process completely. The amount needed is 7 mol % G_{D1a}, 4 mol % G_{M1} and only 1.4 mol % G_{T1b}.

From these experiments we derived further evidence that G_{D1a} is bend back to the membrane surface. The inhibition of the dehydration process is mainly caused by charge-charge-repulsion between neighboured bilayers thus allowing hydration of the membrane surface. The same effect could be obtained with phosphatidic acid (data not shown) where a conformational effect can be excluded. With G_{M1} and even more clearly marked with G_{T1b} we have to assume an additional effect. We conclude that the G_{M1} and G_{T1b} head group protrude out into the water phase thus acting as a hydrated spacer between adjacent bilayer membranes. G_{T1b} which has the largest headgroup and in addition is most highly charged has the strongest potency to keep a membrane surface hydrated.

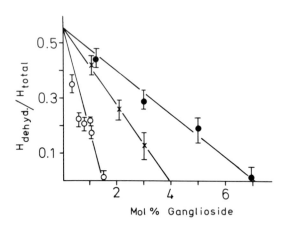

Fig. 7: The fraction of DMPE in the dehydrated phase is given as function of ganglioside content for G_{D1a} (●-●-●), G_{M1} (x-x-x) and G_{T1b} (o-o-o).

This work has been supported by a grant from the Deutsche Forschungsgemeinschaft under contract Ga 233/10. We like to thank Mrs. A. Minde for the preparation of the manuscript.

Literature

Galla, H.-J; Hartmann, W. (1980). Excimer-forming lipids in membrane research. Chem. Phys. Lipids, 27,199-219.

Goins, B., Masserini, M., Barisas, B. G. and Freire, E. (1986). Biophys. J., 49, 849-856.

Hresko, R. C., Sugár, J. P., Barenholz, Y. and Thompson, T. E. (1986). Lateral distribution of a pyrene-labeled phosphatidylcholine in phosphatidylcholin bilayers: Fluorescence phase and modulation study. Biochemistry, 25, 3813-3828.

Lazarovici, P. and Yavin, E. (1985). Tetanus toxin interaction with human erythrocytes. II. Kinetic properties of toxin association and evidence for a toxin-ganglioside macromolecular complex formation. Biochim. Biophys. Acta, 812, 532-542.

Maggio, B., Cumar, F.A. and Caputto, R. (1980). Configuration and interaction of the polar head group in gangliosides. Biochem. J., 189, 435-440.

Ollmann, M., Schwarzmann, G., Sandhoff, K. and Galla, H.-J. (1987). Pyrene labeled gangliosides: micelle formation in aqueous solution, lateral diffusion and thermotropic behaviour in phosphatidylcholine bilayers. Biochemistry, in press.

Probst, W., Nobius, D. and Rahmann, H. (1984). Cell. Mol. Neurobiol., 4, 157-176.

Rahmann, H. and Hilbig, R. (1983). Phylogenetical aspects of brain gangliosides in vertebrates. J. Comp. Physiol., 151, 215-224.

Seddon, J. M., Cevc, G. and Marsh, D. (1983). Calorimetric studies of the gel-fluid and lamellar- inverted hexagonal phase transitions in dialkyl- and diacyl-phosphatidylethanolamines. Biochemistry, 22, 1280-1289.

Spiegel, S. (1985). Fluorescent derivatives of ganglioside GM1 function as receptors for cholera toxin. Biochemistry, 24, 5947-5952.

Fehrenbach et al. (Eds.), Bacterial Protein Toxins, Zbl. Bakt. Suppl. 17
© Gustav Fischer, Stuttgart, New York, 1988

Interaction of Diphteria Toxin (Fragment B) with Natural Membranes

P. Falmagne[1], R. Wattiez[1], V. Cabiaux[2], A. Phalipon[3], M. Kaczorek[3],
P. M. Tulkens[1, 4] and J.-M. Ruysschaert[2]

[1]Laboratoire de Chimie biologique, Université de l'Etat à Mons, B-7000 Mons
[2]Laboratoire de Chimie physique des Macromolécules aux Interfaces, Université Libre de Bruxelles, B-1050 Bruxelles
[3]Unité des Applications du Génie Génétique, Institut Pasteur de Paris, 28, rue du Dr Roux, F-75724, Paris Cédex 15
[4]Laboratoire de Chimie Physiologique and ICP, Université Catholique de Louvain, B-1200 Bruxelles

ABSTRACT

Diphtheria toxin fragment B contains several domains of interaction with lipid bilayers. Most of these domains are included in CB1, the cyanogen bromide peptide located in the middle region of fragment B. At low pH (4.5), CB1 is able to promote the destabilization of model membranes as well as to induce the lysis of sheep erythrocytes and rat liver lysosomes. CB1 is also toxic to Vero cells at a concentration of $3.10^{-7}M$. Site-directed mutagenesis was used to investigate which of these functional domains of fragment B is responsible for the interaction of diphtheria toxin with eukaryotic cell membranes.

KEYWORDS

Diphtheria toxin fragment B, Cyanogen bromide peptide CB1, Natural membranes, Lipid–associating domains, Site–directed mutagenesis.

INTRODUCTION

Fragment B (Mr 37240) of diphtheria toxin (Mr 58390) mediates, via acidic endosomes, the internalization of the toxin molecule into the cytoplasm of sensitive eukaryotic cells where the toxin fragment A (Mr 21150) catalytically inhibits protein synthesis by ADP–ribosylation of elongation factor 2 and kills the cell (Olsnes and Sandvig, 1985; Pappenheimer, 1982).

The transmembrane transport of fragment A takes place in a cellular compartment where the receptor-bound toxin is exposed to pH lower than 5.3 (Draper and Simon, 1980; Sandvig and Olsnes, 1980). In these conditions of acid pH, fragment B changes its conformation (Blewitt, Chung and London, 1985), exposes hydrophobic regions cryptic at pH 7.2 and inserts itself into the membrane (Hu and Holmes, 1984; Montecucco, Schiavo and Tomasi, 1985).

Structural analysis of the amino-acid sequence of fragment B has revealed the presence of at least four different domains of interaction with the lipid bilayer (Falmagne and co-workers, 1984, 1985; Lambotte and co-workers, 1980).

1. Three amphiphilic alpha-helical hydrophilic surface lipid-associating domains, or surface-seeking domains (residues 16-30, 44-63, 173-184). These domains specifically interact with the charged phospholipid headgroups and are inserted in the bilayer in a way that most likely induces its destabilization.
2. Two adjacent amphiphilic alpha-helical hydrophobic transverse lipid-associating domains (residues 133-151, 153-172) which would be involved in the pore formation observed in black lipid membranes (Deleers and co-workers, 1983; Kayser and co-workers, 1981).
3. An extremely hydrophobic membrane-penetrating segment (residues 225-246) which has all the properties of a signal sequence. It also contains a cluster of four prolyl residues. Using conformational analysis based on computer-assisted modeling, it has been demonstrated that the "cis-trans" isomerization of Pro 242 and 245 induced by low pH – but not by neutral pH – profoundly changes the conformation of this segment in a way that uncovers the hydrophobic region and promotes its insertion into a lipid layer; this low pH-driven process leads to the destabilization of the lipid matrix (Brasseur and co-workers, 1986).
4. A strongly cationic site (residues 247-281) which includes the disulfide bridge of fragment B and constitutes at least a large part of the P-site (Cabiaux and co-workers, 1985).

Most of these domains – particularly the transmembrane domains and the membrane-penetrating segment – are included in CB1 (Mr 13070), the cyanogen bromide peptide of fragment B located in its middle region. On the other hand, CB1 does not include the C-terminal region of fragment B involved in the toxin binding to its receptors. Like diphtheria toxin and fragment B, CB1 has been shown to induce, at low pH, pore formation in planar lipid bilayers (Deleers and co-workers, 1983; Kayser and co-workers, 1981) and fusion and aggregation of small unilamellar vesicles of phospholipids, especially if the latter contain phosphatidylinositol, as is the case for asolectin (Cabiaux and co-workers, 1984, 1985; Falmagne, Cabiaux and Ruysschaert, 1986). The other regions of fragment B have no such destabilizing effects on model membranes.

In the present work, we show that CB1 kills Vero cells with a cytotoxic dose of 3.10^{-7}M and is able to induce, at low pH but not at neutral pH, the lysis of sheep erythrocytes and of lysosomes of rat liver cells, at about the same concentration. In a further attempt to identify which functional domains of CB1 are actually involved in membrane destabilization, we used site-directed mutagenesis to create two different kinds of fragment B mutants. In the first mutants, Pro 242 and 245 of the membrane-penetrating segment were replaced by two alanines to eliminate the predicted low pH-induced conformational change; in the second mutants, Ile 171 and 172 of the transmembrane domains were substituted by two lysyl residues to destroy its amphiphilic character.

INTERACTION WITH NATURAL MEMBRANES

Fig. 1 shows that CB1 has a toxic activity on African green monkey kidney (Vero) cells. A 3 h. incubation of Vero cells with 10^{-6}M CB1 led to a 75% decrease of protein synthesis, 50% reduction being obtained with 3.10^{-7}M CB1. That the cytotoxicity of CB1 is not due to the presence of traces of diphtheria toxin was demonstrated by the fact that CB1 had the same toxic activity on Vero cells in

the presence of 10^{-8}M fragment B. At this concentration, fragment B is absolutely non-toxic but perfectly able to compete with diphtheria toxin for the cell
surface receptors, as shown in Fig. 1 (inset), and to increase the cytotoxic
dose of the toxin by at least one order of magnitude. CB1, therefore, was not
contaminated by diphtheria toxin. The absence of contaminating fragment A was
confirmed by automated amino acid microsequence analysis.

In the presence of NH_4Cl (10mM), the cells were completely protected from the
cytotoxic effect of CB1 (Fig. 1). As it is well established that CB1 requires a
low pH to destabilize model membranes, the protective effect of NH_4Cl suggests
that CB1 exerted its cytotoxic activity from a cellular compartment where it was
exposed to a low pH and not directly on the pericellular membrane.

A direct pH-dependent destabilizing effect of CB1 on natural membranes was
demonstrated by incubating variable concentrations of CB1 with rat liver cell
lysosomes and sheep erythrocytes at neutral and low pH. Fig. 2 shows that a 15
min incubation of lysosomes from rat liver cells with increasing concentrations
of CB1, at 25°C and pH 4.5, induced a significant decrease of the structural
latency of the lysosomal marker enzyme N-acetyl-beta-glucosaminidase (E.C.
3.2.1.29). No effect on the lysosomal enzyme was observed at pH 7.0 (Fig. 2,
inset). Interestingly enough, the effect of CB1 on the lysosomal membrane at pH
4.5 was quantitatively equivalent to that obtained with similar concentrations
of Triton X-100, a non-ionic detergent currently used to suppress the structural

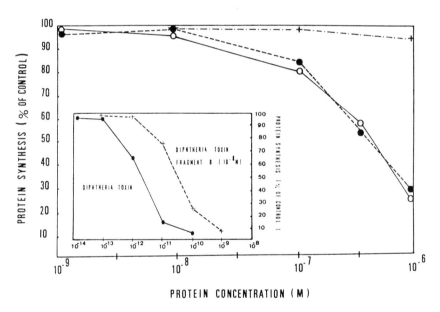

PROTEIN CONCENTRATION (M)

Fig. 1: Protein synthesis inhibition in Vero cells treated with CB1. Vero cells
were incubated for 3 h at 37°C in Dulbecco's modified Eagle's medium containing
10% fetal calf serum and 20 mM Hepes buffer pH 7.2 with increasing concentrations of CB1 alone (O), or CB1 plus 10^{-8}M fragment B (●), or CB1 plus NH_4Cl
(10 mM) (+). The ability of the cells to incorporate ^{14}C-leucine during 30 min
is expressed as percent of the control values (no CB1 added). Inset: Protein
synthesis inhibition in Vero cells intoxicated with diphtheria toxin in the
absence (●) or in the presence (+) of 10^{-8}M fragment B.

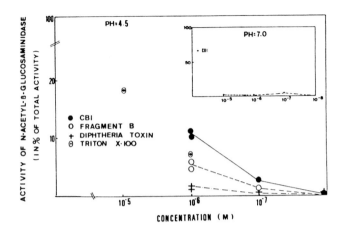

Fig. 2: CB1-induced release of the structural latency of N-acetyl-beta-glucosa-minidase from lysosomes of rat liver. Rat liver homogenates were prepared at 0°C in isotonic (0.25 M) sucrose buffered at pH 7.4 with 3 mM imidazole. Incubation was carried out at 25°C for 15 min in isotonic media with increasing concentrations of CB1 (●), fragment B (O), diphtheria toxin (+) or Triton X-100 (⊖) in 100 mM citrate buffer pH 4.5 - 0.15 M NaCl. Inset: incubation in the presence of CB1 in 50 mM Hepes buffer pH 7.0 - 0.15 M NaCl. The activity of the enzyme was determined according to Sellinger and co-workers (1960) and is expressed as the percent of the activity measured in the presence of 0.2% Triton X-100 (total activity).

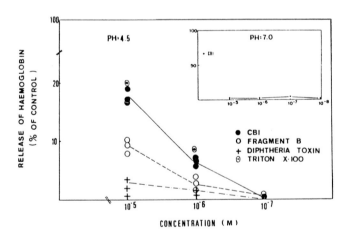

Fig. 3.: CB1-induced release of haemoglobin from sheep erythrocytes. Erythrocytes from defibrinated sheep blood were incubated for 30 min at 37°C with increasing concentrations of CB1 (●), fragment B (O), diphtheria toxin (+) or Triton X-100 (⊖) in 50 mM cacodylate-HCl buffer pH 4.5 - 0.15 M NaCl. Inset: incubation in the presence of CB1 in 50 mM Hepes buffer pH 7.0 - 150 mM NaCl. Erythrocytes were sedimented by centrifugation and the release of haemoglobin was measured from the A_{411} of haemoglobin in the supernatant fluid and expressed in percent of the amount released in the presence of 0.2% Triton X-100.

latency of lysosomal enzymes in homogenates. In the same experimental conditions, at low pH, fragment B had lesser effect than CB1 and diphtheria toxin
had no significant effect, a situation similar to that already observed with
black lipid membranes (Kayser and co-workers, 1981).

As shown in Fig. 3, CB1 is also capable, at low pH but not at neutral pH (Fig. 3
inset), to induce the release of haemoglobin from sheep erythrocytes after a 30
min incubation at 37°C. Here too, at pH 4.5, fragment B had a lesser effect and
diphtheria toxin did not show any significant effect.

These results clearly suggest that CB1 has on the stability of natural membranes
an effect comparable to that it has on model membranes, in similar conditions.
Thus some of the domains identified in the region of fragment B corresponding to
CB1 must be responsible for the interaction of diphtheria toxin with eukaryotic
cell membranes and for their resulting destabilization. At the low pH of the
endosome, such a destabilization could play an important role in the fragment B-
mediated transmembrane transfer of fragment A through the endosomal membrane
into the cytosol.

FRAGMENT B MUTANTS: SITE-DIRECTED MUTAGENESIS

The entire gene coding for the wild type fragment B was first reconstructed by
cloning in a puc 18 vector (pTarB; Fig. 4.a.). In this vector, the tox B gene
is under the control of the lac promoter and the coded protein contains an
additional N-terminal sequence of 8-9 amino acid residues. To reduce the length
of this extra sequence and to obtain a high level of protein expression, the
tox B gene was then cloned into the expression vector pKK 233-2. An ATG initiation codon was provided to the tox B gene by cloning of the gene into the unique
restriction site Nco I of pKK 233-2, using a 6- mer Nco linker to maintain the
translational reading frame. In this construction, the tox B gene is under the
control of the strong promoter p trc - a trp lac fusion promoter - inducible by
isopropylthiogalactoside (IPTG) (pKKB; Fig. 4.b.).

For site-directed mutagenesis, the fragment EcoRI-KpnI of pTarB containing the
tox B gene was cloned in the coliphage M13mp18 containing the selectable am4
marker that gives enhanced yields of mutants (Carter, Bedouelle and Winter,
1985). Four 15-16 mer oligonucleotides were synthesized that were designed to
introduce the following mutations:
  (1) Ile 171 ⟶ Lys (2) Ile 171 ⟶ Lys (3) Pro 242 ⟶ Ala (4) Pro 242 ⟶ Ala
                         Ile 172 ⟶ Lys   Pro 245 ⟶ Ala
 Mutagenesis was directed by annealing the single-stranded M13 recombinant to the
oligonucleotide which then served as a primer for the synthesis of the complementary strand using DNA polymerase I. After ligation, the resulting heterodu-
plexes were used to transform E. coli. Replication in vivo produced recombinant
M13 progeny possessing either mutant or wild type genotypes. Mutants were identified by hybridization using the ^{32}P labelled mutagenic oligonucleotide as a
probe. In principle, the mutagenic oligonucleotide forms a more stable duplex
with a mutant clone with perfect match than with a wild type clone bearing a
mismatch. The mutant is detected by forming a duplex at a low temperature where
both mutant and wild type DNAs interact, then carrying out washes at increasingly higher temperatures until only mutant DNA molecules hybridize. Fig. 5 shows
the screening performed on mutants in which Ile 171 was substituted by Lys. To
verify that the desired mutation had actually been produced, the single stranded
DNA was sequenced by the dideoxy chain-termination method. The ClaI-KpnI 870 bp

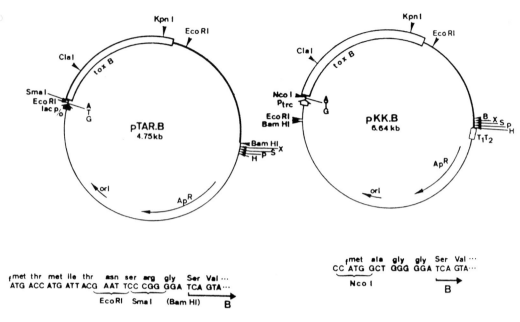

Fig. 4: (a) Construction of pTarB; (b) construction of pKKB.

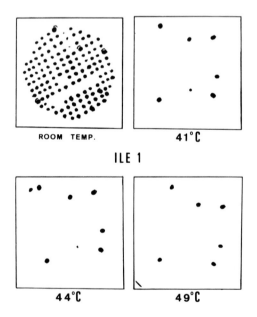

Fig. 5: Screening of mutant Ile 171 ⟶ Lys. Hybridization of ^{32}P labelled mutagenic oligonucleotide with the E. coli clones as a function of temperature.

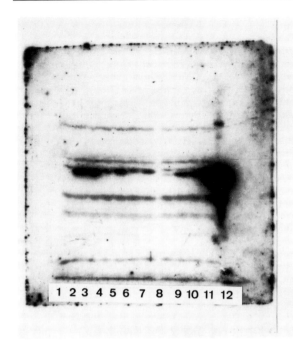

1 TG 1

2 pKKB n.i.

3 pKKB i.

4 pKKB 364 n.i.   Ile 171 → Lys

5 pKKB 364 i.

6 pKKB 364.5 n.i.   Ile 171→Lys
                     Ile 172→Lys

7 pKKB 364.5 i

8 pKKB 435 n.i.   Pro 242→Ala

9 pKKB 435 i.

10 pKKB 435.8 n.i.   Pro 242→Ala
                      Pro 245→Ala

11 pKKB 435.8 i.

12 DTB

Fig. 6: Western blot analysis showing the expression of wild type and mutant pKKB by TGI in the presence (i.) or in the absence (n.i.) of IPTG.

fragment of the mutants were then cloned in the expression vector (pKKB) from which the ClaI–KpnI fragment containing the tox B wild type gene had been deleted. The constructions were tested by hybridization with the ^{32}P-labelled oligonucleotide using pKKB wild type as a negative control. The four mutated pKKB were also sequenced by the Maxam–Gilbert procedure using isolated double stranded DNA.

The expression of the wild type fragment B and of the four fragment B mutants was studied in E. coli TGI. The expression was induced by adding IPTG (final concentration: 5mM) to a culture of TGI at A_{660nm}= 0.3. After 30 min of induction, 1 ml of the culture was centrifuged and the total proteins were characterized by PAGE-SDS. Immunoblotting showed that a protein with an apparent molecular weight of 38000 daltons was expressed by TGI transformed either with pKKB or with the mutants (Fig. 6). No degradation or proteolysis was observed 30 min after addition of IPTG. Fragment B was indeed localized in the cytoplasm of E. coli and its concentration evaluated at 10 mg/litre of a culture at A_{660nm}= 1. Moreover, the expression of fragment B was non toxic for E. Coli since the growth of TGI transformed with the tox B gene and the four mutants was identical to the growth of nontransformed TGI even two hours after the addition of IPTG (not shown).

The next step will be the purification of the modified fragments B produced by E. coli, the reconstitution of the corresponding toxins by linking these fragments B to normal fragment A via a disulfide bridge and the study of the biological activity of these mutant toxins.

REFERENCES

Blewitt, M.G., L.A. Chung, and E. London (1985). Effect of pH on the conformation of diphtheria toxin and its implications for membrane penetration. Biochemistry, 24, 5458–5464.

Brasseur, R., V. Cabiaux, P. Falmagne, and J.-M. Ruysschaert (1986). pH dependent insertion of a diphtheria toxin B fragment peptide into the lipid membrane : a conformational analysis. Biochem. Biophys. Res. Commun., 136, 160–168.

Cabiaux, V., M. Vandenbranden, P. Falmagne, and J.-M. Ruysschaert (1984). Diphtheria toxin induces fusion of small unilamellar vesicles at low pH. Biochim. Biophys. Acta, 775, 31–36.

Cabiaux, V., M. Vandenbranden, P. Falmagne, and J.-M. Ruysschaert (1985). Aggregation and fusion of lipid vesicles induced by diphtheria toxin at low pH : Possible involvement of the P site and the NAD+ binding site. Bioscience Rep., 5, 243–250.

Carter, P., H. Bedouelle, and G. Winter (1985). Improved oligonucleotide site-directed mutagenesis using M13 vectors. Nucleic Acids Res., 13, 4431–4443.

Deleers, M., N. Beugnier, P. Falmagne, V. Cabiaux, and J.-M. Ruysschaert (1983). Localization in diphtheria toxin fragment B of a region that induces pore formation in planar lipid bilayers at low pH. FEBS Lett, 160, 82–86.

Draper, R.K., and M.I. Simon (1980). The entry of diphtheria toxin into the mammalian cell cytoplasm : Evidence for lysosomal involvement. J. Cell Biol., 87, 849–854.

Falmagne, P., C. Capiau, V. Cabiaux, M. Deleers, and J.-M. Ruysschaert (1984). Fragment B of diphtheria toxin : Correlation between amino acid sequence and lipid binding properties. In : J.E. Alouf, F.J. Fehrenbach, J.H. Freer and J. Jeljaszewicz (Eds.), Bacterial Protein Toxins. FEMS Symposium n° 24, Seillac, France, June 1983, Academic Press London, pp. 139–146.

Falmagne, P., C. Capiau, P. Lambotte, J. Zanen, V. Cabiaux, and J.-M. Ruysschaert (1985). The complete amino acid sequence of diphtheria toxin fragment B. Correlation with its lipid binding properties. Biochim. Biophys. Acta, 827, 45–50.

Falmagne, P., V. Cabiaux, and J.-M. Ruysschaert (1986). Diphtheria toxin–lipid interactions. Fusion of lipid vesicles at low pH. In : P. Falmagne, J.E. Alouf, F.J. Fehrenbach, J. Jeljaszewicz and M. Thelestam (Eds.), Bacterial Protein Toxins. 2d European Workshop, Wépion, Belgium 1985, Gustav Fischer Verlag, Stuttgart, pp. 93–100.

Hu, V.W., and R.K. Holmes (1984). Evidence for direct insertion of fragments A and B of diphtheria toxin into model membranes. J. Biol. Chem., 259, 12226–12233.

Kayser, G., P. Lambotte, P. Falmagne, C. Capiau, J. Zanen, and J.-M. Ruysschaert (1981). A CNBr peptide located in the middle region of diphtheria toxin fragment B induces conductance change in lipid bilayers. Biochem. Biophys. Res. Commun., 99, 358–363.

Lambotte, P., P. Falmagne, C. Capiau, J. Zanen, J.-M. Ruysschaert, and J. Dirkx (1980). Primary structure of diphtheria toxin fragment B : Structural similarities with lipid–binding domains. J. Cell Biol., 87, 837–840.

Montecucco, C., G. Schiavo, and M. Tomasi (1985). pH dependence of the phospholipid interaction of diphtheria-toxin fragments. Biochem. J., 231, 123–128.

Olsnes, S., and K. Sandvig (1985). Entry of polypeptide toxins into animal cells. In : I. Pastan and M.C. Willingham (Eds.), Endocytosis, Plenum Publishing Corp., pp. 195–234.

Pappenheimer, A.M., Jr. (1982). Harvey Lect. Ser., 76, 45–73.

Sandvig, K., and S. Olsnes (1980). Diphtheria toxin entry into cells is facilitated by low pH. J. Cell Biol., 87, 828–832.

Sellinger, O.Z., H. Beaufay, P. Jacques, A. Doyen, and C. de Duve (1960). Tissue fractionation studies. 15. Intracellular distribution and properties of N-acetylglucosaminidase and galactosidase in rat liver. Biochem. J., 74, 450-456.

Fehrenbach et al. (Eds.), Bacterial Protein Toxins, Zbl. Bakt. Suppl. 17
© Gustav Fischer, Stuttgart, New York, 1988

Studies on the Insertion of Diphtheria Toxin into Biological Membranes

C. Montecucco[1], E. Papini[1], G. Schiavo[1], R. Rappuoli[2] and M. Tomasi[3]

[1]Centro C.N.R. Biomembrane e Dipartimento di Scienze Biomediche Sperimentali, Universita' di Padova, I-Padova
[2]Centro Ricerche Sclavo, Via Fiorentina 1, I-53100 Siena
[3]Laboratorio di Biologia Cellulare, Istituto Superiore di Sanita', I-Roma

SUMMARY

Acidic pHs induce a conformational change of diphtheria toxin that enables it to interact with the hydrocarbon chains of phospholipids. This structural transition has been followed in liposomal model systems by hydrophobic photolabelling and in vivo by toxicity assays on low pH treated cells. At neutral pH the toxin interacts with the bilayer surface and this interaction is proposed to contribute to the toxin binding to cells. At acidic pHs the toxin also interacts hydrophobically with the fatty acid chains and the pKa of this interaction is higher for protomer B than for the enzymic A chain. This suggests that protomer B is the first part of the toxin that at low pH inserts into the membrane wherefrom it assists the penetration of chain A.

INTRODUCTION

The process of cell killing by diphtheria toxin (DT) may be divided into three main steps: a) binding to the cell plasma membrane, b) membrane translocation and c) block of protein synthesis by modification of EF-2. While detailed information on the last step are available, we know very little on the first two passages (1,2).

DT binds to sensitive cell lines with an association constant around 10^9 liters/mole and binding is inhibited by polyphosphates (3-6). The number of receptors varies from the thousands of HeLa cells to the hundreds of thousand of highly sensitive cell lines such as Vero cells (3-7). There are evidence that a protein is involved in this saturable high affinity binding site (8). It also appears that a low affinity non-saturable site(s) is present since crm 45, which lacks a 12 kDa COOH-terminal fragment involved in receptor binding, is also fixed by cells (3). The toxin-receptor complex appears to enter into a coated pit where it is endocytosed (9,10).

All the available evidence indicate that DT enters the cytoplasm from a low pH endosomal compartment (1,7). A very strong support to this idea is provided by the finding that cellular protein synthesis is stopped after a short incubation with the toxin at low pH (11-13). This experiment is particularly important because it has opened the possibility to test several paramenters for their influence on the toxin membrane translocation. Thus it has been shown that a transmembrane pH gradient is required and that there appears to be no influence of the transmembrane potential (14). The pH dependence of the phenomenon has also been investigated (15) and found to be in good agreement with that determined for the hydrophobic photolabelling of diphtheria toxin incubated with liposomes (16) and with the one determined by following the intrinsec fluorescence of the protein (17). These results speak in favour of the relevance of liposomal model systems to study the role of the lipid interaction of DT in its binding to cell and in its membrane translocation.

We have investigated in detail the interaction of diphtheria toxin with the lipid bilayer with different techniques also employing several toxin mutants altered either in their fragment A or fragment B. We report below some evidence that DT binds at neutral pH to the lipid bilayer surface of negatively charged liposomes. At low pH the toxin interacts with the fatty acid chains of phospholipids and the pKa of this interaction, as monitored by hydrophobic photolabelling, is higher for fragment B than for protomer A.

METHODS

The pH dependence of the interaction of DT with liposomes of dipalmitoyl phosphatidylcholine (DPPC, 90%) and dipalmitoyl phosphatidic acid (DPPA, 10%) was followed by turbidity and fluorescence energy transfer as reported elsewhere (Papini et al., submitted). Hydrophobic photolabelling was performed as before (16) in a 125 mM NaCl, 10 mM NaPi, 10 mM NaCitrate, 1.5 mM EDTA, pH 7.4 buffer. Block of protein synthesis on Vero cells treated with DT at low pH was performed essentially as described by Sandvig & Olsnes (13).

RESULTS and DISCUSSION

Lipid interaction of diphtheria toxin at neutral pH.

The interaction of diphtheria toxin with liposomes of different lipid composition was monitored by hydrophobic photolabelling with liposomes doped with trace amounts of two different radioactive photoreactive phosphatidylcholines: PC I (tritium labelled), that reacts only with those regions of a protein interacting with the polar superficial region of the lipid bilayer, and PC II (^{14}C labelled), that probes deeper, hydrophobic, interactions of the toxin with the hydrocarbon chains of phospholipids. The reaction of these probes with a protein is triggered by illumination, it is rather unspecific and results in the covalent attachment of the reagent, and hence of its radioactivity, to the lipid-interacting protein. Essentially, this method is a semi-quantitative assay of the interaction of a protein with the lipid bilayer at two different levels: hydrophilic and superficial with PC I, deeper and hydrophobic with PC II (18).

Figure 1 shows that DT is labelled with the surface probe, but not with the deeper one at neutral pH when DT is incubated with liposomes of asolectin or DPPC-DPPA. This result extends the observations of Alving et al. (19) and

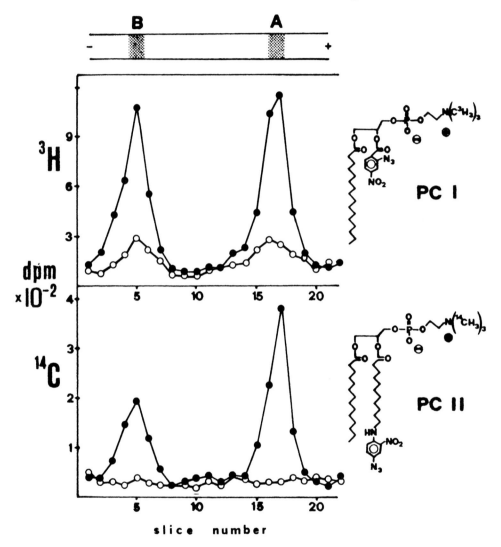

Fig. 1. Pattern of labelling of DT incubated and illuminated with asolectin liposomes doped with PC I and PC II (formulae in the right panels) at neutral pH (open symbols) and pH 4.5 (closed symbols). The radioactivity associated to the two toxin fragments was determined after electrophoresis (Coomassie blue staining profile shown in the top panel), gel slicing and counting.

indicates that the toxin interacts with the polar head groups of phospholipids without altering the orientation of the fatty acid chains. Unfortunately it is difficult to determine by hydrophobic photolabelling the association constant for this lipid binding that appears to be a weak one (19). However, as discussed elsewhere (20), this interaction may be relevant for the binding of DT to cells. It has been suggested that lipid adsorption may be the first step in the association of DT to cell and that the lipid-bound toxin is then trasported laterally to reach its protein receptor; at this stage the association of DT to the cell is the product of its lipid binding and its protein binding (20), as shown in fig. 2.

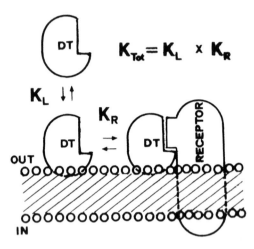

Fig. 2. Schematic model for DT binding to the cells. Details in the text.

Such a model accounts for the non-specific non-saturable binding of DT to cells (3,4) as due to lipid binding and for the saturable high affinity binding site as due to the binding both to the protein and to the lipid components. The model of fig. 2 would also explain the protective effect, with respect to DT intoxication, of both proteases and of phospholipase C, which removes the phosphate head group from phospholipids (21,22). Moreover it provides a rationale for the difficult isolation of the DT receptor by affinity chromatography on immobilized-DT columns because the operation with detergent solubilized membranes relies only on the association of DT to the protein and lacks the additional effect of lipid binding. A low K_R is not surprising in the light of the consideration that cells are unlikely to have suicide tendencies and hence there has been no evolutive pressure to improve the cell ability to bind DT. It is more likely that the DT structure has been improved for its ability to parasitize cellular surface structures. A simple way to reach this goal is the fusion in the DT molecule of two functional abilities: the ability to bind to a protein and the ability to bind to the phospholipid head groups; neither of the two abilities taken alone would confer good cell binding to DT, while the two together are responsible for the high cell association constants of DT to all sensitive cell lines (7).

Low pH lipid interaction of diphtheria toxin.

        Several line of evidence indicate that DT undergoes a pH-driven
conformational change, that enables the toxin to interact with the hydrocarbon
chain of lipids (16,17) and alter the conductance of the lipid bilayer (23,24).
The range of pH were the transition occurs is between 5 and 6 (16,17). We have
recently confirmed these observations by following the change of turbidity and
the fusion of liposomes of DPPC-DPPA incubated with DT at different pHs.
However, all these measurements could not discriminate between the role of the
two toxin protomers. Figure 1 shows that this limitation does not hold for
hydrophobic photolabelling, which is based on the analysis of the distribution
of radioactivity bound to the toxin chains after their separation by SDS-PAGE.
It clearly appears from fig. 1 that DT at low pH becomes able to interact with
the hydrocarbon chains of phospholipids and that this interaction is mediated
by both DT protomers. This hydrophobic interaction of both DT chains is not in
agreement with the model put forward by Kagan et al. (24) for the DT membrane
translocation. As shown in fig. 3, panel I, this model suggests that protomer B
penetrates into the membrane at low pH forming a protein channel that allows
the passage of the hydrophilic fragment A in an extended form. The results of

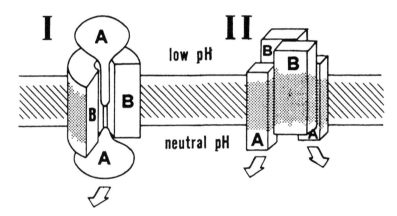

Fig. 3. Suggested models for the membrane translocation of diphtheria toxin.
Model I envisages a B protein channel that allows the passage across the
membrane of the enzyme A without contact with lipids. Model II suggests that
protomer B forms in the membrane a protomer A translocating unit, either alone
or together with a cellular membrane protein, that allows the passage of A with
its polar residues facing a hydrophilic cleft on the translocating unit and its
hydrophobic residues in contact with the hydrocarbon chains of lipids.

our hydrophobic photolabelling experiments (16) as well as those of other
laboratories (25,26) rather support model II of fig. 3, where both DT chains
enter into contact with the lipid bilayer. If a dimer or a larger aggregate is
the membrane penetrating form of DT, then a proper alignment of the B
fragments could create a hydrophilic surface able to interact with the
hydrophilic residues of the A chain, while its hydrophobic residues would be
exposed to the hydrocarbon chains of lipids (including those of the photoactive

phospholipids). In such a way the hydrophilic residues of chain A would be shielded from the contact of the hydrophobic milieu of the inner part of the lipid bilayer thus effectively reducing the energetic cost of the membrane translocation process. The hydrophilic cleft of protomer B could also provide a kind of nucleation center for protein segments 20-30 residues long with the result of transferring segment by segment protomer A across the lipid bilayer as suggested by Singer et al. (27). In a less simplified view the A chain translocating unit could be formed by protomer B in association with a yet unknown cell membrane protein as suggested by the existence of DT resistant cell mutants apparently defective in membrane translocation (28).

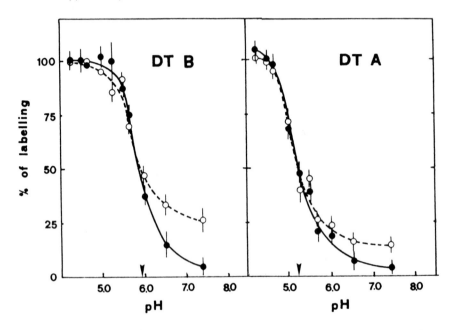

Fig. 4. pH dependence of the labelling with PC I (open symbols) and with PC II (closed symbols) of DT fragment B (left panel) and fragment A (right panel).

As shown in fig. 4, the pKa of the low-pH driven lipid interaction of protomer B is higher (5.9) than that of protomer A (5.2). This measure is particularly reliable since it is obtained for the two chains at the same time, on the same conditions, on the same gel lines. One direct consequence of this finding is that fragment B is the first part of the toxin that inserts into the endosomal membrane as the pH of the endosomal lumen lowers because of the ATPase inward proton pumping activity. The insertion of B assists the one of the enzymic A chain, as suggested by its higher pKa value when part of the intact toxin (5.2) as compared to its isolated state (4.9).

These results, obtained in model systems have been paralleled by experiments on the intoxication of Vero cells, a kidney fibroblast cell line highly sensitive to DT. Cells were incubated with the toxin, the pH was lowered to different values and the block of protein synthesis was was determined (13).

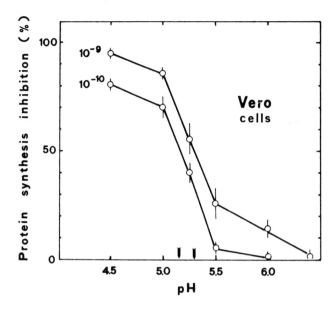

Fig. 5. pH dependence of the block of protein synthesis of Vero cells incubated with diphtheria toxin for five minutes at the pHs indicated.

Fig. 5 shows that the pKa of Vero cells is clearly below 5.5. This result suggest that the penetration of fragment B into the membrane is not the rate limiting step of cell intoxication. Moreover it provides a strong support for the actual biological relevance of studies performed with liposomes, a system that is amenable to several manipulations not allowed with cells.

References

1. Olsnes, S. and Sandvig, K. (1987) in "Immunotoxins" (Fraenkel, A.E., Ed.), Martinus Nijhoff Publising, in press
2. Ward, W.H.J. (1987) Trends. Biochem. Sci. **12**, 28–31
3. Boquet, P. and Pappenheimer, A.M. (1976) J. Biol. Chem. **251**, 5770–5778
4. Chang, T. and Neville, D.M. (1978) J. Biol. Chem. **253**, 6866–6871
5. Middlebrook, J.L., Dorland, R.B. and Leppla, S.H. (1978) J. Biol. Chem. **253**, 7325–7330
6. Didsbury, J.R., Moehring, J.M. and Moehring, T.J. (1983) Mol. Cell. Biol. **3**, 1283–1294
7. Neville, D.M. and Hudson, T.H. (1986) Ann. Rev. Biochem. **55**, 195–224
8. Eidels, L., Proia, R.L. and Hart, D.A. (1983) Microbiol. Rev. **47**, 596–620
9. Moya, M., Dautry-Varsat, A., Goud, B., Louvard, D. and Boquet, P. (1985) J. Cell Biol. **101**, 548–5598.
10. Morris, R.E., Gersten, A.S., Bonventre, P.F. and Saelinger, C.B. (1985) Infect. Immun. **50**, 721–727

11. Sandvig, K. and Olsnes, S. (1980) J. Cell Biol. **87**, 828–832
12. Draper, R.K. and Simon, M.I. (1980) J. Cell Biol. **87**, 849–854
13. Sandvig, K. and Olsnes, S. (1981) J. Biol. Chem. **256**, 9068–9076
14. Sandvig, K., Tonnessen, T.I., Sandl, O. and Olsnes, S. (1986) J. Biol. Chem. **261**, 11639–11644
15. Olsnes, S. and Sandvig, K. (1986) J. Biol. Chem. **261**, 1553–1561
16. Montecucco, C., Schiavo, G. and Tomasi, M. (1985) Biochem. J. **231**, 123–128
17. Blewitt, M.G., Chung, L.A. and London, E. (1985) Biochemistry **24**, 5458–5464
18. Montecucco, C. (1987) Methods Enzymol., in press
19. Alving, C.R., Iglewski, B.H., Urban, K.A., Moss, J., Richards, R.L. and Sadoff, J.C. (1980) Proc, Natl. Acad. Sci. U.S.A. **77**, 1986–1990
20. Papini, E., Colonna, R., Schiavo, G., Cusinato, F., Tomasi, M., Rappuoli, R. and Montecucco, C. (1987) F.E.B.S. Lett. **215**, 73–78
21. Moehring, T.J. and Crispell, J.P. (1974) Biochem. Biophys. Res. Commun. **60**, 14461452
22. Olsnes, S., Carvajal, E., Sundan, A. and Sandvig, K. (1985) Biochim. Biophys. Acta **846**, 334–341
23. Donovan, J.J., Simon, M.I., Draper, R.K. and Montal, M. (1981) Proc. Natl. Acad. Sci. U.S.A. **78**, 172–176
24. Kagan, B.L., Finkelstein, A. and Colombini, M. (1981) Proc. Natl. Acad. Sci. U.S.A. **78**, 4950–4954
25. Zalman, L.S. and Wisnieski, B.J. (1984) Proc. Natl. Acad. Sci. U.S.A. **81**, 3341–3345
26. Hu, V. and Holmes, R.K. (1984) J. Biol. Chem. **259**, 12226–12233.
27. Singer, S.J., Maher, P.A. and Jaffe, M.P. (1987) Proc. Natl. Acad. Sci. U.S.A. **84**, 1015–1019
28. Moehring, J.M. and Moehring, T.J. (1979) Somat. Cell. Genet. **5**, 453–468

Fehrenbach et al. (Eds.), Bacterial Protein Toxins, Zbl. Bakt. Suppl. 17
© Gustav Fischer, Stuttgart, New York, 1988

Pore Formation by Staphylococcus Aureus Alpha-Toxin: a Study using Planar Bilayers

G. Menestrina

Dipartimento di Fisica, Universita' di Trento I-38050 Povo, Trento

ABSTRACT

Staphylococcus aureus α-toxin interacts with planar lipid membranes by opening ionic pores which can be directly observed in voltage clamp experiments as discrete current steps. The aggregation of several toxin monomers is required for the formation of one pore. Single channel conductance depends linearly on the solution conductivity suggesting that the pores are filled with aqueous solution and have an average diameter of 10 ± 1 Å. These pores are open all the time in a solution containing only monovalent cations at physiological pH, but undergo a dose and voltage dependent inactivation in the presence of divalent cations as well as at low pH. The inhibiting efficiency follows the sequence H > Zn > Tb > Ca > Mg > Ba suggesting that binding of these cations to carboxyl groups of the protein may be involved in the inactivation.

KEY WORDS

Staphylococcus aureus; α-toxin; ionic channel; divalent cations; inactivation; planar lipid membranes.

INTRODUCTION

Staphylococcus aureus α-toxin is a cytolytic exotoxin secreted as a single water-soluble polypeptide of 33,000 daltons molecular weight (Freer and Arbuthnott, 1983; Freer and others, 1973). The polypeptide is strongly surface active: it inserts into preformed lipid monolayers increasing their surface pressure (Freer and others, 1973; Bukelew and Colacicco, 1971) and forms itself monolayers at an air-water interface (Bukelew and Colacicco, 1971), suggesting that it can undergo a hydrophilic to amphiphilic transition. This toxin causes erythrocyte lysis in three distinct steps: binding to the cell membrane followed by ion leakage and finally hemoglobin release (Cassidy and others, 1974; Harshman, 1979). The molecular events leading to membrane damage are not yet fully understood; it has been proposed that α-toxin oligomerizes on the cell surface forming an amphiphilic hexamer that inserting into the lipid bilayer generates a transmembrane channel responsible for ion leakage (Füssle and others, 1981; Arbuthnott and others, 1973; Freer, 1982). A colloid-osmotic shock then follows the leakage of ions and leads to the lysis of the membrane and eventually to the death of the cell.

In order to test this hypothesis we have studied the effects of S.aureus α-toxin on planar lipid membranes comprised of purified phospholipids. We have found that the toxin actually forms ionic channels of well defined conductance in the lipid bilayer. This model system proves to be quite useful for the elucidation of a number of properties of these pores such as average diameter, water content, oligomeric composition and interaction with divalent cations, which are all physiologically relevant.

MATERIALS AND METHODS

Planar phospholipid bilayer membranes were prepared by the apposition of two monolayers on a Teflon septum containing a hole of about 0.2 mm diameter separating two buffered salt solutions (Montal and Mueller, 1972). The monolayers were comprised of egg phosphatidylcholine (PC). Bathing solutions, 4 ml on each side, contained various amounts of KCl or NaCl, as specified in the text, 1 mM EDTA (Merck) and were buffered by 10 mM Tris (Calbiochem) at pH 7.0. Staphylococcus aureus α-toxin was a kind gift of Dr. K.D.Hungerer of the Behringwerke laboratories (Marburg,D) and was used without further purification. Amounts of toxin from a stock aqueous solution was added to one compartment only (cis side) to a final concentration ranging 5 to 250 μg/ml and the addition was followed by a vigorous mixing of the solutions with magnetic bars. The transmembrane potential was clamped to the desired value and the current flowing through the membrane continously recorded, the details have been given elsewhere (Menestrina, 1986).

RESULTS AND DISCUSSION

Pores are large and filled with water

The addition of small amounts of S.aureus α-toxin to the solution bathing a planar bilayer produces, under voltage clamp conditions, a stepwise increase of the current flowing through the membrane (Fig. 1a). These current steps are quite homogeneous in size and their amplitude represents the ionic conductance of just one toxin lesion. The conductance value is actually rather large, for example it is 180 pS with KCl 0.2 M, and this is a strong indication that ionic channels are formed by this toxin, the incorporation pattern is in fact quite similar to that observed with other well known pore forming proteins such as hemocyanin (Menestrina and Antolini, 1981), porin (Benz and others, 1980) and colicin (Davidson and others, 1984).

In Table 1 the mean conductance of the α-toxin channel is reported for three different concentrations of KCl in the bathing solution together with the conductivity of the solution and the ratio between the two values. It appears that the conductance of the channel varies almost linearly with the conductivity of the

solution suggesting that the pores are filled with water. By means
of a simple model and assuming a cylindrical shape of the pore, its
radius can be estimated from the values in the right column of
Table 1 in 5 Å. The pore diameter can thus be calculated to be 10 Å
in good agreement with the finding that α-toxin at lytic

TABLE 1   Average Conductance of α-Toxin Pores

G^a (pS)	σ^b (mS/cm^{-1})	$R^c * 10^9$ (cm)	C^d (M)
750	85.0	8.8	1
180	21.3	8.5	0.2
75	6.6	11.4	0.05

a: G = single channel condutance
b: σ = solution conductivity
c: R = ratio G/σ
d: C = KCl concentration

concentrations (20 µg/ml) releases sucrose (8.8 Å effective
diameter) but not inulin (diameter 30 Å) from resealed erythrocyte
ghosts (Füssle and others, 1981).

Pores result from an aggregation mechanism

One major question on the α-toxin lesion regards its oligomeric
nature. It is generally agreed that the channel is formed by a
toxin hexamer, biochemical evidences leave little or no doubt about
that (Bhakdi and others , 1981; Füssle and others, 1981; Tobkes and
others, 1985), however it is not yet clear wether the hexamer is
formed before its insertion into the bilayer or it is formed by the
aggregation of monomers already incorporated into the lipid film.
We addressed this question by measuring the pore formation rate as
a function of toxin concentration in solution since a power
dependence larger than one between these two variables would favour
the second of the two hypothesis. The results are shown in Fig. 1b
in a double logarithmic plot, the straight line drawn has a slope
2.4 suggesting that an aggregation of preinserted monomers is
indeed involved. These results are consistent with published data
on toxin binding and hemolysis of erythrocytes (Bhakdi and others

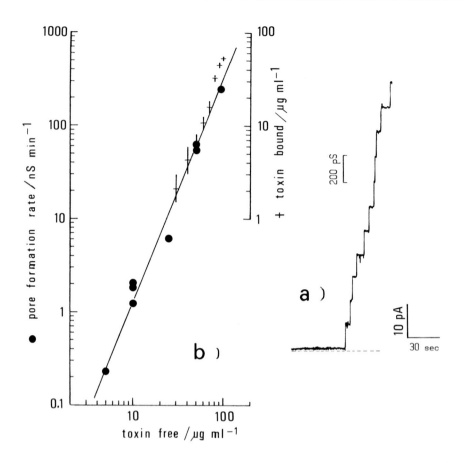

Fig. 1: a) Current steps following the addition of 20 μg/ml of α-toxin to one side of a PC planar bilayer clamped at +40 mV which are due each to the opening of a new ionic channel in the membrane. Bathing solution was 0.2 M KCl symmetrical.The dashed line indicates zero of current.
b) circles: double logarithmic plot of the rate of conductance increase, due to channel formation, versus the concentration of α-toxin used in a PC membrane bathed by 0.1 M KCl; vertical bars: same kind of plot for the amount of toxin bound to human erythrocytes, adapted from Bhakdi and others (1984).

1984) which are also reported on the figure for comparison.

Pores are closed by divalent cations

In a solution containing relatively high concentrations of

monovalent cations (≥0.1 M) α-toxin channels remain open all the
time after their incorporation, irrespectively of the applied
voltage (see Fig. 1a). If however divalent cations such as Ca++
are added to the solution the current flowing through the channels
after the application of a voltage jump decreases from an initial

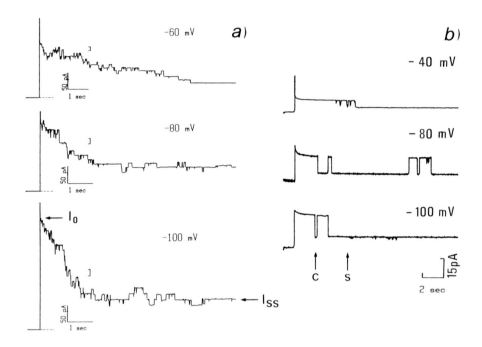

Fig. 2: a) Current relaxations after the application of voltage pulses from a 0 mV holding
potential to a PC membrane containing about 20
α-toxin channels. Applied voltages are
indicated. Bathing solution was 0.1 M KCl plus
40 mM CaCl$_2$, α-toxin was 5 µg/ml. Vertical
bars indicate a conductance of 200 pS; dashed
lines indicate zero of current. The initial
fast transient is due to the charging of the
membrane capacity. Initial and steady-state
current are indicated as Io and Iss
respectively.
b) same kind of experiment but with a membrane
containing only one channel; the solution was
0.1 M NaCl plus 50 mM CaCl$_2$, toxin was added at
1 µg/ml. Two closed states of different
lifetime, closed and shut, are indicated by c
and s respectively.

large value (Io, which corresponds to all the channels open) to a
lower steady state one (Iss), Fig. 2a. Both the extent of the

relaxation and its rate are larger the larger the applied potential. The ratio Iss/Io is in general a sigmoidal function of the applied voltage and the current relaxations can always be described as the sum of two exponential components whose time constants are bell shaped functions of the final voltage (see Fig. 3b).

The elementary events leading to this decrease can be better understood looking at Fig. 2b. Here voltage steps of increasing amplitudes have been applied to a membrane containing just one α-toxin channel, in the presence of Ca++. After the onset of voltage the channel, which was open at 0 mV, enters fast fluctuations between an open and a closed state and finally becomes completely closed or shut. The single channel experiment offers an immediate explanation to the many channel current relaxation i.e. ionic channels which are open at 0 mV tend to close at the onset of voltage producing the current decrease, the channels then reopen when the potential is clamped again to 0 mV.

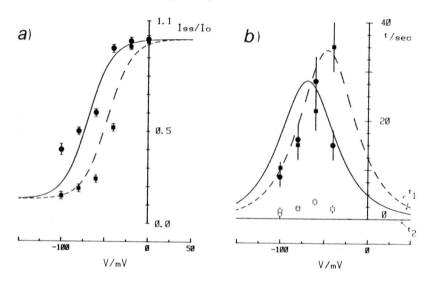

Fig.3 Channel inactivation measured by the ratio Iss/Io (in part a) and the two time constants τ_1 and τ_2 necessary to describe the relaxation (in part b) as a function of voltage for two different Mg++ concentrations. Complete inactivation would correspond to a value of Iss/Io equal to zero. Mg++ concentrations are 50 mM, circles and solid lines, 6r 100 mM, squares and dashed lines and are added to a 0.1 M KCl solution. Empty points are for the faster time constant τ_2 . Theoretical lines are drawn according to a binding-inactivating model (Menestrina, 1986).

The existence of two closed states, closed and shut, which merges from the single channel trace is in good agreement with the finding

that the current decay in many channel experiments is adequately described as the sum of two purely exponential components of different time constant.
Inhibition effects can be observed in the presence of a number of divalent cations as well as at low pH suggesting that protons can also effectively block the α-toxin channels. The extent of channel inactivation, given by the ratio Iss/Io, and the two time constants describing the relaxation are a function of both the concentration of the divalent cation added and the applied voltage. This is shown in Fig. 3 for the case of Mg++.
The combined effects of voltage and cation concentration can be understood on the basis of a simple model, which has been used to draw the theoretical lines in Fig.3 , based on a specific binding of the cations to the channel (Menestrina, 1986). From this model an intrinsic binding constant can be estimated for each inactivating cation; we have found the following sequence of binding constants to hold: H+ > Zn++ > Ca++ > Mg++ > Ba++; this sequence and the absolute values of the affinity constants suggest that a carboxyl group on the protein could be the substrate for cation action. It is noteworthy that this sequence is the same as that observed for the protective effects of the same cations on whole cells by Pasternak and others (1985).

REFERENCES

Arbuthnott, J.P., J.H.Freer, and B.Billcliffe (1973). Lipid-induced polymerization of Staphylococcal α-toxin. J.Gen.Microbiol., 75, 309-319.
Benz, R., J.Ishii, and T.Nakae (1980). Determination of ion permeability through the channels made of porins from the outer membrane of Salmonella typhimurium in lipid bilayer membranes. J.Membrane Biol., 56, 19-29.
Bhakdi, S., R.Füssle, and J.Tranum-Jensen (1981). Staphylococcal α-toxin: oligomerization of hydrophilic monomers to form amphiphilic hexamers induced through contact with deoxycholate detergent micelles. Proc.Natl.Acad.Sci.USA, 78, 5475-5479.
Bhakdi, S., M.Muhly, and R.Füssle (1984). Correlation between toxin binding and hemolytic activity in membrane damage by staphylococcal alpha-toxin. Infect.Immun., 46, 318-323.
Bukelew, A.R., and G.Colacicco (1971). Lipid monolayers. Interaction with Staphylococcal α-toxin. Biochim.Biophys.Acta, 233, 7-16.
Cassidy, P., A.R.Six, and S.Harshmann (1974). Biological properties of Staphylococcal α-toxin. Biochim.Biophys.Acta, 332, 413-425.
Davidson, V.L., K.R.Brunden, W.A.Cramer, and F.S.Cohen (1984). Studies on the mechanism of action of channel-forming colicins using artificial membranes. J.Membrane Biol., 79, 105-118.
Freer, J.H. (1982). Cytolytic toxins and surface activity. Toxicon, 20, 217-221.
Freer, J.H., J.P.Arbuthnott, and B.Bilcliffe (1973). Effects of Staphylococcal α-toxin on the structure of erythrocytes membranes. J.Gen.Microbiol., 75, 321-332.
Freer, J.H., and J.P.Arbuthnott (1983). Toxins of Staphylococcus aureus. Pharmac. Ther., 19, 55-106.
Füssle, R., S.Bhakdi, A.Sziegoleit, J.Tranum-Jensen, T.Kranz, and Wellensiek, H.J. (1981). On the mechanism of membrane damage by Staphylococcus aureus α-toxin. J.Cell.Biol., 91, 83-94.

Harshman, S. (1979). Action of staphylococcal α-toxin on membranes: some recent advances. Mol.Cell.Biochem., 23, 142-152.

Menestrina, G. (1986). Ionic channels formed by Staphylococcus aureus alpha-toxin: voltage dependent inhibition by di and trivalent cations. J. Membrane Biol., 90, 177-190.

Menestrina, G., and R.Antolini (1981). Ion transport through hemocyanin channels in oxidized cholesterol artificial bilayer membranes. Biochim.Biophys.Acta, 643, 616-625.

Montal, M., and P.Mueller (1972). Formation of bimolecular membranes from lipid monolayers and a study of their electrical properties. Proc.Natl.Acad.Sci.USA, 69, 3561-3566.

Pasternak, C.A., C.L.Bashford, and K.J.Micklem (1985). Ca++ and the interaction of.pore formers with membranes. J.Biosci., 8,273-291.

Tobkes, N., B.A.Wallace, and H.Bayley (1985). Secondary structure and assembly mechanism of an oligomeric channel protein. Biochemistry, 24, 1915-1920.

Fehrenbach et al. (Eds.), Bacterial Protein Toxins, Zbl. Bakt. Suppl. 17
© Gustav Fischer, Stuttgart, New York, 1988

Interaction of Tetanus and Botulinum Toxins with Membranes

C. Montecucco[1], G. Schiavo[1], Z. Gao[2], E. Bauerlein[2], B. R. Dasgupta[3] and P. Boquet[4]

[1]Centro C. N. R. Biomembrane e Dipartimento di Scienze Biomediche Sperimentali,
 Universita' di Padova, I-Padova
[2]Max Planck Institut für Biochemie, Martinsried bei München, F.R.G.
[3]Food Research Institute, University of Wisconsin, Madison, U.S.A.
[4]Institut Pasteur, 28, rue du Docteur-Roux, F-75724 Paris Cédex 15

The Clostridial neurotoxins have been shown to bind polysialogangliosides of the G_{1b} series with various methods, including toxin fixation to t.l.c. plates, to plastic or to paper (1-5).

Because of the importance of membrane binding in the intoxication process, we have decided to further investigate this point on ganglioside-containing liposomes, a model system more closely related to the synaptosomal membranes than micellar or plastic or silica adsorbed gangliosides.

We have used here ASA-PE, a new photoactivatable phosphatidylethanolamine analogue carrying a ^{125}I-p-azido-salicyl group coniugated to the amino group. On illumination it generates a reactive intermediate that can form covalent bonds with protein regions interacting with the hydrophilic surface of the lipid bilayer. As a result these parts of the protein become radioactively labelled and can be identified by autoradiography or counting after electrophoresis or chromatography.

Table 1 reports the amount of radioactivity associated with the toxin bands on the gel as estimated after autoradiography and integration of the spots; the data are expressed as percentage of the maximally labelled sample. This method of membrane hydrophilic photolabelling cannot provide a quantitative estimation of the strenght of association of a protein with the membrane. On the other hand it is very sensitive and can detect even very loose associations.

Tetanus toxin and botulinum toxin type A are poorly labelled in the presence of liposomes made of egg lecithin or egg lecithin plus mixed gangliosides while both toxins are heavily labelled with asolectin vesicles.

The interaction with the negative lipid-containing asolectin liposomes involves both the heavy and the light chains. When bovine brain gangliosides are included there is a further increase in labelling; however, this increase is much lower than the one expected on the basis of the idea that gangliosides are the only lipids involved in the binding of the toxins to the nerve plasma membrane.

Table I

Radioactivity bound to the toxin chains after incubation and illumination in the presence of liposomes of the indicated composition containing the surface probe ^{125}I-ASA-PE

	H chain	L chain
- Tetanus toxin:		
egg lecithin	15	11
egg lecithin + gangliosides	10	9
asolectin	76	90
asolectin + gangliosides	100	92
- Botulinum toxin type A:		
egg lecithin	6	1
egg lecithin + gangliosides	10	3
asolectin	80	7
asolectin + gangliosides	100	18

From the present studies botulinum and tetanus toxins appear to absorb to the surface of liposomes containing negative lipids and negligeably to that of zwitterionic lipid vesicles. This interaction is mediated via both the heavy and light chains of the toxins. As it appears from the amount of labeling, that provides a semi-quantitative extimation of the binding strenght, both botulinum and tetanus toxins are absorbed more efficiently on the surface of polysialoganglioside-containing liposomes. This result was espected on the basis of previous studies that have demonstrated the ability of these neurotoxins to bind to gangliosides (1-5). However these results open the possibility that the membrane lipid binding of the botulinum and tetanus toxins is due not only to the G1b gangliosides but also to an interaction with negative lipids; binding is not restricted to the ganglioside binding fragment.

The present results provide a rationale for the known lack of ganglioside specificity of these toxins of the kind shown by cholera toxin for G_{M1} (1-5) and for the weaker binding of tetanus toxin to the oligosaccharide with respect to the intact ganglioside molecule (6). It also explains the finding that TeTx binds to gangliosides more strongly than its fragment C does (7)

REFERENCES

1. Simpson, L.L. & Rapport, M.M. (1971) J. Neurochem. 18, 1751
2. Kitamura, M., Iwamori, M. & Nagai, Y. (1980) Biochim. Biophys. Acta 628, 328
3. Critchley, D.R., Nelson, P.G., Habig, W.H. & Fishman, P.H. (1985) J. Cell Biol. 100, 1499
4. Kamata, Y.,Kozaki, S., Sakaguchi, G., Iwamori, M. & Nagai, Y. (1986) Biochim. Biophys. Res. Commun. 140, 1015
5. Holmgren, J., Elwing, H., Fredman, P. & Svennerholm, L. (1980) Eur. J. Biochem. 106, 371
6. Habermann, E., Goretzki, K & Albus, U. (1985) Proc. 7th International Tetanus Conference, Nistico' et al. Eds, p. 179, Gangemi Editore, Roma
7. Helting, T., Zwisler, O. & Wiegandt, H. (1977) J. Biol. Chem. 252, 194

Fehrenbach et al. (Eds.), Bacterial Protein Toxins, Zbl. Bakt. Suppl. 17
© Gustav Fischer, Stuttgart, New York, 1988

Localisation of a Cholera Toxin Binding Component in the Nuclei of Mouse Intestinal Cells by the Post Embedding Immunogold Technique.

M. E. Parkinson[1], C. G. Smith[2], S. van Heyningen[1] and P. B. Garland[2]

[1]Department of Biochemistry, University of Edinburgh, Hugh Robson Building, George Square, EH8 9XD. Scotland
[2]Unilever Research, Colworth House, Sharnbrook, Bedford. MK44 1LQ, U.K.

ABSTRACT

A cholera toxin binding component (probably GM1 Ganglioside) has been located in the chromatin of intestinal cell nuclei. Cholera toxin binds with high affinity ($Kd=10^{-9}M$) and specificity to ganglioside GM1. Localisation involved a sandwich of cholera toxin, antitoxin antibody and gold labelled second antibody on mouse intestine, previously embedded in hydrophilic resin. There was a sparse distribution of gold amongst the microvilli, clusters in the cytoplasm, in vesicle-like structures and most surprisingly, a distribution of gold accross the chromatin of the nuclei. All binding could be abolished by preincubating the toxin with ganglioside GM1. Anti-GM1 antibody also bound to the nucleus, indicating the presence of the ganglioside or a similar molecule in the nucleus.

KEYWORDS

cholera toxin, GM1 ganglioside, mouse intestine, post embedding immunogold

INTRODUCTION

Previous studies on the immunocytochemical localisation of GM1 ganglioside used peroxidase conjugated anti-cholera toxin antibody (Hansson, 1977), or the preembedding immunogold technique (Ackerman, 1980). However, both these studies have concentrated on the external GM1 molecules located at the outer surface of the plasma membrane. The only evidence for the intracellular location of GM1 has been demonstrated by biochemical fractionation techniques (Keenan, 1972). Cholera toxin has been shown to bind to GM1 almost exclusively, on the cell surface (Hollenberg,1974). Therefore cholera toxin is a natural probe for GM1 ganglioside and using it to locate GM1 intracellularly may give some indication of the physiological role of the ganglioside. Some gangliosides have altered expression in cancer cells (Feizi, 1985) implicating them in growth regulation. Recently, it has been shown, using cholera toxin B subunit (the ganglioside binding site), that the ganglioside may be a bimodal growth regulator of cells, acting synergistically with EGF (Speigel , 1987). Therefore, the possible location of GM1 ganglioside in the nuclei of mouse intestinal cells may reflect some aspect of this physiologically observed action.

RESULTS

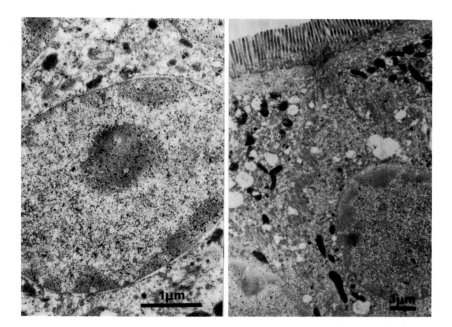

Fig.1. The binding of the B subunit of cholera toxin
(1 µg/ml in Dulbeccos PBS pH 7.4)

Fig.2. The binding of anti -GM1 antibody
(1/100 in PBS buffer)

The results indicate that the predominant binding site for the cholera toxin is the heterochromatin near the nuclear envelope. Prior treatment with pronase abolishes this chromatin binding site. Preabsorption of the toxin with GM1 ganglioside abolishes all binding on both the nucleus and microvilli. Further work is underway to identify this cholera toxin binding component within the nucleus.

REFERENCES

Ackerman, G. A., K. W. Wolken, and F. B. Gelder. (1980). Surface Distribution of Monosialoganglioside GM1 on Human Blood Cells and the Effect of Exogenous GM1 and Neuraminidase on Cholera Toxin Surface labelling. J. Histochem. Cytochem., 28, 1100-1112.

Feizi, T. (1985). Demonstration by Monoclonal antibodies that Carbohydrate Structures of Glycoproteinsand Glycolipids are Onco-Developmental antigens. Nature. 314, 53-57.

Hansson, H. A., J. Holmgren, and L. Svennerholm. (1977). Ultrastructural Localisation of Cell Membrane GM1 Ganglioside by Cholera Toxin. Proc. Natl. Acad. Sci. U. S. A., 74, 3782-3786.

Hollenberg, M. D., P. H. Fishman, V. Bennet, and P. Cuatrecasas. (1974). Cholera Toxin and Cell Growth; Role of Membrane Gangliosides.Proc. Natl. Acad. Sci. U. S. A., 71, 4224-4228.

Keenan, T. W., D. J. Morre and C. M. Huang. (1972). Distribution of Gangliosides among subcellular Fractions from Rat Liver and Bovine mammary Gland. Febs. Letts., 24,204-208.

Speigel, S and P. H. Fishman. (1987). Gangliosides as Bimodal Regulators of Cell Growth. Proc. Natl. Acad. Sci. 84, 141-145.

Fehrenbach et al. (Eds.), Bacterial Protein Toxins, Zbl. Bakt. Suppl. 17
© Gustav Fischer, Stuttgart, New York, 1988

Biological Activities of Cholera Toxin Covalently Conjugated to Liposomes

M. Pescarmona, S. Di Carlo, B. Calzecchi-Onesti and M. Tomasi

Istituto Superiore di Sanità, Laboratorio di Biologia Cellulare, Viale Regina Elena, I-299-00161 Roma

We covalently conjugated cholera toxin (CT) to liposomes in order to obtain a compound whose properties are not simply the mere sum of the single components (1).

Cholera toxin has the unique ability to recognize the oligosaccharide portion of the monosialoganglioside GM1 because of its high affinity constant (Ka 10^{-9}M) (2). The thikness of CT from the polar head group is approximately 18 Å (3). Thus two distinct vesicles, one bearing conjugated CT and the other one containing GM1, upon binding of CT to GM1, are at 18 Å distance. In these conditions the fusion might be possible.

As a recipient membrane we used human erythrocytes (HE) which were preloaded by GM1. The incubation procedures are similar to that described by Facci et al. (4). Briefly 5 x 10^{-5}M, was incubated with HE for 1 hour at 37°C in 20mM sodium phosphate, 150 mM NaCl, pH 7.4 (PBS). At the end of incubation HE were washed twice in PBS and then incubated with 1% (w/v) Bovine Serum Albumin fatty acid-free. This procedure is essential to remove the GM1 absorbed to the external surface but not the one inserted into the lipid bilayer. Incubation of liposomes conjugated with CT (LIP-CT) with HE containing GM1 (HE-GM1) produces an evident agglutination. The phenomenon appears dependent on the number of the vesicles (LIP-CT) added to HE-GM1. A typical experiment gave the following data: 20 μg of CT conjugated to 1 mg of lipids agglutinate 50 μl of 0,6% HE-GM1 (v/v) up to 125 serial dilution.

However when the mixture LIP-CT and HE-GM1 was incubated at 37°C for 30' the lysis was evident (Fig. 1). Since the lysis was also induced by liposomes but at 9 folds higher concentration, the results indicate that the lytic activity of LIP-CT seems likely due to the fact that CT brings about nearly erythrocyte surface a local high concentration of liposomes.

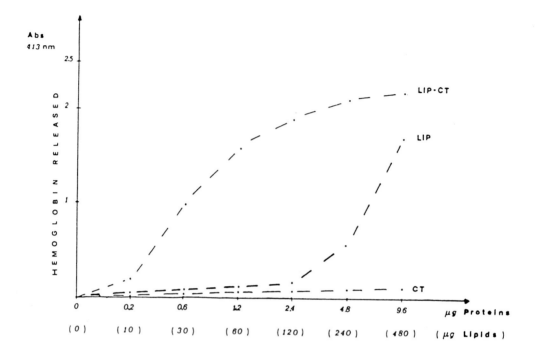

Fig. 1   The ratio between CT and lipids was 1 mg protein to 50 mg
lipids. The lipid composition was: phosphatidylcholine
(45%), cholesterol (45%), phosphatidylethanolamine (10%).

REFERENCES

1)   Fiani, M.L., Grimaldi, P., Sargiacomo, M. and Tomasi, M. (1986).
Zentral. Bakt. Mikro Hyg. Supplement 15, 111-112.

2)   Fishman, P.H. (1982).
J. Membrane Biol., 69, 85-97.

3)   Dwyer, J.D. and Bloomfield, V.A. (1982).
Biochemistry 21, 3229-3231.

4)   Facci, L., Leon, A., Toffano, G., Sonnino, S;, Ghidoni, R., Tettamenti
G. (1984).
J. Neurochem. 42, 299-305.

Fehrenbach et al. (Eds.), Bacterial Protein Toxins, Zbl. Bakt. Suppl. 17
© Gustav Fischer, Stuttgart, New York, 1988

Staphylococcal Exfoliative Toxins: Interaction with Liposomes

Y. Piémot[1], V. Cabiaux[2] and H. Monteil[1]

[1]Laboratoire de Toxinologie Bactérienne, Institut de Bactériologie 3, rue Koeberlé, F-67000 Strasbourg
[2]Lab. Chimie-Physique des Macromolécules aux Interfaces, Campus CP 206/2, Boulevard du Triomphe, B-1050 Bruxelles

ABSTRACT

Staphylococcal exfoliative toxins A and B (ETA and ETB) are toxins responsible for splitting within the epidermis. At acidic pH, ETA becomes more hydrophobic and is able to cause aggregation or fusion of azolectin liposomes, whereas ETB does not. At neutral pH, ETA and ETB have no action on such liposomes. Differential calorimetry reveals interactions between dipalmitoylphosphatidyl-choline liposomes and ETA or ETB at neutral or acidic pH. Thus lipids -ET interactions may be involved in the mode of action of exfoliative toxins.

KEYWORDS

Exfoliative toxin, liposomes, mode of action, fluorescence, calorimetry.

The exfoliative toxins A and B (ETA and ETB) are produced by Staphylococcus aureus. Histologically, they cause a splitting within the epidermis between the stratum granulosum and the stratum spinosum (Wuepper and co-workers, 1975). Clinically this injury leads to the appearance of a Nikolsky sign or to cutaneous blisters. Apart from man, few animal species are sensitive to these toxins : mouse, gold hamster and rhesus monkey. There is no difference between the A and B toxins concerning either their microscopic or their macroscopic action. As yet the molecular mechanism of both toxins remains unknown.

The cohesiveness between superficial keratinocytes is in part related to the presence of lipids (Schaefer, 1985). We therefore tried to assess the inte-raction of exfoliative toxins A and B with lipids.

When ETA is added to an ANS (8-anilinonaphtalene 1-sulfonate) solution at pH 4.3, fluorescence parameters of ANS are modified, indicating an enhancement of the hydrophobicity of the solution. This effect is not observed either at pH 4.3 with ETB or at pH 7.3 with ETA and ETB.

The incubation of azolectin liposomes with ETA and ETB shows an increase of the absorbance at 550 nm for ETA only at pH 4.3. At neutral pH, no modification of the absorbance is noted either with ETA or with ETB. Thus ETA produces an aggregation an/or fusion process at acidic pH. Both processes, aggregation and fusion of liposomes, occur as demonstrated by energy transfer between two fluorescent probes (rhodamine and NBD) (Cabiaux and co-workers, 1985) and the importance of these processes is related to ETA concentration.

Using differential calorimetry techniques, we were able to show that ETA and ETB could interact with small unilamellar vesicles of dipalmitoylphosphatidyl-choline at pH 4.3 and also at pH 7.3.

A low pH could modify ETA structure and hence expose a hydrophobic region at the surface of the molecule. This region could be responsible for the interaction between ETA and azolectin liposomes. Since this effect occurs only for ETA and only at acidic pH, its involvement in vivo remains questionable. However, as shown by differential calorimetry, the nature of lipids could play a role, since both exfoliative toxins interact with dipalmitoylphosphati-dylcholine liposomes.

REFERENCES

Cabiaux, V., M.Vandenbranden, P.Falmagne, and J.M.Ruysschaert (1985). Aggregation and fusion of lipids vesicles induced by diphtheria toxin at low pH: possible involvement of the P site and the NAD+ binding site. Biosci.Rep., 5, 243-250.
Schaefer, H. (1985). La couche cornée. In : INSERM (Ed.), Cours de Biologie de la peau, 27-29 mars 1985. Hôpital E.Herriot, U.INSERM 209, Lyon, France, pp. 5-10.
Wuepper, K.D., R.L.DIMOND, and D.KNUTSON (1975). Studies of the mechanism of epidermal injury by a staphylococcal epidermolytic toxin. J.Invest.Dermatol., 65, 191-200.

Fehrenbach et al. (Eds.), Bacterial Protein Toxins, Zbl. Bakt. Suppl. 17
© Gustav Fischer, Stuttgart, New York, 1988

Botulinum Type A and E Neurotoxins Form Channels in Lipid Vesicles at Low pH

C. C. Shone, P. Hambleton and J. Melling

Vaccine Research and Production Laboratory, PHLS Centre for Applied Microbiology and Research, Porton Down, Salisbury, Wiltshire SP4 OJG, England

The mechanism by which Clostridium botulinum type A neurotoxin is internalised is not clearly understood but the process may resemble that of receptor-mediated endocytosis (Dolly and others, 1984). During the latter process endosomal vesicles develop an acidic pH before delivering their contents to the target organelle, usually the lysosome. Several toxins (diphtheria, tetanus and botulinum type C_1 (Donovan and Middlebrook, 1986) and B neurotoxins (Hoch and others, 1985) have been shown to form channels in lipid bilayers at low pH which may allow the toxin or an active fragment to be transported from the endosome into the cytosol. In this study we show that botulinum type A neurotoxin is able to form channels in lipid vesicles at low pH and that this property of the toxin is retained in a 50 kDa fragment (H_2 fragment) representing the NH_2-terminus of the heavy subunit (Shone and others, 1987)

To study the interaction of the neurotoxin with lipid bilayers, liposomes of defined phospholipid composition were used. Lipid vesicles were loaded with potassium phosphate and the release of potassium ions monitored with an ion selective electrode.

At pH 4.0 both intact botulinum type A neurotoxin and its H_2 fragment released K^+ from phosphatidyl choline/phosphatidyl glycerol liposomes containing potassium phosphate. The purified heavy subunit also evoked K^+ release from vesicles but the light subunit of the neurotoxin was ineffective. No release of K^+ from vesicles was observed with formaldehyde-inactivated neurotoxin. The channels formed by the neurotoxin and the H_2 fragment were also found to be large enough to permit the release of NAD entrapped within lipid vesicles.

Release of K^+ ions from liposomes was highly pH dependent. Optimal release was observed at pH 4.5 which rapidly decreased as the pH was raised and was undetectable above pH 6.0. Below pH 4.5 the isolated H_2 fragment was less efficient at releasing K^+ than the intact toxin.

In addition to phosphatidyl choline/phosphatidyl glycerol vesicles, efficient K^+ release was also observed from vesicles made with phosphatidyl inositol or phosphatidyl serine (Table 1). Poor release of K^+, however, was obtained from vesicles made with phosphatidyl choline/phosphatidyl ethanolamine or with 100% phosphatidyl choline which may indicate the requirement of an overall net negative charge on the phospholipid for channel formation to occur. Some evidence that phospholipid structure is important for the formation of membrane channels was obtained from studies with liposomes containing the negatively charged lipids, dicetyl phosphate and cardiolipin. With the former, channel formation by the toxin was virtually absent and with the latter it was greatly reduced (Table 1).

TABLE 1. Release of K^+ from Liposomes of Phospholipid Composition by Botulinum Type A and E Neurotoxins.
(K^+ released by 0.2 nmol of botulinum neurotoxin at pH 4.5)

Phospholipid composition of liposomes	Percentage of K^+ released by toxin A	E
PtdCho:PtdGro (1:1)	> 95	> 95
Soybean (100%)	63 +16	nd
PtdCho (100%)	< 5	< 5
PtdCho:PtdEtn (1:1)	< 5	< 5
PtdCho:PtdIns (1:1)	> 95	> 95
PtdCho:PtdSer (1:1)	> 95	nd
PtdCho:Cardiolipin (2:1)	31 +6.6	nd
PtdCho:Dicetylphos.(2:1)	< 5	nd

It is not clear from the present study whether or not a conformational change occurs within the H_2 fragment as the pH is lowered which enables membrane binding. Any conformational change which may occur is readily reversible since acid-pulsed toxin was unable to form membrane channels at pH 7.2. The latter result is in contrast to findings with diphtheria toxin which appears to undergo an irreversible conformational change at low pH.

Similar pore formation in lipid vesicles was observed at low pH with single-chain botulinum type E neurotoxin (Table 1). As found for type A neurotoxin, K^+ release was only observed from vesicles composed of negatively charged phospholipids. Conversion of the single chain toxin to the dichain form with trypsin caused only a slight increase in the channel forming activity of the neurotoxin.

The relevance, if any, of the membrane channel-forming activities observed with botulinum type A and E neurotoxins to their potent neuroparalytic activity is not clear. If indeed these toxins are internalised by a process resembling receptor-mediated endocytosis then the low pH which develops in the endosomal vesicle should induce these toxins to embed themselves in the lipid bilayer. Whether or not this process is the first stage in the transport of either the whole toxin or an active fragment from the endosome into the cytosol, however, has yet to be determined.

Dolly, J.O., Black, J., Williams, R.S. and Melling, J. (1984) Acceptors for botulinum neurotoxin reside on motor nerve terminals and mediate its internalizaton. Nature 307 457-460

Donovan J.J. and Middlebrook, J.L. (1986) Ion-conducting channels produced by botulinum toxin in planar lipid membranes. Biochemistry 25 2872-2876

Hoch, D.H., Romero-Mira, M., Ehrlich, B.E., Finkelstein, A., DasGupta, B.R. and Simpson, L.L. (1985) Channels formed by botulinum, tetanus, and diphtheria toxins in planar lipid bilayers. Proc. Natl. Acad. Sci. USA. 82 1692-1696

Shone, C.C., Hambleton, P., and Melling, J. (1987) A 50-kDa fragment from the NH_2-terminus of the heavy subunit of Clostridium botulinum type A neurotoxin forms channels in lipid vesicles. Eur. J. Biochem. (in the press)

Toxins as Virulence Factors

Fehrenbach et al. (Eds.), Bacterial Protein Toxins, Zbl. Bakt. Suppl. 17
© Gustav Fischer, Stuttgart, New York, 1988

Sequence Homologies Among the Enzymically Active Portions of ADP-Ribosylating Toxins

D. M. Gill

Tufts University School of Medicine, Department of Molecular Biology and Microbiology, 136 Harrison Avenue, Boston, MA, Ø2111, U.S.A.

ABSTRACT

The enzymic portions of four ADP-ribosylating toxins have significant sequence homology. The greatest similarity is between cholera toxin A1 and pertussis toxin S1. Diphtheria toxin fragment A and the third domain of Pseudomonas exotoxin A also have substantial homology. The residues in common are mostly situated in or near the NAD binding site but a few of them may be concerned with recognizing the protein substrates, possibly the G domain which is well conserved among all of the GTP-binding substrates. A region of four-fold similarity exists close to the N-terminal ends where there are 18 identities between members of the two pairs. This suggests that all four toxins have a common ancestor.

KEYWORDS

Cholera toxin, Pertussis toxin, Diphtheria toxin, Pseudomonas aeruginosa exotoxin A, heat-labile enterotoxin, ADP-ribosylation, protein sequence, crystal structure, NAD binding site, GTP-binding proteins.

INTRODUCTION

About one half of all known A-B type toxins are ADP-ribosyl transferases and, except for those that modify actin, all choose GTP binding proteins as their major targets. How and why did this happen?

Apart from some homologies between the A1 fragment of cholera toxin and subunit 1 of pertussis toxin (Locht and Keith, 1986; Nicosia and others, 1986), the toxins have been considered to be independent proteins. However, it was not easy to believe that the concentration on a single kind of chemical modification and the restriction to G proteins were both the result of convergent evolution. It was appropriate to look again among the enzymically active portions of the ADP-ribosylating toxins for sequence homologies which could reflect a common origin. The four sequences available are for Pseudomonas aeruginosa exotoxin A (PsT) which is a single chain whose enzymically active portion extends to the C terminus from somewhere between residue 385 and 405 (Hwang and others, 1987), diphtheria toxin (DT) whose enzymically-active fragment A is N terminal, Bordetella pertussis toxin (PT) and cholera toxin (CT) both of which have A5B subunit structures. The

LT, A1	1:	G R	
		N D D - - K L Y R A D S R P P D E I K Q S G L M P R	:25
CT, A1	1:		:25
PT, S1	1:	D D P P A T V V R Y D S R P P E D V F Q N G F T A - W	:26

LT, A1		N Y	
		G Q S E Y F D - - R G T Q M N I N L Y D H A R G T - - O T G F V R H D D G	:58
CT, A1		G N N D - I V D S S K S F V M E N F S S Y H - -	:58
PT, S1		G A D D V D S - R S C Q V G S N - - S A	:49
DT, A			:41
PsT	425:	G A H R Q L E - E R G Y V - - G T F L E A A Q S I V F G G V R A R S Q	:460

LT, A1		L A S Y L I N	
		Y V S T S I S L R S A H L V G Q T I L S - T Y I Y - V I A T A P N M F	:98
CT, A1		F V S T S S S R Y T E V L E H R M Q E A V E A E - G H S - I G Y I T E V R A D - - N E	:98
PT, S1		T Q G N Y D D D W K G F Y S T D N K Y D A A G Y S V D N E	:96
DT, A		D - - - L D A I W R G F Y I A G D P A L A Y G Y A Q D Q E	:70
PsT		E R A G R G T G H F	:486

DT, A	146:	S V E Y I N N W E Q A - K A L S V E L E	:164
PsT	551:	R L E T I L G W P L A E R - - T V V I P	:568

enzymically active unit of B. pertussis toxin is its subunit 1. The active unit of cholera toxin is the N terminal fragment A1 of its subunit A. The cholera toxin sequence used represents several closely related varieties of cholera toxin and heat labile enterotoxins of enteric bacteria, which seem to have diverged quite recently (cf. Finkelstein and others, 1987).

RESULTS AND DISCUSSION

The eye proved to be more discerning than the computer and detected substantial regions of similarity (Fig. 1). There are somewhat more extensive homologies between CT and PT than were reported before, and there are also homologous sequences between DT and PsT which had been missed entirely (Gray and others, 1984). It is not surprising to find homologies within these pairs because CT and PT catalyse modifications of very similar proteins (Gs$\propto$ and Gi$\propto$ respectively) while DT and PsT ADP-ribosylate the same substrate, EF2. More surprisingly, close to the N terminus in each case is a region of common homology where, at 18 positions, one or both of the CT/PT pair have the same residue as one or both of the DT/PsT pair. In Fig. 1 these common residues are indicated by bold outlining. Elsewhere in the protein such "four-fold" correspondences happen infrequently enough to be attributed to chance and there is no other cluster that comes close to this degree of homology. Thus, the common region may well represent an ancestral sequence which has evolved relatively slowly because of functional constraints. Slow change in this region is also evident from the sequences of CT and porcine E. coli heat labile enterotoxin which are identical between positions 28 and 54 (or between 22 and 54 if we ignore the conservative replacement of gln-27 by asn). This is the longest stretch of identity between these two toxins: elsewhere there is an amino acid difference on average every 5 residues or less.

The probable locations of residues that PsT has in common with other toxins were identified on the three dimensional structure of PsT domain III (Allured and others, 1986). The published structure is slightly incomplete and when this led to uncertainty the best fit alignment was determined between the regions of helical and sheet structure in the 3D model and the regions of helical and sheet structure predicted from the primary sequence by the Chou-Fasman method. In Fig. 2, small circles and squares indicate the residues boxed lightly in Fig. 1 while the large circles indicate residues surrounded with heavy boxes. It is evident that the majority of shared residues either line the NAD pocket (the large cleft to the right of the view in Figure 2) or participate in its construction. A few of the common residues, however, are distant from the pocket and may be concerned with the binding of protein rather than NAD. This is particularly the case for the

> Fig. 1 (opposite): Sequence comparisons between four ADP-ribosyl transferases. Boxes enclose pairs of residues identical or conservatively substituted between CT and PT and between DT and PsT. Heavy boxes enclose residues where one or both of the top pair is identical to one or both of the lower pair, but conservative changes are not included. The top three sets describe one continuous sequence for each toxin; the four-fold common region consitutes the second set. Sequence data were taken from Mekalanos and others (1983) for CT; Locht and Keith (1986), and Nicosia and others (1986) for PT; Ratti and others, (1983), and Greenfield and others, (1983) for DT; Gray and others, (1984) for PsT. The residues of a porcine LT (Spicer and Noble, 1982) are shown at the top when they differ from CT.

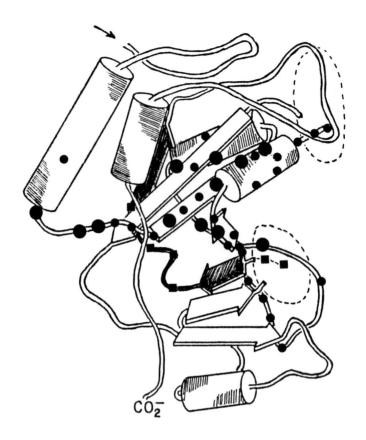

Fig. 2:   Probable locations of conserved
                          residues of Pseudomonas exotoxin A.
The drawing of the C-terminal third domain of PsT is taken
from Allured and others, 1986). The arrow indicates the
N-terminal side (residue 405). Areas enclosed by dashes are
uncertain. Common residues between 425 and 486 are indicated
by circles: the small circles are equivalent to the light
outlining in Figure 1, large circles to the heavy outlining.
The approximate location of common residues between positions
552 and 567 are indicated by small squares: for further
clarity the protein backbone has been heavily shaded in this
region.

N-terminal end of the common region (residues 425-435 of PsT) and for this
reason the common region is considered to consist of putative protein and NAD
binding portions.

Figure 3 summarizes these conclusions and relates them to additional
information about the four toxins. Fig. 4 shows their probalble evolutionary
relationship. Overall the four enzymically active regions have remarkably
similar structural organizations and sizes. Starting from the amino ends, we
can distinguish the following functional regions.

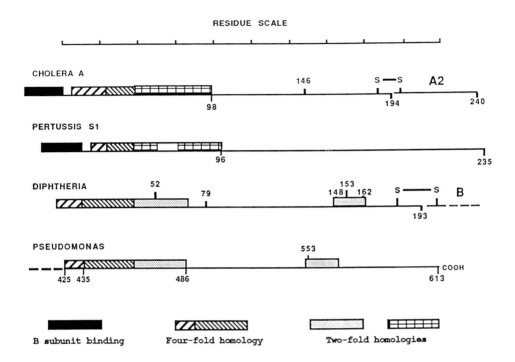

Fig. 3. Functional regions of the ADP-ribosyl transferases.
Numbers written above the lines refer to residues discussed
in the text.

1. An amino terminal region of homology between CT and PT. This is concealed
in cholera holotoxin but is available to antibodies in isolated subunit A and
may therefore form contact with the ring of B subunits (Duffy, Kurosky and
Lai, 1985). The equivalent region of PT may likewise lie at the interface
between S1 and one of the other five subunits of pertussis holotoxin. The
region is absent in diphtheria toxin, and the corresponding residues are quite
heterologous in PsT: both of these toxins have covalent A–B connections which
do not involve subunit–subunit binding.

2. The amino terminal portion of the common region which may be involved in
binding a feature common at least to Gs and EF2 (much of the region is absent
in PT: has it been displaced to positions 70–81?). An obvious candidate
would be the G domain (GTP-binding site), which is conserved to a considerable
degree between EF2, Gi and Gs, while the remainder of the target molecules
are dissimilar (Kohno and others, 1986).

3. The carboxy terminal portion of the common domain, starting with the
sequence HXXG or HG, consists of two segments that are involved in forming the
NAD site. The two segments are separated in DT and PsT by five non-conserved
residues.

4. Immediately adjacent to the common region are stretches of near identity between CT and PT and between DT and PsT but without any evident similarity between the pairs. Perhaps these residues are involved in binding to specific areas on the target proteins that differ between Gs/Gi and EF2, and therefore most probably lie outside the G domains. Within this region is the sole mutation in the non-toxic protein CRM197 (gly-52 → glu: Giannini and others, 1984) which inactivates the enzymic function of the toxin. This mutation also results in an altered binding to cellular receptors (Mekada and Uchida, 1985). Further downstream is one of the two mutational changes in fragment A of CRM228, namely gly-79 → asp; the other change is at residue 162 but it is not known which change inactivates the enzyme (Kaczorek and others, 1983).

5. A further region of homology exists between DT (147-163) and PsT (552-567). The common residues are represented in Fig. 2 by square symbols and appear to be near the NAD binding site. There are several observations which support this assignment. The segment contains glutamic acid residues (in DT glu-148, in PsT glu-553) that react covalently with nicotinamide when the non-covalent toxin.NAD complexes are uv irradiated (Carroll and Collier, 1984) and are therefore close to the active center. Chemical modification of trp-153 results in enzyme inactivation (Michel and Dirkx 1977). Along with gly-79, glu-162 is changed (to lys) in the enzymically inactive CRM228. The truncated diphtheria toxin, CRM1 (Holmes, 1976), which probably terminates near residue 160 (Zucker and Murphy, 1974), is enzymically inactive.

It has not been possible to find such a region in CT or PT, and this absence may relate to the poorer binding of NAD by these toxins. Reported Km(NAD) values are CT: 3 mM to 4 mM (Gill, 1982; Galloway and van Heyningen, 1987), PT: 25 μM (Moss and others, 1983), DT: 5 μM (Goor and Maxwell, 1970) or 1 μM (Chung and Collier, 1977), PsT: 2.5 μM (Lory and Collier, 1980). Nevertheless, arg-146 may be close to the active site for it slowly becomes ADP-ribosylated when cholera toxin has no other substrate (Lai, Xia and Salotra, 1983). (Modification of tryptophan inactivates cholera toxin {deWolf and others, 1981} but the particular tryptophan involved has not been identified).

6. The carboxy-terminal region of CT and DT must be sufficiently exposed to allow access by the proteases that nick these toxins beneath their disulfide bridges and release the active peptides from fragment A2 and fragment B respectively. The region 160-193 seems to be particularly exposed in DT since most monoclonal antibodies raised against the A fragment recognize the C terminal 20%. One of these antibodies neutralizes enzymic activity (Zucker, Murphy and Pappenheimer, 1984). The carboxy-terminal region of CT is likewise exposed to antibodies (Duffy, Kurosky and Lai, 1985). There is no disulfide bridge in PT but the question poses itself whether PT's C-terminal forty or fifty residues might be dispensable too.

The newly discovered botulinal exoenzyme C3, which is suspected to constitute the A component of an A-B toxin, may well be related to the other four toxins. It has about the same size [24,000 Mr (Aktories, Weller and Chhatwal, 1987) or 26,000 (Rubin and others, 1987)] and its target protein p21.bot binds GTP.

It may seem surprising that relatively limited sequences are assigned to the binding of protein substrates. it is worth noting, however, that the active regions of these toxins have approximately the same size (20,000-26,000) as the smallest known NAD glycohydrolases, which are not known to bind to any proteins. Bacterial examples include the NAD glycohydrolases of Pseudomonas putida: 23,500 (Mather and Knight 1972) and of Bacillus subtilis: 24,000-26,000 (Everse, Everse and Kaplan, 1975). The mammalian plasma membrane NAD glycohydrolases vary greatly in size between species but the smallest class, which includes the bovine, ovine and porcine enzymes, has a molecular size of 25,000 (Swislocki and others, 1967, Schuber and Travo, 1976).

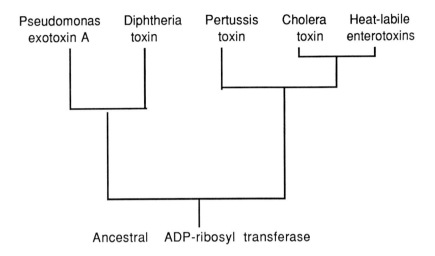

Fig. 4. Possible evolutionary relationships between the enzymic regions of ADP-ribosylating toxins. Other regions of the toxin molecules may have evolved independently.

REFERENCES

Aktories, K, U. Weller and G.S.Chhatwal (1987). Clostridium botulinum type C prodcues a novel ADP-ribosyltransferase distinct from botulinum C2 toxin. FEBS Letters, 212, 109–113.
Allured, V.S., R.J.Collier, S.F.Carroll and D.B.McKay (1986). Structure of exotoxin A of Pseudomonas aeruginosa at 3.0-Angstrom resolution. Proc. Natl. Acad. Sci., 83, 1320–1324.
Carroll, S.F. and R.J.Collier (1984). NAD binding site of diphtheria toxin: Identification of a residue within the nicotinamide subsite by photochemical modification with NAD. Proc. Natl. Acad. Sci., 81, 3307–3311.
Chung, D.W. and R.J.Collier (1977). The mechanism of ADP-ribosylation of elongation factor 2 catalysed by fragment A from diphtheria toxin. Biochim. Biophys. Acta, 483, 248–257.
DeWolf, M.J.S., M.Fridkin, M.Epstein, and L.D.Kohn (1981). Structure-function studies of cholera toxin and its A and B protomers: modification of tryptophan residues. J. Biol. Chem., 256, 5481–5488.
Duffy, L.K., A.Kurosky, and C-Y.Lai (1985). Cholera toxin A subunit: functional sites correlated with regions of secondary structure. Arch. Biochem. Biophys., 239, 549–555.
Everse, J., K.E.Everse and N.O.Kaplan (1975). The pyridine nucleosidases from Bacillus subtilis and Neurospora crassa. Isolation and structural properties. Arch. Biochem. Biophys., 169, 702–713.
Finkelstein, R.A., M.F.Burks, A.Zupan, W.S.Dallas, C.O.Jacob and D.S.Ludwig (1987). Epitopes of the cholera family of enterotoxins. Rev. Infect. Dis. 9, 544–561.
Galloway T.S. and S.van Heyningen (1987). Binding of NAD by cholera toxin.

Biochem. J., 244, 225-230.

Giannini, G., R.Rappuoli, and G.Ratti (1984). The amino acid sequence of two non-toxic mutants of diphtheria toxin. Nucleic Acid Res., 12, 4063-4069.

Gill, D.M. (1982). Cholera toxin catalysed ADP-ribosylation of membrane proteins. In: O.Hayaishi and K. Ueda (Eds.), ADP-ribosylation reactions, Academic Press, New York, pp. 593-621.

Goor, R.S. and E.S.Maxwell (1970). The diphtheria toxin-dependent adenosine diphosphate ribosylation of rat liver aminoacyl transferase II. J. Biol. Chem., 245, 616-623.

Gray, G.L. D.H.Smith, J.S.Baldridge, R.N.Harkins, M.L.Vasil, E.Y.Chen, and H.L.Heynecker (1984). Cloning, nucleotide sequence and expression in Escherichia coli of the exotoxin A structural gene of Pseudomonas aeruginosa. Proc. Natl Acad. Sci., 81, 2645-2649.

Greenfield, L., M.J. Bjorn, G.Horn, D.Fong, G.A.Buck, R.J.Collier and D.A.Kaplan (1983). Nucleotide sequence of the structural gene for diphtheria toxin carried by Corynebacterium diphtheriae. Proc. Natl. Acad. Sci., 80, 6853-6857.

Holmes, R.K. (1976). Characterization and genetic mapping of nontoxigenic (tox) mutants of corynebacteriophage beta. J. Virol., 19, 195-207.

Hwang, J., D.J.Fitzgerald, S.Adhya, and I.Pastan (1987). Functional domains of Pseudomonas exotoxin identified by deletion analysis of the gene expressed in E. coli. Cell, 48, 129-136.

Kaczorek, M., F.Delpeyroux, N.Chenciner, R.E.Streeck, J.R.Murphy, P.Boquet and P.Tiollais (1983). Nucleotide sequence and expression of the diphtheria tox228 gene in Escherichia coli. Science, 221: 855-858.

Kohno, K., T.Uchida, H.Ohkubo, S.Nakanishi, T.Nakanishi, T.Fukui, E.Ohtsuka, M.Ikehara and Y.Okada (1986). Amino acid sequence of mammalian elongation factor 2 deduced from the DNA sequence: homology with GTP binding proteins. Proc. Natl. Acad. Sci., 83, 78-4982.

Lai, C-Y. Q-C.Xia and P.T.Salotra (1983). Location and amino acid sequence around the ADP-ribosylation site in the cholera toxin active subunit A1. Biochem. Biophys. Res. Commun., 116, 341-348.

Locht, C. and J.M.Keith (1986). Pertussis toxin gene: nucleotide sequence and genetic organization. Science, 232, 1258-1264.

Lory, S. and R.J.Collier (1980). Expression of enzymic activity by exotoxin A from Pseudomonas aeruginosa. Infect. Immun. 28, 494-501.

Mather I.H. and M.Knight (1972). A heat-stable NAD glycohydrolase from Pseudomonas putida KB1. Biochem. J., 129, 141-152.

Mekada, E., and T.Uchida (1985). Binding properties of diphtheria toxin to cells are altered by mutation in the fragment A domain. J. Biol. Chem., 260, 12148-12153.

Mekalanos, J.J., D.J.Swarz, G.D.N.Pearson, N.Harford, F.Groyne and M.de Wilde (1983). Cholera toxin genes: nucleotide sequence, deletion analysis and vaccine development. Nature, 306, 551-557.

Michel, A. and J.Dirkx (1977). Occurence of tryptophan in the enzymically active site of diphtheria toxin fragment A. Biochim. Biophys. Acta, 491, 286-295.

Moss, J., S.J.Stanley, D.L.Burns, J.A.Hsia, D.A.Yost, G.A.Myers and E.L.Hewlett (1983). Activation by thiol of the latent NAD glycohydrolase and ADP-ribosyltransferase activities of Bordetella pertussis toxin (islet activating protein). J. Biol. Chem., 258, 11879-11882.

Nicosia, A., M.Perugini, C.Franzini, M.C.Casagli, M.G.Borri, G.Antoni, M. Almoni, P. Neri, G. Ratti and R.Rappuoli (1986). Cloning and sequencing of the pertussis toxin genes: operon structure and gene duplication. Proc. Natl. Acad. Sci., 83, 4631-4635.

Ratti, G., R.Rappuoli, and G.Giannini (1983). The complete nucleotide sequence of the gene coding for diphtheria toxin in the corynephage omega (tox+) genome. Nucleic Acid Res., 11, 6589-6595.

Rubin, E.J., D.M.Gill, P.Boquet and M.R.Popoff (1987). Functional modification of a p21ras-like protein when ADP-ribosylated by exoenzyme C3 of Clostridium botulinum. Submitted.

Schuber, F. and P.Travo (1976). Calf spleen NAD glycohydrolase. Solubilization, purification, and properties of the enzyme. Eur. J. Biochem., 65, 247-255.

Spicer, E.K. and J.A.Noble (1982). Escherichia coli heat-labile enterotoxin. Nucleotide sequence of the A subunit gene. J. Biol. Chem., 257, 5716-5721.

Swislocki, N.I. M.I.Kalish, F.I.Chasalow and N.O.Kaplan (1967). Solubilization and comparative properties of some mammalian diphosphopyridine nucleosidases. J. Biol. Chem., 242, 1089-1094.

Zucker, D.R. and J.R.Murphy (1984). Monoclonal antibody analysis of diphtheria toxin-I. localization of epitopes and neutralization of toxicity. Mol. Immunol., 21, 785-793.

Zucker, D.R. J.R.Murphy and A.M. Pappenheimer (1984). Monoclonal antibody analysis of diphtheria toxin-II. Inhibition of ADP-ribosyl transferase activity. Mol. Immunol., 21, 795 800.

Fehrenbach et al. (Eds.), Bacterial Protein Toxins, Zbl. Bakt. Suppl. 17
© Gustav Fischer, Stuttgart, New York, 1988

Bacterial Cytolysins as Virulence Factors

W. Goebel, S. Kathariou, J. Hacker, T. Chakraborty, M. Leimeister-Wächter, A. Ludwig, J. Hess, M. Kuhn and W. Wagner

Institut für Genetik und Mikrobiologie, Universität Würzburg, Röntgenring 11, D-8700 Würzburg

ABSTRACT

Genetic, biochemical and pathogenesis studies on the hemolysins (cytolysins) of Escherichia coli and Listeria monocytogenes are described. Four major protein domains are characterized by site-directed mutagenesis in HlyA as being essential for hemolytic activity, transport and toxicity of E. coli hemolysin. The effect of hemolysin toxicity in a mouse peritoneum model is directly dependent on the amount of extracellular hemolysin and structural features of HlyA and is not caused by the concomitant release of LPS observed during secretion of hemolysin in E. coli. Expression of hemolysin and hence toxicity is influenced by hly-specific sequences and by the E. coli background.

SH-activated hemolysin of L. monocytogenes (listeriolysin) appears to be essential for survival but not for entrance of these bacteria in mammalian host cells. Listeria species may produce more than one type of hemolytic activity. Clones with genetic determinants expressing hemolytic phenotype in E. coli, which was not caused by the SH-activated cytolysins, were identified in E. coli gene libraries of L. monocytogenes and Bacillus cereus.

KEYWORDS

E. coli hemolysin, listeriolysin, toxicity and virulence, functional domains.

INTRODUCTION

Synthesis of hemolysins has been reported throughout a broad spectrum of gram-negative and gram-positive bacterial species. The in vitro action of hemolysins ultimately causes physical damage to a variety of eukaryotic cells. Such bacterial proteins possessing a membrane-damaging action, often on different types of mammalian cells have also been termed "cytolysins".

Hemolytic Escherichia coli strains are predominantly found among isolates from patients with pyelonephritis. The genetics and biochemistry of this hemolysin have been extensively studied (for review see Hacker and Hughes, 1985; Cavalieri et al., 1984). It has been shown in several animal model systems that this hemolysin is an important virulence factor (Marre et al., 1986; Hacker et al., 1987). Listeria monocytogenes is a gram-positive bacterium which is able to enter and multiply within phagocytic cells (macrophages and monocytes). It can cause septicemia and meningitis with a high rate of mortality (Gray and Klinger, 1966). All known virulent strains produce hemolysin (listeriolysin), whereas non-hemolytic Listeria strains are avirulent. Listeriolysin has therefore been implicated as an important virulence factor in infections caused by L. monocytogenes. Studies using non-hemolytic transposon mutants of L. monocytogenes support this assumption (Gaillard et al., 1986; Kathariou et al., 1987). In this communication we summarize some recent data on the structural and functional aspects of hemolysins from E. coli and L. monocytogenes and describe the implication of these findings for virulence.

A. E. coli hemolysin - a structural and functional analysis

Four genes (hlyC, hlyA, hlyB and hlyD) determine synthesis and secretion of E. coli hemolysin (Hacker and Hughes, 1985). These four genes are located either on large transmissible plasmids or on the chromosome. In the latter case the hly genes are part of larger inserts, 70 kb to 100 kb in size, which carry short directly repeated sequences at their ends (Knapp et al., 1986). Homologous recombination between the two direct repeats leads to deletions which remove these inserts precisely. These deletion mutants can be used as suitable hosts for introducing cloned hly genes from other E. coli strains to study their virulence (see below).
Active hemolysin is secreted by E. coli in the active growth phase. It consists of the HlyA gene product which does not seem to be proteolytically processed during secretion (Welch et al., 1985). However HlyC, a cytoplasmic protein, is necessary to render HlyA hemolytically active. Active hemolysin is sensitive to phospholipase C suggesting that phospholipid(s) may be involved in the activation step catalyzed by HlyC. Activated Hly A (HlyA*) and non-activated HlyA are secreted with the same efficiency by a specific transport system consisting of at least the two gene products, HlyB and HlyD.
Release of lipopolysaccharide (LPS) from the outer membrane is observed during secretion of HlyA and HlyA* (Fig. 1). LPS may be directly associated with HlyA* (transport vesicles?) since extracellular active hemolysin is isolated from the supernatant in large complexes the apparent molecular mass of which exceeds by far the known molecular weight of HlyA (110 kDa) or of a dimeric form of HlyA (Fig. 2). HlyA seems to be the only protein in these complexes (Fig. 2).
Four major functional domains have been recognized on the HlyA protein (mainly by site-directed mutagenesis and analysis of fusion proteins with various parts of HlyA and PhoA) which are essential for hemolytic activity and transport.

(A) The N-terminal end, which may form an amphiphilic helix (similar to target sequences on nuclear proteins which are imported into organelles). This part of HlyA is membrane active and fusion proteins consisting of 50 amino acids (or even less) of the N-terminal end of HlyA and the leader-less PhoA exhibit alkaline phosphatase activity in E. coli suggesting that the PhoA part is transported to the periplasm probably using the

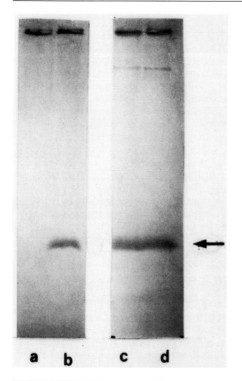

Fig.1: Release of LPS during transport of HlyA. Supernatants from late log phase cultures were concentrated 10 fold and 50 ul aliquots were applied to SDS-PAGE. Supernatants from (a) E. coli 5K, (b) LPS from E. coli 5K, (c) pANN202-812, (d) E. coli 5K, pANN202-812B (hlyC⁻). LPS was detected by immunoblotting with LPS antibodies.

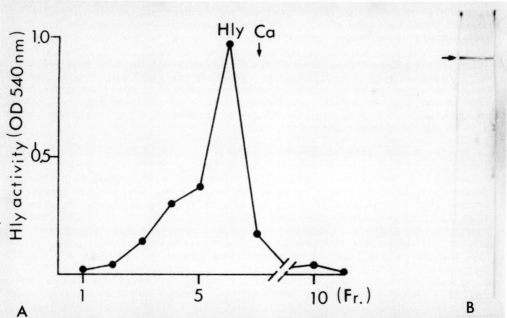

Fig. 2: Hemolytic activity after separation of E. coli 5K, pANN202-812 on sephacryl S400 (A). SDS-PAGE (B) shows the HlyA protein (Mr 110 kDa) from the peak fraction of hemolytic activity. Ca indicates position of catalase (Mr 240 kDa).

N-terminal HlyA sequence as a membrane anchor (Erb et al., 1987). It seems likely that this part of Hly A may be also anchored in the membrane during synthesis of HlyA until the C-terminal end of HlyA is completed. A HlyA mutant in which amino acids 9 to 37 at the N-terminal end are removed by oligonucleotide-directed mutagenesis (Ludwig, unpublished results) is still fully hemolytically active and is transported by the HlyB/HlyD system but becomes rather unstable intracellularly when the transport of the mutant HlyA protein is impaired (e.g. in the absence of a functional HlyB/HlyD system).

(B) The C-terminal end carries the essential signal sequence for transport of HlyA by HlyB/HlyD. A protein consisting of PhoA lacking its own N-terminal signal sequence but possessing the last 60 amino acids of the C-terminal end of HlyA fused to the C-terminal end of PhoA is transported by an "activated" HlyB/HlyD system (Hess et al. manuscript in preparation) but transport of such a fusion protein is more efficient if the N-terminal end of HlyA is also fused to this protein. A similar construct consisting of only the last 24 amino acids from the C-terminal end of HlyA is not transported by HlyB/HlyD suggesting a minimal length for the C-terminal transport signal sequence of HlyA between 24 and 60 amino acids.

(C) The hydrophobic domain between amino acids 299 to 327 in HlyA was removed by oligonucleotide-directed mutagenesis. In another construct hydrophobic sequence was interrupted by introducing two charged amino acids in positions 313 and 314 (Ludwig et al., 1987). Both HlyA mutants were non-hemolytic (in the presence of HlyC) but the HlyA proteins were transported by HlyB/HlyD with the same efficiency as wild-type HlyA and LPS was released in similar amounts upon secretion. Binding of these mutant HlyA proteins to granulocytes was not impaired but preliminary data suggest that the association of these mutant HlyA proteins with phospholipid(s) no longer occured (Wagner, W. et al., unpublished data).

(D) A region consisting of 11 repeats of a consensus sequence (Leu X Gly Gly X Gly Asn Asp) was recognized between amino acids 748 and 849 on HlyA. Removal of one internal repeat by oligonucleotide-directed mutagenesis lead to the loss of hemolytic activity (Ludwig, unpublished results). It is speculated that this region of HlyA is essential for the binding of HlyA to the membrane of the target cells.

B. Virulence of E. coli hemolysin

Virulence of hemolysin was recently demonstrated with cloned hemolysin determinants from different origins in rat, mouse and chicken embryo systems (Marre et al., 1987).Injection of the manipulated E. coli strains into the mouse peritoneum allows the measurement of the level of toxicity exerted by the hemolysin. We have used as E. coli hosts for introducing the various wild-type and mutant hly determinants spontaneously occuring Hly⁻ mutants of O6 and O18 strains which arise by deletion of the chromosomal inserts carrying the hly genes (strains 536-21 and 764-2). As previously shown, E. coli K-12 strains carrying the recombinant plasmid pANN202-312 which derives from the natural plasmid pHly152 exhibits a rather weak hemolytic phenotype. Strain 536-21 transformed with this recombinant plasmid shows low toxicity for mice. Recombinant plasmids carrying the same hlyC-upstream region of pANN202-312 as expression site but the hly genes from two chromosomal hly determinants pANN5311-018 and pANN5311-06) exhibit in the same host strain (536-21) higher titers of extracellular hemolytic activity and significantly higher levels of toxicity for mice (Table 1).

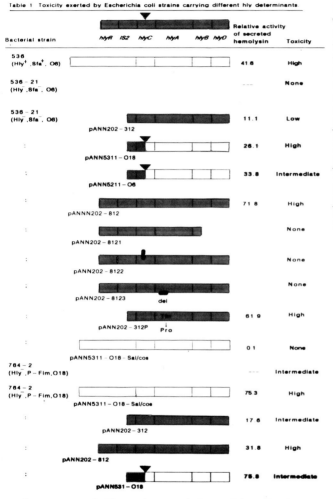

Table 1 Toxicity exerted by Escherichia coli strains carrying different hly determinants

For the toxicity test, 5 mice were used in each test and for each plasmid at least three tests were performed. High toxicity means all mice were killed within 24 h (5/5); none is (0/5); low (1(2)/5) and intermediate (2(3)/5). ( ) indicates a single BamHI site present in all hly determinants which was used for the construction of hybrid hly determinants. Dark bars represent hly sequences from pHly152, light bars those from E. coli 018 strain 764 and dotted bars those from E. coli 06 strain 536.

Parameters influencing toxicity of hemolysin

The recent discovery of a cis acting activator site (hlyR) in pHly152 upstream of the expression region present in pANN202-312 allows the construction of pHly152-derived recombinant plasmids which synthesize and secrete large amounts of hemolysin in E. coli K-12. The difference between pANN202-312 (hlyR⁻) and its hlyR⁺ homolog pANN202-812 was about 100fold based on the amount of HlyA protein synthesized. The difference was only 7 to 10fold in 536-21 but this increase in extracellular hemolysin lead to a high level of toxicity (Table 1), suggesting that the amount of extracellular hemolysin is critical for toxicity. This conclusion is further supported by the fact that 536-21 which carries plasmid pANN202-8121 (hlyB⁻ and hlyD⁻ and hence can not secrete hemolysin) was non-toxic

although it synthesized large amounts of intracellular active hemolysin.
As mentioned above, secretion of hemolysin (and inactive HlyA) is
accompanied by the release of substantial amounts of LPS. To test whether
the observed toxicity was directly caused by hemolysin or indirectly by
the concomitant release of LPS we have used two recombinant plasmids which
do not synthesize active hemolysin but still secrete wild-type levels of
HlyA and release concomitantly LPS. Mutant plasmid pANN202-8122 carries a
defective hlyC gene, and pANN202-8123 carries the above described deletion
in hlyA which removes the hydrophobic domain in HlyA. Both mutant plasmids
when introduced into 536-21 were unable to cause toxicity, suggesting that
hemolysin exhibits the toxic effect directly (Table 1).
The amount of extracellular hemolysin (measured in vitro), although
essential for toxicity, does not strictly correlate with the toxicity
exerted in mice. We therefore tested whether structural differences in the
HlyA proteins may be responsible for the observed differences.
Comparison of the amino acid sequences of HlyA proteins from the pHly152-
encoded and various chromosomal determinants shows in all chromosomal HlyA
proteins, exhibiting high to intermediate toxicity, in amino acid position
3, Pro and only in the pHly152-derived HlyA protein, exhibiting low
toxicity, Thr in this position (Hess et al., 1986). We changed in pANN202-
312 by site-directed mutagenesis Thr into Pro and obtained a hemolysin
(pANN202-312P in Table 1) and a higher level of toxicity in the mouse
model, suggesting that structural features of HlyA may also influence the
biological function of hemolysin.
As described above, pANN202-812 (hlyR$^+$) expressed about 100 times more
HlyA in E. coli K-12 than pANN202-312 (hlyR$^-$) but only 10 times more in
the O6 strain 536-21 and even less in the O18 strain 764-2 (Table 1)
suggesting a host influence on the expression of the hly genes. This was
further substantiated by the recent isolation of chromosomal mutants of E.
coli K-12 in which expression of pANN202-812 is significantly decreased
(almost to the level of pANN202-312). The recombinant plasmid pANN5311-O18
Sal/cos was poorly expressed in 536-21 (O6) and the toxicity of this
manipulated strain was low. The same recombinant plasmid introduced into
the strain 764-2 (O18) expressed high hemolytic activity in vitro and
exhibited high toxicity. These data indicate that the host background is
modulating the expression of hly determinants and hence may also influence
in toxicity.
The level of toxicity exerted by the described wild-type and mutant hly
genes in the mouse peritoneum-system correlated with the virulence which
these hly genes exhibited in the rat pyelonephritis system (Marre et al.,
1986).

C. Hemolysin of L. monocytogenes and its involvement in virulence

Virulent strains of Listeria monocytogenes produce a SH-activated
cytolysin, termed listeriolysin. Like other SH-activated cytolysins,
listeriolysin cross reacts immunologically with antiserum against
streptolysin O (SLO). We have recently described the isolation of
listeriolysin-negative mutants from L. monocytogenes Sv1/2a obtained
mutagenesis with transposon Tn916 (Kathariou et al., 1987). These mutants
were avirulent in mice and unable to survive in mouse peritoneal
macrophages but can still enter the macrophages and even non-professional
phagocytes such as 3T6 cells (an embryonic mouse fibroblast cell line)
(Kuhn et al., 1987). Avirulent, nonhemolytic L. innocua strains and the
avirulent but hemolytic L. seeligeri strains were unable to enter these

cells (Fig. 3). Interestingly, even the strongly hemolytic L. ivanovii which exhibits reduced virulence in mice was unable to penetrate 3T6 cells (Fig. 3). This indicates that hemolysin in the mouse may be necessary for survival but not for the entrance of virulent Listeria in mammalian cells. The isolation of mutants from virulent L. monocytogenes strains, which were still hemolytic but lacked another extracellular 60 kDa protein and were unable to enter 3T6 cells, further supports this assumption (Goebel et al., 1987).

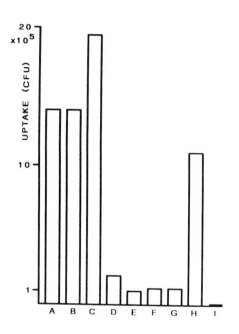

Fig. 3: Invasion of different Listeria strains in 3T6 cells. Invasion assays were performed essentially as described (Isberg and Falkow, 1985).Each column represents the mean value of two experiments. (A) L. monocytogenes Sv1/2a (Mackaness). (B) L.monocytogenes Sv1/2a (EGD), (C) L. monocytogenes Sv4b, (D) L. monocytogenes Sv3a, (E). L. innocua Sv6b, (G) L. ivanovii , (H) L. monocytogenes 1/2a (Mackaness) Hly⁻(Tn916), (I) B. subtilis

As recently pointed out by Kathariou et al. there is an apparent lack of direct correlation between the levels of cytolytic in vitro activity and virulence of L. monocytogenes strains (Fig. 4). A hyperhemolytic mutant of a L. monocytogenes Sv4b strain which produced about 10 times more hemolysin than the parental strain did not exhibit increased virulence. Although these data do not exclude the possibility that the level of listeriolysin synthesized in vitro may not reflect the level in vivo, they suggest that either lysis of host cell membranes (phagosomal membrane?) is not itself the key factor in virulence or that this lysis is brought about even by the low amounts of hemolysin produced by many weakly hemolytic virulent strains.

As recently shown (Kathariou et al. , 1987) extracellular listeriolysin from L. monocytogenes is a 58 kDa protein that cross reacts with anti SLO. L. ivanovii secretes in large amounts protein of similar Mr which likewise cross reacts with anti SLO. No such protein was observed in supernatants of various L. seeligeri strains and no cross reactivity with anti SLO was observed, indicating that the hemolysin of L. seeligeri is unrelated to listeriolysin (Goebel et al., 1987).

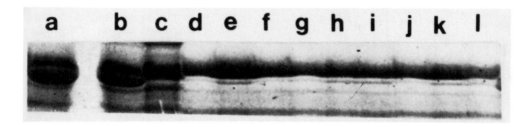

Fig. 4: Lack of correlation between the amount of listeriolysin produced in vitro and virulence of L. monocytogenes strains. Virulence tested in a mouse model is identical for all L. monocytogenes but the amount of listeriolysin (Mr = 56 kDa) secreted into the culture supernatant (indicated by the arrow) is apparently quite different among these strains. The relatively constant upper band represents the 60 kDa protein also mentioned in the text. (a) L. monocytogenes NCTC7973, (b) L. monocytogenes Sv1/2a (Mackaness, SLCC5764), (c) to (l) L. monocytogenes "EGD" strain collection from different laboratories

More than one type of hemolytic E. coli clones was detected in a L. monocytogenes gene library constructed in E. coli. The first type carried recombinant plasmids with a common 2.0 kb fragment coding for a 23 kDa protein which did not cross react with anti-SLO or anti-listeriolysin antibodies. The second type of hemolytic clones was detected by using anti- SLO to screen the gene bank. One of these clones carried a plasmid with a 9 kb insert of Listeria DNA which encoded several polypeptides one of which, a protein of 61 kDa, was found to be cross reacting with anti SLO. Subcloning of this fragment resulted in more strongly hemolytic colonies. The recombinant plasmids of these subclones expressed a smaller protein, not cross reacting with anti SLO which caused a CAMP effect with S.aureus suggesting that this protein may represent a CAMP-like factor similar that of B-type Streptococci. The other type of subclone expressed the 61 kDa protein which cross reacted with anti- SLO but was not hemolytic. The latter type may represent the actual "listeriolysin" clone. The same difficulties observed in cloning the gene for SH-activated listeriolysin in E. coli was encountered by us in a similar attempt to clone the gene for the SH-activated cereolysin from Bacillus cereus in E. coli. As reported (Kreft et al., 1983) several strongly hemolytic clones were identified in a cosmid gene library of B. cereus constructed in E. coli. All of these clones carried two adjacent genes (cerA and cerB) which did not encode the expected cereolysin (Gilmore et al, to be published).

As recently shown (Gilmore, M., personal communication) the isolated CerB protein has sphingomyelinase activity. E. coli K-12 carrying cerB was weakly hemolytic and could replace Staphylococcus aureus (known to produce a sphingomyelinase) in a CAMP assay with S. agalactiae. Comparison of the amino acid sequence of CerA (deduced from the DNA sequence of cerA) with the published 26 amino acids from the N-terminal end of phospholipase C from B. cereus (Otnaess et al., 1977) indicates complete homology with amino acids 39 to 65 of CerA (Fig. 5).Assuming that the first 38 amino

```
121   GGATATTCTAGTCATAGGTTAACCGGACGACATCATAGGATCCTAACAAAATGTTTACAA   180
            190              210              230

181   TAATTCAATTATAAAATGGAGGATTTTATATGAAAAAGAAAGTACTTGCTTTAGGCGCAG   240
                      rbs        MetLysLysLysValLeuAlaLeuGlyAlaA
            250              270              290

241   CTAGTACATTAGTTGCTCCATTACAAAGTGTTGCATTTGCTCATGAAAATGATGGGGGAC   300
      laIleThrLeuValAlaProLeuGlnSerValAlaPheAlaHisGluAsnAspGlyGlyG
            310              330              350

301   AGAGATTTGGAGTTATTCCGCGCTGGTCTGCTGAAGATAAACATAAAGAAGGCGTGAATT   360
      lnArgPheGlyValIleProArgTrpSerAlaGluAspLysHisLysGluGlyValAsnS
            370              390              410

361   CTCATTTATGGATTGTAAACCGAGCAATTGATATTATGTCTCGTAATACAACACTTGTAA   420
      erHisLeuTrpIleValAsnArgAlaIleAspIleMetSerArgAsnThrThrLeuValL
            430              450              470

421   AACAAGATCGAGTTGCACTATTAAATGAATGGCGTACTGAGTTAGAGAACGGTATTTATG   480
      ysGlnAspArgValAlaLeuLeuAsnGluTrpArgThrGluLeuGluAsnGlyIleTyrA
            490              510              530
```

Fig. 5: DNA sequence of the 5´region of cerA and the deduced amino-acid sequence of the N-terminal part of CerA compared to the published (Otaness et al. 1977) first 26 amino acids (underlined) or the mature phospholipase C of B. cereus. (rbs) indicates putative ribosome binding site of mRNA for CerA.

acids of the primary gene product of CerA represents a pre-pro sequence, this data strongly suggest, that CerA is identical with phospholipase C. It thus appears that a strong hemolytic phenotype can be obtained in E. coli by the cloning of the two adjacent phospholipase genes (sphingomyelinase and phospholipase C), and a weak hemolytic phenotype by cloning a sphingomyelinase gene (cerB) or a "CAMP-like" protein (hemolytic clone type II of L. monocytogenes).
It is interesting to note that the listeriolysin-negative transposon mutants of L. monocytogenes were completely non-hemolytic, suggesting that these additional "hemolytic" activities of L. monocytogenes become only apparent in an E. coli background or that inactivation of the listeriolysin gene by insertion of a transposon blocks also expression of these activities.

Cavalieri, S.J., G.A. Bochach, and I.S. Snyder (1984) Escherichia coli hemolysin: Characteristics and probable role in pathogenicity. Microbiol. Rev., 48, 326-343

Erb, K., M. Vogel, W. Wagner, and W. Goebel (1987) Alkaline phosphatase which lacks its own signal sequence becomes enzymatically active when fused to N-terminal sequences of E. coli hemolysin (HlyA). Mol. Gen. Genet. (in press)

Felmlee, T., S. Pellet, E.Y. Lee, and R.A. Welch (1985) Escherichia coli hemolysin is released extracellularly without cleavage of a signal peptide. J. Bact., 163, 88-93

Gaillard, J.L., P. Berche, and P. Sansonetti (1986) Transposon mutagenesis as a tool to study the role of hemolysin in the virulence of Listeria monocytogenes. Inf. Immun. 52, 50-55

Goebel, W., S. Kathariou, M. Kuhn, Z. Sokolovic, J. Kreft, S. Köhler, D. Funke, T. Chakraborty and M. Leimeister-Wächter (1987) Hemolysin from Listeria - biochemistry, genetics and function in pathogenesis. Infection (in press)

Gray, M.L., and A.H. Klinger (1966) Listeria monocytogenes and listeric infections. Bact. Rev., 30, 309-382

Hacker, J., and C. Hughes (1985) Genetics of Escherichia coli hemolysin. Current Topics of Microbiology and Immunology, 166, 1-162. Ed. W. Goebel, Springer Verlag, Heidelberg

Hacker, J., H. Hof, L. Emödy, and W. Goebel (1987) Influence of cloned Escherichia coli hemolysin genes, S-fimbriae and serum resistance on pathogenicity in different animal models. Microbial Pathogenesis, 1, 533-547

Hess, J., M. Vogel, W. Wels, and W. Goebel (1986) Nucleotide sequence of a plasmid-encoded hemolysin determinant and its comparison with a corresponding chromosomal hemolysin sequence. FEMS Letters, 34, 1-11

Isberg, R.R. and S. Falkow (1985) A single genetic locus encoded by Yersinia pseudotuberculosis permits invasion of cultured cells by Escherichia coli K-12. Nature, 317, 262-264

Kathariou, S., P. Metz, H. Hof, and W. Goebel (1987) Tn916-induced mutations in the hemolysin determinant affecting virulence of Listeria monocytogenes. J. Bact., 169, 1291-1297

Knapp, S., J. Hacker, T. Jarchau, and W. Goebel (1987) Large unstable inserts in the chromosome affect the virulence properties of the uropathogenic Escherichia coli O6 strain 536. J. Bact., 168, 22-30

Kreft, J., H. Berger, M. Härtlein, B. Müller, G. Weidinger, and
    W. Goebel (1983) Cloning and expression in Escherichia coli and
    Bacillus subtilis of the hemolysin determinant from
    Bacillus cereus. J. Bact., 155, 681-689

Kuhn, M., S. Kathariou, and W. Goebel (1987) Hemolysin supports
    survival but not entry in mammalian cells of the intracellular
    bacterium Listeria monocytogenes. Inf. and Immun. (submitted)

Ludwig, A., M. Vogel, and W. Goebel (1987) Mutations affecting
    activity and transport of haemolysin in Escherichia coli.
    Molec. Gen. Genet., 206, 238-245

Marre, R., J. Hacker, W. Henkel, and W. Goebel (1987) Influence
    of cloned Escherichia coli hemolysin genes, S-fimbriae and
    serum resistance on pathogenicity in different animal models.
    Microbial Pathogenesis, 1, 533-547

Otnaess, A.B., C. Little, K. Sletten, R. Wallin, S. Johnsen,
    R. Flengsrud, and H. Prydz (1977) Some characterisitcs of
    phospholipase C from Bacillus cereus. Eur. J. Biochem.,
    79, 459-468

The authors like to thank Dr. Hof for experimental help and many
fruitful discussions and E. Appel for editorial assistance. This
work   was   supported   by   grants   from   the   Deutsche
Forschungsgemeinschaft (SFB 105 - A12 and SFB 165 - B4).

Fehrenbach et al. (Eds.), Bacterial Protein Toxins, Zbl. Bakt. Suppl. 17
© Gustav Fischer, Stuttgart, New York, 1988

Intracellular Life Style of Shigella Flexneri

P. J. Sansonetti, B. Baudry, P. Clerc, A. T. Maurelli, X. Nassif, A. Ryter

Service des Entérobactéries, Unité INSERM 199, Institut Pasteur, 28, rue du Dr Roux, F-75724 Paris Cédex 15

ABSTRACT

A major step in the virulence of Shigella flexneri is the capacity of this enteric pathogen to invade cells of the human colonic mucosa. Most of the attributes necessary are encoded by a 220 kbases plasmid. Sequences have been detected which are required for the bacterium to direct its own phagocytosis. This process involves polymerization of actin and accumulation of myosin at the site of entry. Transmembrane signalling is currently unknown. In a further step bacteria are allowed to grow intracellularly through their plasmid encoded capacity to lyse the membrane of the phagocytic vacuole. Finally, Shigella flexneri performs early and efficient killing of host-cells through shut-off of cellular respiration and fermentation. This mechanism appears independent of the production of Shiga-like toxin.

KEYWORDS

Shigella flexneri, entry into cells, intracellular multiplication, cell-killing.

INTRODUCTION

The primary step in the pathogenesis of bacillary dysentery is invasion of the human colonic mucosa (La Brec and co-workers, 1964). The invasive process encompasses complex fetures which include penetration into epithelial cells, intracellular multiplication, spreading to adjacent cells and to the conjunc-tive tissue of the intestinal villus (Formal, Hale and Sansonetti, 1983). This sequence of events leads to a strong inflammatory reaction which causes ulcera-tions and abscesses but may also prevent systemic dissemination of the pathogen. Therefore, the overall invasive process can be considered as the integration of two steps : one of invasion of individual epithelial cells and one of tissue invasion. The former requires the ability of the bacterium to induce its own phagocytosis by cells which are non professional phagocytes. It can be approximated in vitro by infecting monolayers of mammalian cells such as Henle intestinal or HeLa cells. The second step of tissue invasion requires survival of the bacteria within tissues, elicitation of the inflammatory reaction and tissue destruction. It can be studied in more definitive assays such as the Sereny test (Sereny, 1957), and the rabbit ligated ileal loop (Formal and co-workers, 1961).

LOCATION OF GENETIC SEQUENCES NECESSARY FOR INVASIVENESS IN SHIGELLA FLEXNERI.

Plasmids of 140 Mdal are consistently found in S. flexneri (Sansonetti, Kopecko and Formal, 1982). These plasmids are associated with the invasive phenotype, they are largely homologous and certainly derived from a common ancestor. pWR100, the virulence plasmid of S. flexneri serotype 5 has been further studied.

Homology between E. coli and Shigella is so high that they cannot be differentiated on the basis of polynucleotide hybridization. Therefore, conjugal mating between these genera allowed construction of hybrid strains by a stepwise transfer of previously identified virulence-associated genes from S. flexneri 2a Hfr to a rough, avirulent, E. coli K12 recipient (Sansonetti and co-workers, 1983). This process showed that the 140 Mdal plasmid pWR100 was sufficient to confer the ability to invade HeLa cells. In addition, Shigella chromosomal genes are necessary for expression of a full virulence phenotype when hybrids are tested in more definitive assays. These chromosomal segments include the his+ region (45 min), which had already been linked to the expression of the somatic antigen (Formal and co-workers, 1970). A region designated kcp+ which is linked to purE (12 min) had already been shown to be necessary for a positive Sereny test (Formal and co-workers, 1971). Finally, a poorly defined region limited by mtl+ (80 min) and arg+ (87 min) had been shown to be required for survival of strains in the intestinal mucosa (Formal and co-workers, 1965). It must be included in E. coli hybrids which eventually invade the rabbit ileal loop with tissue destruction, elicit a positive Sereny test and cause fluid accumulation.

PHENOTYPIC EXPRESSION OF THE CHROMOSOMAL AND EXTRACHROMOSOMAL VIRULENT LOCI.

Role of plasmid pWR100.

pWR100 encodes functions that are essential for invasion of mammalian cells including entry into cells, intracellular multiplication and killing of host cells.

Recent evidences indicate that S. flexneri penetrates into cells via directed phagocytosis (P. Clerc, P.J. Sansonetti, submitted for publication). This was suggested by the observation that F-actin as well as myosin accumulated underneath the cell membrane at the site of entry. Plasmid DNA sequences involved in entry of S. flexneri into HeLa cells have been cloned in the cosmid vector pJB8 (Maurelli and co-workers, 1985). The cloned inserts which restored invasiveness shared a common sequence of 37 kbases. Expression of one of these recombinant plasmid, pHS4108, has been studied in minicells. It encodes 12 polypeptides which are resolved by two-dimensional electrophoresis (B. Baudry et al.,submitted for publication). Among these, Western blot analysis using the serum of a monkey convalescent from shigellosis revealed that four polypeptides were recognized in the parental virulent strains M90T as well (Maurelli and co-workers, 1985). The same serum recognizes four equivalent polypeptides in all Shigella species and in enteroinvasive E. coli. These four polypeptides are the only protein antigens that are regularly recognized during natural infection in human beings (Hale, Oaks and Formal, 1985). Molecular weights of these polypeptides vary between 78 and 35 Kdal. Their genes are organized in an operon (Baudry et al., submitted for publication). Although their precise role in the entry process is as yet unclear, they may turn out to be essential components of a future Shigella vaccine.

Involvement of pWR100 in intracellular multiplication.
Plasmid associated genes are also needed for efficient intracellular multiplication (Sansonetti and co-workers, 1986). pWR100 endows E. coli K12 with the same replication potential as the wild type S. flexneri M90T. On the other hand, the cosmid recombinant molecule pHS4108 which codes for penetration into cells does not confer on recipient strains the same ability to multiply intracellularly. Upon transfer of this plasmid in BS176, a plasmidless avirulent derivative of M90T, transformants invaded HeLa cells but replicated poorly intracellularly. Intracellular growth was as poor as Salmonella typhimurium C5. Such experiments also demonstrated a lack of correlation between intracellular multiplication and production of Shiga-toxin. A sequential electron microscopic study performed on HeLa cells respectively infected with the four strains already mentioned demonstrated that M90T induced early lysis of the phagocytic membrane after penetration within cells. By 30 min after centrifugation induced penetration, all bacteria were lying freely within the cytoplasm of the cells. Similar observations could be made with E. coli K12 carrying pWR100. On the other hand, BS176 (pHS4108) and S. typhimurium C5 demonstrated late and unefficient ability to lyse the phagocytic membrane. These electron microscopic observations established a clear correlation between plasmid-mediated intracellular multiplication and ability to perform early lysis of the membrane surrounding the phagocytic vacuole. Demonstration of a plasmid mediated contact hemolytic activity produced by virulent shigellae provides a likely candidate for lysis of the phagosome.

Involvement of plasmid pWR100 in early killing of host cells.
Using the continuous macrophage cell-line J774 to study the intracellular fate of both an invasive and a non invasive, plasmidless derivative of S. flexneri M90T, plasmid pWR100 appeared to mediate a very efficient and rapid killing activity on host cells. Expression of this activity required bacteria to be intracellular since macrophages were protected by cytochalasin D. A battery of strains differing in their levels of Shiga-like toxin production demonstrated that inhibition of protein synthesis was not required for early killing. Damage to macrophages rather correlated with the ability of invasive bacteria to rapidly and efficiently lyse the membrane of the phagocytic vacuole (Clerc and co-workers, 1987). Metabolic events mediating early killing have recently been demonstrated to involve rapid drop in intracellular ATP concentration increase in pyruvate concentration and arrest in lactate production (Sansonetti and Mounier, in press). The role of the release of bacteria within the cytosol for subsequent expression of such cytotoxic activity is likely.

Phenotypic expression of chromosomal loci.
Most shigellae seem to encode the O-antigenic determinants at a chromosomal locus closely linked to the histidine genes at 45 min on the map. S. flexneri contains an additional locus next to the proline genes, at 6 min, encoding the type specific antigen (Formal and co-workers, 1970). Expression of a smooth LPS is not necessary for invasion of cells (Formal, Hale and Sansonetti, 1983 ; Okamura and Nakaya, 1977) but rather for intraluminal survival of bacteria and protection against bactericidal activity of the serum within tissues.

Another critical factor for bacterial virulence is the availability of iron which is essential for bacterial growth. The level of free iron is severely restricted in tissues due to the fact that most of ferric ions are chelated both in the intracellular and extracellular compartments. Extracellular iron is attached to high-affinity iron-binding proteins : lactoferrin or transferrin. Pathogenic bacteria multiply in such hostile conditions if they produce siderophores which may scavenge iron from binding proteins.

S. flexneri produces the hydroxamate type siderophore aerobactin (Payne and co-workers, 1983). Recent studies with the E. coli K 12-S. flexneri hybrids showed that one of the chromosomal segments located between mtl+ and arg+ which allowed bacteria to multiply successfully within the mucosa of the rabbit ileal loop contained the genes necessary for synthesis of aerobactin as well as of the ferric-aerobactin outer membrane receptor (Griffiths and co-workers, 1985). In a recent series of experiments (Nassif and co-workers, in press), we have demonstrated that an iuc::Tn10 mutant of S. flexneri M90T which no longer produced hydroxamate was neither impaired in its capacity to grow within the lumen of rabbit ligated intestinal loops nor limited in its capacity to grow intracellularly and kill cells. It was thus concluded that aerobactin production acted as a virulence factor for invasive bacteria at the stage of multiplication within tissues when lying within the extracellular compartment of the intestinal villus.

Finally, when constructing E. coli K12-S. flexneri hybrids, extension of the sequence to LDC- allowed production of fluid within the intestinal loop, thus suggesting that genes encoding or regulating Shiga-toxin production had been transferred (9). It is as yet unclear whether Shiga-toxin production endows bacteria with a higher virulence potential in term of tissue destruction or just codes for enterotoxicity. Production of a tox-mutant is necessary to resolve this critical problem.

REFERENCES

Clerc, P.L., A. Ryter, J. Mounier, and P.J. Sansonetti (1987). Plasmid-mediated early killing of eukaryotic cells by Shigella flexneri as studied by infection of J774 macrophages. Infect. Immun., 55, 521-527.

Formal, S.B., D. Kundel, H. Schneider, N. Kunev and H. Sprinz (1961). Studies with Vibrio cholerae in the ligated loop of the rabbit intestine. Br. J. Exp. Pathol., 42, 504-510.

Formal, S.B., E.H. La Brec, T.H. Kent, and S. Falkow (1965). Abortive intestinal infection with an Escherichia coli-Shigella flexneri hybrid strain. J. Bacteriol., 89, 1374-1382.

Formal, S.B., P. Gemski Jr., L.S. Baron, and E.H. La Brec (1970). Genetic transfer of Shigella flexneri antigens to Escherichia coli K12. Infect. Immun., 1, 279-287.

Formal, S.B., P. Gemski Jr., L.S. Baron, and E.H. La Brec (1971). A chromosomal locus which controls the ability of Shigella flexneri to evoke keratoconjunctivitis. Infect. Immun., 3, 73-79.

Formal, S.B., T.L. Hale, and P.J. Sansonetti (1983). Invasive enteric pathogens. Rev. Infect. Dis., 5, 5702-5707.

Griffiths, E., P. Stevenson, T.L. Hale, and S.B. Formal (1985). Synthesis of aerobactin and a 76,000 dalton iron-regulated outer membrane protein by Escherichia coli K12-Shigella flexneri hybrids. Infect. Immun., 49, 67-71.

Hale, T.L., E.V. Oaks, and S.B. Formal (1985). Identification and antigenic characterization of virulence-associated, plasmid-coded proteins of Shigella spp. and enteroinvasive Escherichia coli. Infect. Immun., 50, 620-629.

La Brec, E.H., H. Schneider, T.J. Magnani, and S.B. Formal (1964). Epithelial cell penetration as an essential step in the pathogenesis of bacillary dysentery. J. Bacteriol., 88, 1503-1518.

Maurelli, A.T., B. Baudry, H. d'Hauteville, T.L. Hale, and P.J. Sansonetti (1985). Cloning of plasmid DNA sequences involved in invasion of HeLa cells by Shigella flexneri. Infect. Immun., 49, 164-171.

Okamura, N., and R. Nakaya (1977). Rough mutant of Shigella flexneri 2a that penetrates culture cells but does not evoke keratoconjunctivitis in guinea-pigs. Infect. Immun., 17, 4-8.

Payne, S.M., D.W. Niesel, S.S. Peixotto, and K.M. Lawlor (1983). Expression of hydroxamate and phenolate siderophores by Shigella flexneri. J. Bacteriol., 155, 949-955.

Sansonetti, P.J., D.J. Kopecko, and S.B. Formal (1982). Involvement of a plasmid in the invasive ability of Shigella flexneri. Infect. Immun., 35, 852-860.

Sansonetti, P.J., T.L. Hale, G.I. Dammin, C. Kapper, H.H. Collins, and S.B. Formal (1983). Alterations in the pathogenicity of Escherichia coli K12 after transfer of plasmids and chromosomal genes from Shigella flexneri. Infect. Immun., 39, 1392-1402.

Sansonetti, P.J., A. Ryter, P. Clerc, A.T. Maurelli, and J. Mounier (1986). Multiplication of Shigella flexneri within HeLa cells : lysis of the phagocytic vacuole and plasmid-mediated contact hemolysis. Infect. Immun., 51, 461-469.

Sereny, B. (1957). Experimental keratoconjunctivitis shigellosa. Acta Microbiol. Acad. Sci. Hung., 4, 367-376.

Fehrenbach et al. (Eds.), Bacterial Protein Toxins, Zbl. Bakt. Suppl. 17
© Gustav Fischer, Stuttgart, New York, 1988

Genetic Analysis of the Role of Toxins and Protein A in the Pathogenesis of Staphylococcus aureus Infections Properties of an Unexpressed Alpha-Toxin Locus from a Clinical Isolate

T. J. Foster[1], M. O'Reilly[1], A. H. Patel[1], P. Nowlan[2] and J. Bramley[3]

[1]Microbiology Department, Moyne Institute, and [2]Wellcome Research Animal Laboratories, Trinity College, Dublin 2, Ireland
[3]Institute for Animal Diseases Research, Compton, Nr. Newbury, Berkshire, U.K.

ABSTRACT

Site-specific mutations in chromosomal genes coding for α-toxin, β-toxin and protein A have been isolated by allele replacement and lysogenic conversion. α-toxin-deficient mutants were less virulent than the wild-type strain after subcutaneous, intraperitoneal and intramammary inoculation of mice. Evidence is presented that protein A contributes to S. aureus virulence in mice to a small but significant degree.

Clinical isolates that do not express α-toxin but which have a defective copy of the α-toxin gene (hly[o]) are frequently isolated from cases of Toxic Shock Syndrome and septicaemia. Combining restriction fragments from cloned hly[o] and hly[+] genes suggests that the genetic basis for the lack of α-toxin production is a mutation(s) located within the hly coding sequence.

KEY WORDS

Allele-replacement mutations, α-toxin, β-toxin, protein A, virulence, silent α-toxin gene.

INTRODUCTION

S. aureus causes a variety of infections in man, including furuncles, endocarditis, osteomyelitis and septicaemia. It is also the major cause of mastitis, the economically important disease of dairy cattle. The organism produces an array of extracellular and cell-bound proteins which may be of importance in infection. These include cytolytic toxins (α-, β-, δ-, γ-toxins, leucocidin), coagulase, protein A, and surface proteins which probably aid colonization of tissues by binding, for example, to fibronectin and collagen.

One approach to studying the role of individual factors in pathogenesis is genetic analysis. Mutants defective in a factor are isolated and tested in experimental infections. Any loss of virulence implicates the missing component as a virulence factor. This approach has been used to study the role of α-toxin, coagulase and protein A in the pathogenesis of S. aureus infections of mice

(Jonsson and others 1985). However, the mutants were isolated following chemical mutagenesis and may have mutations affecting other virulence factors. It is preferable to use mutants which are known to have a single (preferably site-specific) mutation affecting the gene of interest. In this paper we describe the isolation and properties of site-specific mutations in genes coding for α-toxin, β-toxin and protein A by recombinational allele-replacement and by phage integration. Preliminary virulence data from infections of mice is reported.

The α-toxin is considered to be a major virulence factor in S. aureus infections. Paradoxically, there are several reports of recent clinical isolates not expressing this toxin, for example, many of the isolates from cases of Toxic Shock Syndrome (Carlson, 1986; Clyne, de Azavedo and Arbuthnott 1987) and septicaemic patients (Christensson and Hedstrom, 1987). The genetic basis for the failure to express α-toxin is being investigated.

RESULTS

Mutations of S. aureus Defective in α-toxin and Protein A

In a previous paper we described the use of recombinational allele replacement to generate site-specific mutations in the gene coding for α-toxin (hly) of S. aureus 8325-4 (O'Reilly and others 1986). This involved inactivation of the cloned hly gene by insertion of a fragment of plasmid pE194 with an erythromycin resistance (Em^r) marker. The hly$^+$ gene in the chromosome of S. aureus was replaced by the hly::Em^r allele by recombination with a shuttle plasmid carrying the mutant allele. The Hly$^-$ Em^r recombinants were detected after elimanation of the shuttle plasmid by an incompatible tetracycline resistance plasmid.

A similar procedure was used to isolate a substitution mutation in the protein A gene (spa). A 1.2 kb BclI fragment carrying sequences which code for the 5 IgG binding domains of Spa were deleted and replaced by a BglII fragment from a S. aureus conjugative plasmid carrying resistance to ethidium bromide and quaternary ammonium compounds (Patel and others, 1987). A double mutant lacking both α-toxin and protein A was constructed by transducing the hly::Em^r mutation into S. aureus Δspa::Eb^r.

Inactivation of β-toxin.

Expression of β-toxin can be conveniently inactivated by lysogenization with a phage (42E was used here) which probably has its attachment site in the structural gene for the toxin (hlb; Coleman and others, 1986). This is certainly the mechanism of inactivation of lipase by lysogenization with phage 54a (Lee and Iandolo, 1986) where sequencing studies showed that the att site is in the coding sequence for the protein.

Characterization of the hly^o Gene of S. aureus Todd 555.

S. aureus strain Todd 555 was isolated from a case of Toxic ShockSyndrome. It does not produce α-toxin or β-toxin (Clyne, de Azavedo and Arbuthnott, 1987) and is haemolytic on agar plates only when grown in an atmosphere of 20% CO_2, primarily due to production of γ-toxin (Clyne, de Azavedo and Arbuthnott, 1987). Southern blot hybridization of Todd 555 genomic DNA with an intragenic hly gene probe showed extensive DNA homology with the wild-type hly gene. Furthermore, 5 restriction sites spanning the wild-type gene were conserved (Fig. 1). Similar results were obtained in experiments with other Hly$^-$ isolates. The hly^o gene was cloned in plasmid pBR322 in E. coli and transferred back to S. aureus 8325-4 hly::Em^r on a shuttle plasmid. No haemolysis was seen around colonies on blood agar and no immunoreactive protein was detected by immunoblotting. This suggests that the defect in Todd 555 is not associated with a trans-acting regulatory element such as agr (Recsei and others, 1986). This is supported by the fact that a wild type hly$^+$ gene is expressed in Todd 555 when introduced on a shuttle plasmid.

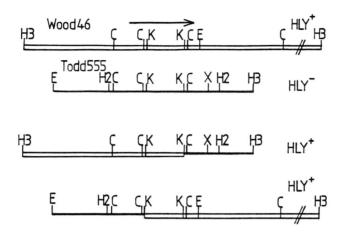

Fig. 1. Restriction maps of hly^+ and hly^o determinants. Structure of hybrid hly genes.
    The upper two diagrams show maps of the hly^+ determinant of strain Wood 46 and the hly^o locus of Todd 555. Hybrid hly determinants are shown below. The arrow shows the position and direction of transcription of the hly gene. Restriction sites are abbreviated as follows: C, ClaI; H3, HindIII; K, KpnI; H2, HincII; X, XbaI.

In addition, no expression could be detected during growth of strain Todd 555 in diffusion chambers implanted in the peritoneal cavity of mice, showing that expression of the gene is not induced by in vivo growth conditions.
    Northern blotting demonstrated that the level of mRNA hybridizing to an hly gene probe was drastically reduced. This could be due to a mutation in the promoter or to mRNA degradation caused by premature termination of translation. The former explanation is less likely because placing strong promoters upstream from the putative coding sequence in hly^o did not stimulate α-toxin production in E. coli or S. aureus.
    The Todd 555 hly^o gene and the hly^+ gene from Wood 46 were cleaved with restriction enzymes and spliced together to form hybrid hly genes (Fig. 1.) These "mix-and-match" experiments suggest that the defect in the Todd 555 hly gene is in the central KpnI fragment which is contained within the coding sequence for the toxin. This will be tested directly by DNA sequencing and by replacing the Wood 46 KpnI fragment with that from Todd 555 and vice versa. Presumably the mutation is one that results in premature translational termination (ie nonsense or frameshift).

Virulence of Mutants Defective in α-toxin and Protein A.
Sha Sha mice were injected subcutaneously with Hly^+ Spa^+, Hly^- Spa^+, Hly^+ Spa^- and Hly^- Spa^- derivatives of strain 8325-4. Strains that produced α-toxin caused a raised, cream coloured oedaematous lesion with a outer reddened area. In contrast, Hly^- strains caused a lesion with a sunken, blackened centre. In mice injected with Hly^+ bacteria neutrophil infiltration was confined to the periphery of the lesion whereas mice infected with Hly^- mutants had lesions with large numbers of neutrophils in close contact with bacteria. Many of these neutrophils were necrotic. The α-toxin-producing strains were at least 10-fold more virulent

than those which lacked the toxin in terms of the number of bacteria required to generate a lesion of equivalent area (Table 1).

Experimental mastitis and peritonitis also showed that α-toxin is an important virulence factor for S. aureus infections of mice. At least four fold more Hly⁻ bacteria were required to kill mice compared to the otherwise isogenic Hly⁺ strains when injected intraperitoneally (Table 2). Also 12/20 mice injected in a mammary gland with Hly⁺ bacteria died within 48h, whereas 20/20 survived infection with the isogenic Hly⁻ strain.

TABLE 1 Subcutaneous Lesions in Sha Sha Mice Caused by
S. aureus mutants.

Inoculum cfu	Mean lesion size (mm^2)			
	Hly^+ Spa^+	Hly^+ Spa^-	Hly^- Spa^+	Hly^- Spa^-
2×10^9			a. 170 b. 183	34^s 103^{ns}
5×10^8			b. 64	53^{ns}
2×10^8	a. 866 b. 843	272^s 219^s	29	0
5×10^7	b. 372	85^s		
2×10^7	a. 63	8^s		
1×10^7	a. 10	0		

a. Mean area of lesions on 6 mice
b. Mean area of lesions on 9 mice
s. Statistically significant according to the Mann-Whitney U-test (p = 5%)
ns. not significant (p = 5%)

TABLE 2 Survival of Laca Mice Inoculated Intraperitoneally
with S. aureus mutants.

Inoculum (cfu)	Number of animals killed			
	Hly^+ Spa^+	Hly^+ Spa^-	Hly^- Spa^+	Hly^- Spa^-
2×10^9			6/6	6/6
1×10^9			4/6	5/6
5×10^8	6/6	5/6	0/6	0/6
2.5×10^8	4/6	0/6		
1.2×10^8	1/6	0/6		

These experiments have also produced some data which suggests that protein A contributes to S. aureus virulence in mouse infections. Spa$^+$ strains generally formed larger skin lesions than the Spa$^-$ counterpart. However, in some comparisons between Hly$^-$Spa$^+$ and Hly$^-$Spa$^-$ strains the differences were not significant at p = 5%. (Table 1).

The data in Table 2 does not show any difference in virulence between Spa$^+$ and Spa$^-$ strains. However, differences were observed when the time of death was measured. Pools of 12 mice were injected intraperitoneally with 5 x 10^8 bacteria (Hly$^+$Spa$^+$ and Hly$^+$Spa$^-$ strains) or 2 x 10^9 bacteria (Hly$^-$Spa$^+$ and Hly$^-$Spa$^-$ strains) and the time of death was measured at four hourly intervals. When compared by the Mann-Whitney U test the Spa$^+$ strains were shown to kill mice significantly more quickly (p = 5%) than the otherwise isogenic Spa$^-$ strain, suggesting that protein A contributes to the virulence of S. aureus.

Role of β-toxin in Pathogenesis.
Preliminary experiments with a β-toxin-deficient mutant (Hlb$^-$) of strain 8325-4 suggested that expression of β-toxin contributes to the ability of the organism to grow in the mammary gland of lactating mice. The number of Hlb$^+$ cells recovered from glands inoculated with about 2 x 10^4 bacteria was 10-fold higher than the Hlb$^-$ strain. There was no difference in the rate of growth of these strains in vitro. These tests were performed with strains that were deficient in α-toxin.

In order to determine if β-toxin is a virulence factor in peritonitis caused by S. aureus in mice, groups of 12 animals were injected intraperitoneally with mutants and the time of death was observed. No differences were found when the death times for the following pairs of strains were analyzed by the Mann-Whitney U test (Hly$^-$Spa$^+$Hlb$^+$ and Hly$^-$Spa$^+$Hlb$^-$; Hly$^+$Spa$^+$Hlb$^+$ and Hly$^+$Spa$^+$Hlb$^-$; Hly$^+$Spa$^-$Hlb$^+$ and Hly$^+$Spa$^-$Hlb$^-$; Hly$^-$Spa$^-$Hlb$^+$ and Hly$^-$Spa$^-$Hlb$^-$). Thus, there is no evidence that β-toxin is a virulence factor in peritonitis caused by S. aureus in mice.

DISCUSSION

We have isolated site-specific mutations in genes coding for virulence factors of S. aureus. These mutations are characterized by having a selectable drug resistance marker at the insertion site which aids in strain construction (eg constructing mutants with two or more lesions by transduction) and also facilitates chromosome mapping (Pattee, 1986). We intend to extend this genetic analysis of virulence to include coagulase and γ-toxin, both of which have been cloned in this laboratory (Phonimdaeng and others, 1987: Cooney, Arbuthnott and Foster, 1987).

So far our studies have been mainly confined to the laboratory strain NCTC8325-4. We intend to study the effect of mutations on the virulence of a bovine mastitis strain. We are currently isolating the Hly$^-$ and Spa$^-$ mutations in one such strain and will test their ability to cause mastitis.

We have demonstrated convincingly that α-toxin is an important virulence factor for S. aureus infections of mice. This is not surprising because α-toxin is the most potent exotoxin of S. aureus and has been strongly implicated as a virulence factor by other studies (eg Adlam and others, 1977). The results with protein A-deficient mutants suggest a role for this factor in experimental infections of mice. In most comparisons the Spa$^+$ strains were more virulent than the Spa$^-$ counterpart. However, a degree of caution must be exercised because differences were not always observed (Table 1).

Our finding that Spa$^-$ mutants have lower virulence is contrary to a previous report that Spa$^-$ mutants of strain SA113 were indistinguishable from the parental strain in the mouse mastitis model (Jonsson and others, 1985). This could be explained by the use of different bacterial strains (which have some differences in expression of extracellular proteins) or by the use of different animal models for virulence. It will be interesting to determine if our Spa⁻ mutants are any less virulent than the Spa⁺ counterpart in causing mouse mastitis.

β-toxin does not seem to have a major role in S. aureus infections of mice. Hlb⁻ mutants were as virulent as Hlb⁺ strains in intraperitoneal tests. However, Hlb⁺ strains grew to a higher titre in the mouse mammary gland which suggests a role in promoting growth in vivo. Perhaps β-toxin has a more significant role to play in the pathogenesis of bovine mastitis.

The precise mature of the mutation(s) that inactivated the α-toxin gene of strain Todd 555 awaits DNA sequence analysis. Genetic experiments suggest that a functional promoter is located 5' to the hly° gene. Thus, failure to initiate transcription is unlikely to be the cause of the lack of toxin synthesis. Construction of hybrid hly°-hly⁺ genes in vitro suggests that the defect is located within the coding sequence. A nonsense or frameshift mutation could lead to degradation of untranslated mRNA and this could explain the drastic reduction in mRNA in Northern blotting experiments.

ACKNOWLEDGEMENT

This research was supported in part by the Wellcome Trust and by the Biotechnology Action Programme of the Commission of the European Communities (contract number BAP-0131-IRL).

REFERENCES

Adlam, C., P.D. Ward, A.C. McCartney, J.P. Arbuthnott, and C.M. Thorley (1977). Effect of immunizing with highly purified alpha and beta toxins on Staphylococcal mastitis in rabbits. Infect. Immun., **17**, 250-256.

Carlson, E. (1986). A CO_2 enhanced hemolytic activity of Staphylococcus aureus associated with toxic shock shydrome: inhibition by agar. J. Infect. Dis., **154**, 186-188.

Christensson, B., and S.A. Hedstrom (1986). Biochemical and biological properties of Staphylococcus aureus septicemia strains in relation to clinical characteristics. Scand. J. Infect. Dis., **18**, 297-303.

Clyne, M., J. de Azavedo and J.P. Arbuthnott (1987). Production of gamma haemolysin by Toxic Shock Syndrome associated strains of Staphylococcus aureus. J. Clin. Microbiol., (manuscript submitted).

Coleman, D.C., J.P. Arbuthnott, H.M. Pomeroy, and T.J. Birbeck (1986). Cloning and expression in Escherichia coli and Staphylococcus aureus of the beta-lysin determinant from Staphylococcus aureus: evidence that bacteriophage conversion of beta-lysin activity is caused by insertional inactivation of the beta-lysin determinant. Microb. Pathog., **1**, 549-564.

Cooney, J., J.P. Arbuthnott and T.J. Foster. In: proceedings of the 3rd European Workshop - Bacterial Protein Toxins (1988) This volume

Jonsson. P., M. Lindberg, I. Haraldsson, and T. Wadstrom (1985). Virulence of Staphylococcus aureus in a mouse mastitis model; studies with alpha haemolysin, coagulase and protein A as possible virulence determinants with protoplast fusion and gene cloning. Infect. Immun., **49**, 765-769.

Lee, C.Y., and J. Iandolo (1986). Integration of staphylococcal phage L54a occurs by site-specific recombination; structural analysis of the attachment sites. Proc. Natl. Acad. Sci. USA., **83**, 5474-5478.

O' Reilly, M., J.C.S. de Azavedo. S. Kennedy, and T.J. Foster (1986). Inactivation of the alpha-haemolysin gene of Staphylococcus aureus by site-directed mutagenesis and studies on expression of its haemolysins. Microb. Pathog., **1**, 125-138.

Patel, A.H., P.Nowlan, E.D.Weavers, and T.J.Foster (1987). Studies on the virulence of protein A-deficient and α-toxin-deficient mutants of Staphylococcus aureus isolated by allele replacement. Infect. Immun., (manuscript submitted).

Pattee, P.A. (1986). Chromosome map location of the alpha-hemolysin structural gene in Staphylococcus aureus NCTC8325. Infect. Immun., 54, 593-596.

Phonimdaeng P., M.O'Reilly, P.W.O'Toole and T.J.Foster (1987). Molecular cloning and expression of the coagulase gene of Staphylococcus aureus. J. Gen. Microbiol. (submitted).

Recsei, P., B.Kreiswirth, M.O'Reilly, P.Schlievert, A.Gruss, and R.P.Novick (1986). Regulation of exoprotein gene expression in Staphylococcus aureus by agr. Mol. Gen. Genet., 202, 58-61.

Fehrenbach et al. (Eds.), Bacterial Protein Toxins, Zbl. Bakt. Suppl. 17
© Gustav Fischer, Stuttgart, New York, 1988

Role of CAMP-Factor (Protein B) for Virulence

F. J. Fehrenbach[1], D. Jürgens[1], J. Rühlmann[1], B. Sterzik[1] and M. Özel[2]

[1]Dept. of Microbiology and [2]Dept. of Virology-Electronmicroscopy, Robert Koch-Institut des Bundesgesundheitsamtes, Nordufer 20, D-1000 Berlin 65

ABSTRACT

This paper summarizes the present knowledge on the main physico-chemical properties of protein B (CAMP-factor), the more general concept of the CAMP-reaction and "CAMP like hemolysis" and the very recent findings on the unspecific binding of protein B to the Fc region of different immunoglobulin classes from various species. Evidence for the role of protein B in group B streptococcal pathogenicity is provided. In addition, preliminary data on the existence of functional domaines for Fc- and lipid-binding sites of protein B based on the characterization of CNBr-peptides are presented.

KEYWORDS: CAMP-factor; protein B; group B streptococci; hemolysis; mechanism; pathogenicity; immunoglobulin Fc-binding; CNBr-peptides; peptide arrangement; functional domaines.

INTRODUCTION

Protein B (CAMP-factor) was first described in 1944 by Christie, Atkins and Munch-Petersen (1) as an extracellular product of group B streptococci. The authors reported on the hemolysis of sheep red blood cells which was obviously caused by the synergistic activity of S. aureus sphingomyelinase and the "CAMP-factor". Meanwhile, a number of similar "CAMP-like" reactions have been described (1-6); see TABLE 1. However, the protein B induced lysis of target cells in vitro which has been studied in detail (7-9) remained rather an epiphenomenon and was not considered to be of relevance in vivo.

RESULTS AND DISCUSSION

Protein B is released from growing cultures of group B streptococci (GBS) during mid to late logarithmic growth phase into the medium and the production of protein B is enhanced in the presence of CO_2. Protein B is a polypeptide and can be purified from the culture supernatant to homogeneity as shown by Jürgens (10). It is isolated together with 4 satellite proteins which are very similar in their physico-chemical properties. Some properties of protein B from GBS type II b (NCTC 8181) are summarized in TABLE 2.

TABLE 1: "CAMP"- and CAMP-like Lytic Reactions

cocytolysin	co-factor	target cells	Lit.:
CAMP-factor (S. agalactiae)	sphingomyelinase (S. aureus)	SRBC	(1)
CAMP-factor (S. agalactiae)	phospholipase-C (Cl. perfringens)	HRBC; MRBC; RRBC	(2)
Streptolysin O "oxidized" (S. pyogenes)	phospholipase-C (Cl. perfringens)	HRBC; MRBC	Sterzik,B.,Jürgens,D., Fehrenbach, F.J. (unpublished)
"CAMP-like factor" (Aeromonas spec.)	sphingomyelinase (S. aureus)	SRBC	(3)
lipase (P. acnes)	phospholipase-C (Cl. perfringens)	HRBC; SRBC	(4)
cholesterol oxidase	phospholipase-C	SRBC	(5)
cholesterol oxidase (Brevibacterium)	phospholipase-D (C. ovis)	SRBC	(6)

Mechanism of lysis

It was widely accepted in the past that co-hemolysis was due to the reaction of protein B (CAMP-factor) with either ceramide generated in the target cell membrane by sphingomyelinase treatment or with a membrane constituent normally not accessible but exposed after enzyme treatment (8). However, it became clear from the work of our laboratory (2) that this view had to be improved in favour of a more general concept of co-hemolysis.

TABLE 2: Physico-chemical and Biological Properties of Protein B (CAMP-factor)

		Lit:
nature of protein B:	polypeptide (monomer)	
mol. wt.:	25.000	(2;10)
pI:	9.1	
heat inactivation (100° C):	$\hat{=}$ 100 % after 5 min < 60 % after 5 min in the presence of 0.1 % SDS	
binding of:	an-) ionic detergents cat-) (charge shift)	(10)
co-hemolysis of:	SRBC; RRBC; HRBC (and RBC of other species)	(2)
antigenic:	inactivated by AB	
unspecific binding of immunoglobulins:	IgG) at the Fc-part IgM)	(11)

Our data revealed (2) that protein B induced co-hemolysis proceeds not only in target cells rich in sphingomyelin (or ceramide) but in a variety of other red blood cell species after treatment with either sphingomyelinases or phospholipases. We have therefore suggested that sphingomyelinases and/or phospholipases create a metastable lipid phase by removing the zwitterionic residue from phospho- or sphingolipids of the outer leaflet of the membrane bilayer (2).

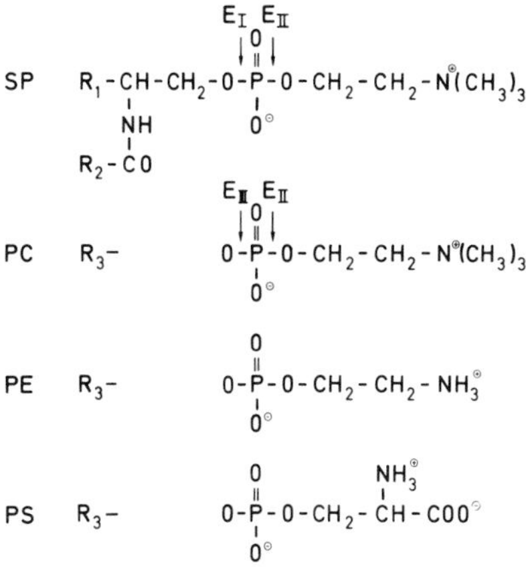

$$SP \quad R_1-CH-CH_2-O-\overset{\overset{\displaystyle E_I \; E_{II}}{\overset{\displaystyle O}{\underset{\displaystyle \|}{\;}}}}{\underset{\displaystyle O^\ominus}{P}}-O-CH_2-CH_2-\overset{\oplus}{N}(CH_3)_3$$
$$\underset{\displaystyle R_2-CO}{\overset{\displaystyle NH}{|}}$$

$$PC \quad R_3- \qquad O-\overset{\overset{\displaystyle E_I \; E_{II}}{\overset{\displaystyle O}{\underset{\displaystyle \|}{\;}}}}{\underset{\displaystyle O^\ominus}{P}}-O-CH_2-CH_2-\overset{\oplus}{N}(CH_3)_3$$

$$PE \quad R_3- \qquad O-\overset{\displaystyle O}{\underset{\displaystyle O^\ominus}{\overset{\displaystyle \|}{P}}}-O-CH_2-CH_2-\overset{\oplus}{N}H_3$$

$$PS \quad R_3- \qquad O-\overset{\displaystyle O}{\underset{\displaystyle O^\ominus}{\overset{\displaystyle \|}{P}}}-O-CH_2-\overset{\overset{\displaystyle \oplus}{\overset{\displaystyle NH_3}{|}}}{CH}-COO^\ominus$$

Fig. 1: Phospho- and sphingolipids involved in the CAMP- and "CAMP-like" hemolysis. Type of substrate (sphingomyelin = SP; phosphorylcholine = PC; phosphorylethanolamine = PE; phosphatidylserine = PS) and site of cleavage by sphingomyelinases (E_I) and phospholipases-D (E_{II}) and -C (E_{III}). R_1 and R_2 saturated and unsaturated long chain fatty acids. R_3 = 1,2-diacyl-sn-glycerol.

Removal of phosphorylcholine and the concomitant release of diglycerides in the target cell membrane results in a change of membrane fluidity and physically in a rounding up of the cells. Protein B then interacts with the metastable lipid phase and probably induces "phase separation" which may result in the destruction of the bilayer. The type of membrane lesion caused by protein B is shown in Fig. 2.
While the true hemolysins contribute to bacterial pathogenicity the CAMP-factor induced lysis which is only observed in vitro was not considered to be of relevance in GBS infections in vivo although protein B inactivating antibodies were found earlier in human and animal sera (11).

Unspecific binding of immunoglobulins by protein B

Very recent work from our laboratory (12) has shown that protein B inactivating antibodies exist that react in a non-immune reaction with protein B. Moreover, monoclonal antibodies lacking any determinant specificity were found to bind also to protein B. Further studies into the mechanism of non-specific binding of immunoglobulins (Ig) to protein B showed that IgG and IgM antibodies of various mammalian species such as human, mouse, rabbit and bovine were capable of binding thereby inactivating the co-hemolytic activity.

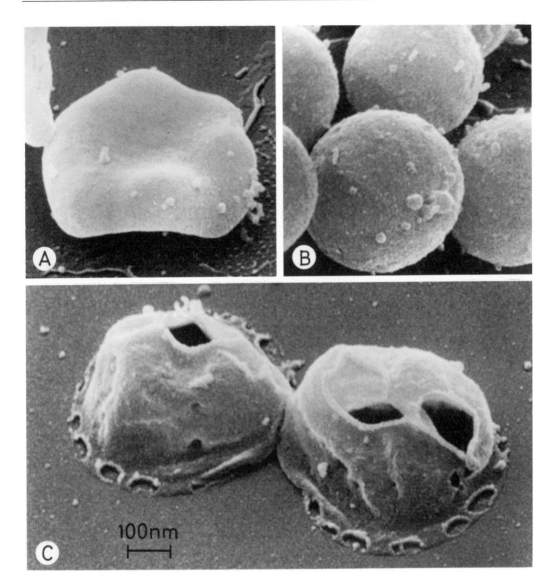

Fig. 2: Scanning electron microscopy of target cells (SRBC) at different stages in the CAMP-reaction. SRBC control (A); After sphingomyelinase treatment SRBC show a spherical morphology (B); Lysis of sphingomyelinase treated SRBC by protein B (CAMP-factor) leads to lesions in the cell-membrane (C). Magnification: x 15.000.

TABLE 3: Inhibition of Co-hemolysis by Mono- and Polyclonal Antibodies

antibody (class)	source	inhibition of co-hemolysis
IgG (polyclonal)	human	yes
IgG₁ (monoclonal)	mouse	yes
IgM (polyclonal)	mouse	yes
IgM (monoclonal)	human	yes

The non-immune binding of protein B to Ig's suggested that it may bind in a "protein A-like" way. Since the binding of protein B to immunoglobulins can be detected by inactivation of the co-hemolytic activity it was possible to locate the binding site at the Ig-molecule more precisely using protein A (PA) as a competitor for the Fc-binding site (12). Interestingly, protein B/Ig complex formation was blocked by PA when PA and IgG or IgM were incubated prior to the addition of protein B. Together with the results from gel exclusion chromatography using Fc-fragments for binding of ^{125}I-protein B these data suggested that protein B binds to the Fc-part of immunoglobulins (12). Moreover, we have shown by using an anti-streptolysin O antibody that the anti-SLO/protein B complex retained the capacity to inactivate streptolysin O. Thus, the experiments indicated the binding of protein B to the Fc-part of either IgG or IgM classes leaving the Fab sites of the Ig's active. PA competes with protein B for the Fc-binding site. The inactivation of co-hemolysis, therefore, is due to the binding of protein B (CAMP-factor) to the Fc-site of Ig's.

Protein B in pathogenicity

Although there was no evidence from the literature that protein B was involved in pathogenicity the unspecific binding of protein B to immunoglobulins suggested to us its possible role in GBS infections.

When tissue sections of mice infected with GBS were stained with either FITC- or peroxidase-labelled protein B antibodies, clusters of protein B producing cocci were seen, however, differing in their intensity of staining. Peroxidase positive material was found not only at the surface of GBS but also halo-shaped around the cocci.

It is suggested from bacterial counts in GBS-infected neonates with early and late onset septicemia where up to 10^5 cfu/ml of blood were found in the circulation that considerable amounts of protein B would not only temporarily be exposed on the bacterial cell surface but also shedded into the circulation. Protein B released in systemic infections could thus effectively impair the host immune response and possibly promote spread of infection.

To evaluate this hypothesis we established a model for GBS infections in mice using three different GBS strains (type I a, I b and II b). We were able to demonstrate that mice infected i.p. with sublethal doses of either of the GBS strains and that received seven repeated injections of pure protein B (a total of 900 µg; strain II b) during the first nine hours of infection developed fatal septicemia within 24 hours. Colony counts in these animals were usually 10^8 cfu/ml in the blood. Animals treated in the same way with either PBS or trypsinized protein B recovered. Protein B itself was not pathogenic for mice (12).

Arrangement and functions of CNBr-fragments of protein B

The five polypeptides which remained closely associated during purification by hydrophobic interaction chromatography (10) share also common antigenic properties as shown by immuno-blotting with a rabbit anti protein B antibody. Moreover, CNBr-cleavage of protein B and the four satellite proteins resulted in the formation of a 10- and 15 kDa fragment (Fig. 3).

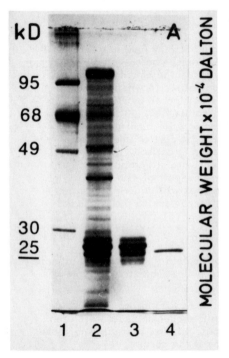

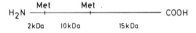

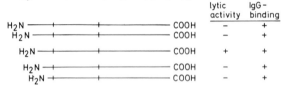

ARRANGEMENT OF THE CNBr - FRAGMENTS OF PROTEIN B **B**

STRUCTURAL RELATIONSHIP BETWEEN PROTEIN B AND THE SATELLITE PROTEINS

Fig. 3A: Characterization of protein B and the satellite proteins by analytical SDS-PAGE (T = 12 %; C = 2,6 %). Slots 1 - 4 represent: marker proteins (1); culture supernatant of strain NCTC 8181, type II b (2); protein B + satellite proteins (3) and purified protein B (4).

Fig. 3B: Arrangement of the CNBr-fragments of protein B. Structural and functional relationship between the satellite proteins and protein B. Protein B remains the only one which is lytically active although all peptides share common antigenic properties and exhibit non-immune binding of IgG or IgM.

Additionally, smaller fragments of about 2 kDa representing the heterogenic N-terminal sequence of protein B and the satellite proteins were found (see J. Rühlmann, poster abstract in this book). The arrangement of the CNBr-fragments is shown in Fig.3B.

It was found that all the 15 kDa-fragments derived from the four satellite proteins and protein B exhibited Fc-binding properties. With the exception of protein B neither the satellite proteins nor their CNBr-fragments were active in co-hemolysis (Fig. 3B). It is obvious from Fig. 2 that the satellite proteins and protein B represent a considerable amount of the extracellular proteins released during streptococcal growth and infection. Although heterogenic molecular species they share common biological properties (Fc/Ig-binding) which may be important for streptococcal pathogenicity.

REFERENCES

1. Christie, R., N.E.Atkins, and E.Munch-Petersen (1944). A note on a lytic phenomenon shown by group B streptococci. Austr.J.Exp.Biol.Med.Sci. 22, 197-200

2. Fehrenbach, F.J., C.M.Schmidt, B.Sterzik, and D.Jürgens (1984). Interaction of amphiphilic bacterial polypeptides with artificial membranes. In: J.E.Alouf, F.J.Fehrenbach, J.H.Freer, J.Jeljaszewicz (Eds.), Bacterial Protein Toxins, Academic Press. Inc., Ltd., London/U.K., pp. 317-324

3. Figura, N., and P.Guglielmetti (1987). Differentiation of mobile and mesophilic Aeromonas strains into species by testing for a CAMP-like factor. J.Clin.Microbiol, 25, 1341-1342

4. Kar Choudhury, T.K. (1978). Synergistic lysis of erythrocytes by Propionibacterium acnes. J.Clin.Microbiol., 8, 238-241

5. Patzer, E.J., R.R.Wagner, and Y.Barenholz (1978). Cholesterol oxidase as a probe for studying membrane organisation. Nature, 274, 394-395

6. Linder, R., and A.W.Bernheimer (1982). Enzymatic oxidation of membrane cholesterol in relation to lysis of sheep erythrocytes by corynebacterial enzymes. Arch. Biochem.Biophys., 213, 395-404

7. Doery, H.M., B.J.Magnusson, J.M.Cheyne, and J.Gulasekharam (1963). A phospholipase in staphylococcal toxin which hydrolyses sphingomyelin. Nature, 198, 1091-1092

8. Bernheimer, A.W., R.Linder, and L.S.Avigad (1979). Nature and mechanism of action of the CAMP protein of group B streptococci. Infect.Immun., 23, 838-844

9. Sterzik, B., and F.J.Fehrenbach (1985). Reaction components influencing CAMP-factor induced lysis. J.Gen.Microbiol., 131, 817-820

10. Jürgens, D., F.Y.Y.I.Shalaby, and F.J.Fehrenbach (1985). Purification and characterization of CAMP-factor from S. agalactiae by hydrophobic interaction chromatography and chromatofocusing. J.Chromatogr., 348, 363-370

11. Brown, J., R.Farnsworth, L.W.Wannamaker, and D.W.Johnson (1974). CAMP-factor of group B streptococci: Production, assay and neutralization by sera from unimmunized rabbits and experimentally infected cows. Infect.Immun., 9, 377-383

12. Jürgens, D., B.Sterzik, and F.J.Fehrenbach (1987). Unspecific binding of group B streptococcal cocytolysin (CAMP-factor) to immunoglobulins and its possible role in pathogenicity. J.Exp.Med., 165, 720-732

Fehrenbach et al. (Eds.), Bacterial Protein Toxins, Zbl. Bakt. Suppl. 17
© Gustav Fischer, Stuttgart, New York, 1988

Bacterial Toxins and Enzymes Showing Biological Activity towards Phagocytic Cells: an Overview

C. G. Gemmell

Department of Bacteriology, University of Glasgow, Royal Infirmary, Glasgow G4 OSF, Scotland

ABSTRACT

The host's inflammatory response to invasion by a bacterial pathogen forms the first line of defence against infection. Any breaches in this response, consisting as it does of a number of related and sequential activities of the reticuloendothelial system (RES), is likely to result in infection and pathological damage. Key factors in the pathogen – RES interaction include the biological activity of various exotoxins. Each stage of phagocytic cell function (chemotaxis, ingestion, killing and release of inflammatory mediators) can be influenced by a number of bacterial toxins. As well as providing new information about bacterial pathogenicity, their study provides more understanding of phagocytic cell function.

KEY WORDS

phagocytic cells; chemotaxis; chemiluminescence; ingestion and killing; mediators of inflammation; bacterial toxins

INTRODUCTION

The virulence potential of pathogenic bacteria is varied; some possess only one or more structural components which are associated with colonization of body surfaces or resistance to host defense mechanisms whereas others can elaborate one or more soluble exoproducts with specific or non-specific toxicological properties. The characteristics of the infections caused by this spectrum of pathogens is influenced by their virulence factor armamentarium. Only by studying how each virulence factor interacts with the host can one reach any understanding of the underlying molecular mechanism of action. This review will be restricted to those bacterial exoproducts which have been shown to interact with the primary line of host defence, namely the reticuloendothelial system (RES). I shall concentrate on this aspect of non-specific immunity since the interaction of bacterial toxins with the cells associated with specific immunity was well-reviewed by Alouf (1986). However in order to understand how bacterial toxins and enzymes interact with the RES (and in particular the polymorphonuclear leukocytes) it is necessary to provide some background to the basic physiology of the cells involved.

The nature of the inflammatory response to infection is now well-understood with the recognition that the process comprises cell release from the bone marrow, entry into the peripheral circulation, translocation from the blood vessels to the tissues (diapedesis), chemotaxis towards the focus of infection, opsonophagocytosis (opsonisation, attachment and ingestion), degranulation and killing by the polymorphonuclear leukocytes and monocytes and final eradication of the pathogen. Each of the latter steps will be described in some detail before specific examples of bacterial toxins which can interfere with the efficiency of the inflammatory response are given.

Chemotaxis

One of the earliest events accompanying the acute inflammatory response is an increase in the adherence of circulating PMN to the vascular endothelium close to the focus of infection. The cells leave the circulation and guided towards the bacteria by chemotaxis. Chemotaxis is defined as directed movement of cells in response to substances in the environment. Chemotaxis must be clearly distinguished from undirected, random motility in which movement occurs with equal probability in all directions. Chemotactic factors are released in the vicinity of the invading microorganisms and can be derived from the interaction between microorganisms and the host or from the microorganisms themselves. However, the principal mechanism by which microbes generate chemotactic stimuli for phagocytes is activation of the complement system by either the classical or alternative pathway. During activation, C3 and C5 are cleaved and among other fragments C3a and C5a are formed. These soluble chemotactic factors appear to interact with specific receptor sites on the PMN surface, and trigger a complex series of events involving serine esterase activation, fluxes of calcium, sodium and potassium ions, changes in surface charge and metabolic activation. The chemotactic signal is translated into movement of the cell.

Opsonization and attachment

Having arrived at the site of inflammation, phagocytes must recognize what to attack. Certain bacteria can be recognized and phagocytized without further modifications of the surface of the bacteria. However, recognition and phagocytosis can be greatly enhanced by coating the microorganisms with certain serum proteins (opsonization). Specific antibody of the IgG1 and IgG3 subclasses and the activated third component of the complement system (C3b) may act as opsonins. Activation of C3 can be promoted by specific antibody acting in concert with C1, C4 and C2 activation (classical pathway) or via the alternative complement pathway. On the surface of the phagocytic cell receptors are present for the Fc component of immunoglobulin and for the C3b molecule. These receptors interact with the opsonins on the surface of a microorganism to facilitate ingestion.

Ingestion

When particle-associated opsonins bind to receptor sites on the surface of the phagocyte, a series of changes is initiated in the cell which leads to particle ingestion. Cellular pseudopods surround the particle as a result of the sequential and circumferential interaction of receptors on the phagocyte surface with IgG or C3b ligands distributed diffusely over the particle surface. In this way, the phagocyte membrane moves around the particle until it is fully enclosed within a phagocytic vacuole.

Degranulation

Degranulation is the secretion of lysosomal enzymes into phagosomes. This process plays an important role in killing and digestion of phagocytosed microorganisms. The fusion of granules with the phagosomes takes place following the complete engulfment of the particles.

Respiratory burst

The respiratory or metabolic burst is a marked increase in metabolic activity taking place when phagocytes are exposed to appropriate stimuli. The respiratory burst occurs with perturbation of the plasma membrane and is independent of the process of ingestion. The metabolic burst consists of a sharp increase in oxygen consumption, superoxide (O_2^-) and hydrogen peroxide (H_2O_2) formation and hexose monophosphate shunt activity. This is accompanied by the emission of light (chemiluminescence). After perturbation of the plasma membrane of the phagocyte, a membrane-associated enzyme system, NADPH-oxidase, is activated. This system catalyzes the one-electron reduction of oxygen to O_2, using NADPH as electron donor. The O_2^- can either lose or accept an electron and thus can act either as reductant or as oxidant. When two O_2^- molecules interact, one is oxidized and the other is reduced: $O_2^- + O_2^- + 2H+ \rightarrow O_2 + H_2$). This spontaneous reduction can be catalyzed by the enzyme superoxide dismutase. Further reaction of H_2O_2 can result in formation of the highly reactive hydroxyl radical (OH^-).

NADP can be converted back to NADPH by the hexose monophosphate shunt. This is a metabolic pathway in which glucose is oxidized to carbon dioxide and a five-carbon sugar, with NADP serving as electron-acceptor. Because NADPH-oxidase is located in the plasma membrane, and the outside of the plasma membrane becomes the inside of the phagocytic vacuole, the products of the reaction are released in the extracellular fluid or in the phagocytic vacuole. O_2^- that escapes to the cytoplasm is reduced to H_2O_2 by superoxide dismutase and cytoplasmic H_2O_2 is detoxified by catalase and glutathione peroxidase-glutathione reductase systems.

Chemiluminescence by phagocytic cells is a consequence of the generation of oxygen-derived radicals by the metabolic burst and can be amplified by adding a compound (luminol or lucigenin) that emits intense light upon oxidation by oxygen species. Luminol-enhanced chemiluminescence only reflects the myeloperoxidase-mediated metabolic activity of the cell whereas other oxygen species involved in chemiluminescence reactions (O_2^-, H_2O_2, OH^- and $^1O_2$), can be trapped by lucigenin.

Anti-microbial systems

The mechanisms by which phagocytes kill microorganisms may be divided into two broad categories: oxygen-dependent and oxygen-independent systems.

Oxygen-dependent systems

Oxidative mechanisms of killing may be divided into those which are myeloperoxidase-mediated and those which are not. Myeloperoxidase is deposited by degranulation into the phagocytic vacuoles where, in the presence of H_2O_2 and halide ions, it catalyzes the oxidation of halide ions to hypohalide ions by H_2O_2. H_2O_2 is formed during the respiratory burst and chloride ions are present in the phagocytes at a level considerably above that required for participation in myeloperoxidase activity.

Oxygen-independent systems

Bactericidal systems that are independent of the respiratory burst include those based upon acid, lysozyme, lactoferrin and granular cationic proteins. The acidity of the vacuole itself may be bactericidal or bacteriostatic for many microorganisms. Acidification also appears to enhance the function of some antimicrobial enzyme systems (myeloperoxidase-H_2O_2-halide, lysozmye). Lysozyme, a cationic low molecular-weight enzyme, attacks the mucopeptide of cell walls of some bacterial species, resulting in lysis of the microorganisms. Lactoferrin, an iron-binding protein, inhibits the growth of microorganisms by binding the iron required as an essential nutrient for bacterial growth. Cationic proteins are proteins rich in arginine which rapidly affect the ability of bacteria to replicate without destroying their structural integrity. PMN contain also a variety of proteases and hydrolases. These enzymes serve a digestive rather than a microbicidal function.

TOXINS AND PHAGOCYTIC CELL FUNCTION

In the last few years an increasing number of bacterial exoproducts have been demonstrated to exert some antagonistic activity toward polymorphonuclear leukocyte function (Arbuthnott, 1981). Each aspect of phagocyte function (chemotaxis, phagocytosis and metabolic burst) has been analysed with variable results depending upon the exoproduct used. A summary of the products displaying biological activity is presented in Table 1 (for Gram-positive bacteria) and Table 2 (for Gram-negative bacteria).

Table 1   EXOPROTEINS WITH ACTIVITY AGAINST PHAGOCYTIC CELLS

PRODUCER BACTERIUM	TOXIN	BIOLOGICAL ACTIVITY MEASURED		
		CHEMOTAXIS	PHAGOCYTOSIS	OXYGEN METABOLISM
S. AUREUS	α-haemolysin	−	+	+
" "	δ-haemolysin	O	O	O
" "	leukocidin	O	−	O
S. PYOGENES	streptolysin O	−	−	+
" "	streptolysin S	O	O	O
CL. PERFRINGENS	δ-toxin	O	O	O
CL. DIFFICILE	toxin B	O	−	+
B. ANTHRACIS	protective antigen + oedema factor	n.t.	−	−
S. PNEUMONIAE	pneumolysin	−	−	+

+ = stimulation; O = no effect; − = inhibition

Table 2   EXOPROTEINS WITH ACTIVITY AGAINST PHAGOCYTIC CELLS

PRODUCER BACTERIUM	TOXIN	BIOLOGICAL ACTIVITY MEASURED		
		CHEMOTAXIS	PHAGOCYTOSIS	OXYGEN METABOLISM
E. COLI	α-haemolysin	−	−	+
" "	enterotoxin	0	−	0
B. PERTUSSIS	toxin (PT)	−	−	n.t.
Ps. AERUGINOSA	protease	−	0	+
PAST. HAEMOLYTICA	toxin A			
L. PNEUMOPHILA	P2	n.t.	0	−
" "	protease	−	−	−
V. CHOLERAE	enterotoxin	−	0	0

+ = stimulation;   0 = no effect;   − = inhibition

In the earliest studies, several products of staphylococci and streptococci were shown to alter leukocyte structure and function. For example streptolysins O and S induced degranulation of rabbit leukocytes following visible disturbance of subcellular organisation. In one case streptolysin S acted directly on the leukocyte and did not require intracellular absorption of the toxin to produce damage (Van Epps and Anderson, 1974; Anderson and Duncan, 1980). Similarly Staphylococcus aureus releases both α-haemolysin and leukocidin which can affect leukocyte function (Wilkinson, 1980; Woodin, 1970). The haemolysin at doses which were without effect on cell viability was able to inhibit PMN chemotaxis (Russell and others, 1976: Schmeling and others, 1981) enhance PMN aggregation and enhance phagocytic ingestion and killing of Staphylococcus aureus (Gemmell and others, 1982). In addition the toxin caused a dose-dependent stimulus to the respiratory burst of the PMN as soon as the toxin contacted the PMN membrane (Gemmell and others, 1983). Subsequently it has been shown that this toxin induces release of leukotrienes (Suthorp and others, 1987) from the intoxicated PMN and this may explain some of the effects on PMN function. Staphylococcal leukocidin, on the other hand, consists of two protein components, S and F, and induces cell membrane permeability changes in the PMN ultimately leading to its lysis. Enhanced protein secretion and calcium ion accumulation occurred concomitantly with increased ATPase activity and prostaglandin synthesis and release (Ofek, Bergner-Rabinowitz and Ginsberg, 1972). More recently studies with leukocidin have focussed upon its binding to the leukocyte membrane (Noda and others, 1981) and its effect on membrane associated enzymes (Noda and others, 1982).

By way of illustrating the diverse effects produced by a single bacterial pathogen in terms of its interaction with the polymorphonuclear leukocytes, Pseudomonas aeruginosa can both stimulate and repress phagocytic cell function. Originally described as a leukocidin (Scharmann, Jacob and Porstendörfer, 1976) and shown to inhibit phagocytic ingestion and killing, this exoproduct has been renamed as a cytotoxin (but distinct from toxin A) and shown depress PMN chemotaxis as well as phagocytic function (Baltch and others, 1985). Using electron microscopy it was shown that the toxin allowed a low molecular weight marker (ruthenium red) to enter the cell. However ultimately the toxin caused complete dstruction of the PMN. In addition two exoproteases (alkaline protease and elastase) strongly inhibited luminol-enhanced myeloperoxidase-mediated chemiluminescence (Kharazmi and others, 1984) but when these products were tested against the phagocytic activity of human leukocytes, there was a differential inhibition of uptake of Pseudomonas aeruginosa compared to Staphylococcus aureus. No effect was seen on the killing rate of either

organism (Kharazmi and others, 1984, 1986) suggesting that the proteases acted
through an effect on components of the leukocyte cell surface.

A new area of investigation of toxin interaction with the polymorphonuclear
leukocyte has been in terms of phospholipid metabolism. It is well established
that leukocytes upon stimulation generate free arachidonic acid from
phospholipids which is then metabolised to three groups of derivatives ie. the
prostaglandins, the thromboxanes and the leukotrienes which are formed by
oxygenation and further transformation. Several toxins including α-haemolysin
S. aureus and the thiol-activated toxins (streptolysin O alveolysin and
Clostridium perfringens theta toxin) have been shown to generate several
leukotrienes (Bremm and others 1984, 1985; Suttorp and others, 1987). In
particular leukotrienes C4 D4, E4 and B4 were demonstrated in the supernatents
of cells stimulated by sub-lytic doses of each toxin using high pressure liquid
chromatographic analysis. Although similar findings have not been demonstrated
with Streptococcus pneumoniae and its pneumolysin there is evidence that this
toxin also impairs phagocytic cell chemotaxis, respiratory burst and killing
activity (Johnson, Boese-Marrazzo and Pierce, 1981; Paton and Ferrante, 1983).
Stimulation of leukotriene synthesis is recognised as an important pathway
whereby leukocyte locomotion is controlled.
Therefore some of the key functions of the phagocytic cell may be altered by
this toxin-mediated leukotriene release.

CONCLUSIONS

In this review I have tried to place our knowledge of phagocytic cell function
in relation to our awareness that certain bacterial toxins can display a variety
of biological activities thereon. In many cases because we do not fully
understand the molecular basis for toxin action we can only surmise how it might
be acting upon phagocytic cell function. On the other hand for those toxins
that we do know something of their mode of action, the relative crudeness of
some of the phagocytic assays used leaves us in some doubt as to the importance
of the findings. Because of the diversity of findings reported I have only
selected one or two for detailed discussion and refer to the others in the
Tables. Nevertheless the addition of the phagocytic cell to the range of other
cell types (erythrocytes, platelets and tissue culture cells) used to monitor
bacterial toxin action in vitro will undoubtedly help our understanding of the
virulence of several bacterial pathogens. With the development of more
sophisticated methods to study each aspect of phagocytic cell physiology and
biochemistry it would be a useful excercise to compare and contrast the activity
of a range of bacterial exotoxins in this new model system.

References

Alouf, J.E. (1986). Interaction of bacterial protein toxins with host defense
mechanisms. IN: P. Falmagne, J.E. Alouf, F.J. Fehrenbach, J. Jeljaszewicz and
M. Thelestam (Eds.) Bacterial Protein Toxins Zent. fur Bakter. Mikrobiol. Hyg.
Suppl 15, p121-130.

Anderson, B.R. and Duncan, J.L. (1980) Activation of human neutrophil metabolism
by streptolysin O J. Infect. Dis. 142: 680-685.

Arbuthnott, J.P. (1981) Membrane-damaging toxins in relation to interference
with host defense mechanisms. In: F.O'Grady and H. Smith (Eds.), Microbial
perturbation of host defences. Acad. Press Inc. London pp 77-120.

Baltch, A.L., Hammer, M.C., Smith, R.P., Obrig, T.G., Conroy, J.V., Bishop, M.B., Egy, M.A. and Lutz, F. (1985) Effects of Pseudomonas aeruginosa cytotoxin on human serum and granulocytes and their microbicidal, phagocytic and chemotactic functions Infect. Immun. 48: 498–506.

Bremm, K.D., Brom, J., Alouf, J.E., Konig, W., Spur, B., Crea, A. and Peters, W. (1984) Generation of leukotrienes from human granulocytes by alveolysin from Bacillus alvei. Infect. Immun. 44: 188–193.

Bremm, K.D., Konig, W., Pfeiffer, P., Rauschen, I., Theobald, K., Thelestam, M. and Alouf, J.E. (1985) Effect of thiol-activated toxins (Streptolysin O, alveolysin and theta toxin) on the generation of leukotrienes and leukotriene-inducing and - metabolizing enzymes from human polymorphonuclear granulocytes. Infect. Immun. 50: 844–851.

Gemmell, C.G., Peterson, P.K., Landstrom L.A., and Quie, P.G. (1983) Stimulation of particle-induced chemiluminescence in human polymorphonuclear leukocytes by staphylococcal α-toxin. J. Infect. Dis. 147: 729–732.

Gemmell, C.G. Peterson, P.K., Schmeling, D.J. and Quie, P.G. (1982) Effect of staphylococcal α-toxin on phagocytosis of staphylococci by human polymorphonuclear leukocytes. Infect. Immun. 38: 975–980.

Johnson, M.K., Boese-Marrazzo, D. and Pierce, W.A. (1981) Effects of pneumolysin on human polymorphonuclear leukocytes and platelets. Infect. Immun. 34: 171–176.

Kharazmi, A., Doring, G., Hoiby, N. and Valerius, N.H. (1984) Interaction of Pseudomonas aeruginosa alkaline protease and elastase with human polymorphonuclear leukocytes in vitro. Infect. Immun. 43: 161–165.

Kharazmi, A., Eriksen, H.O., Doring, G., Goldstein, W. and Hoiby, N. (1986) Effect of Pseudomonas aeruginosa proteases on human leukocyte phagocytosis and bactericidal activity Acta path. Microbiol immunol. scand. Sect. C 94: 175–179.

Kharazmi, A., Hoiby, N., Doring, G. and Valerius, N.H. (1984) Pseudomonas aeruginosa exoproteases inhibit human neutrophil chemiluminescence. Infect. Immun. 44: 587–591.

Noda, M., Kato, I., Hirayama, T. and Matsuda, F. (1982) Mode of action of staphylococcal leukocidin: effects of the S and F components on the activities of membrane - associated enzymes of rabbit polymorphonuclear leukocytes Infect. Immun. 35: 38–45.

Noda, M., Kato, I., Matsuda, F. and Hirayama, T. (1981) The mode of action of staphylococcal leukocidin. I Relationship between the binding of 125 I-labelled S- and F components of leukocidin to rabbit polymorphonuclear leukocytes and the leukocidin activity. Infect. Immun. 34: 362–367.

Ofek, I., Bergner-Rabinowitz and Ginsburg, I. (1972) Oxygen-stable haemolysins of Group A streptococci V111. Leukotoxic and antiphagocytic effects of streptolysins S and O. Infect. Immun. 6: 459–464.

Paton, J.C. and Ferrante, A. (1983) Inhibition of human polymorphonuclear leukocyte respiratory burst, bactericidal activity and migration by pneumolysin. Infect. Immun. 41: 1212–1216.

Russell, R.J., Wilkinson, P.C., McInroy, R.J., McKay, S. McCartney, A.C and Arbuthnott, J.P. (1976) Effects of staphylococcal products on locomotion and chemotaxis of human blood neutrophils and monocytes. J. Med. Microbiol. 8: 443–449.

Scharmann, W., Jacob, F. and Porstendorfer (1976) The cytotoxic action of leukocidin from Pseudomonas aeruginosa on human polymorphonuclear leukocytes J. gen. Microbiol. 93:   303–308.

Schmeling, D.J., Gemmell, C.G., Craddock, P.R., Quie, P.G. and Peterson,   P.K. (1981) Effect of staphylococcal α-toxin on neutrophil migration and adhesiveness Inflammation 5:   313–321.

Suttorp, N., Seeger, W., Zucker-Reimann, J., Roka, L. and Bhakdi, S. (1987). Mechanism of leukotriene generation in polymorphonuclear leukocytes by staphylococcal alpha toxin. Infect. Immun. 55:   104–110.

Van Epps, D.E. and Andersen, B.R. (1974) Streptolysin O inhibition of neutrophil chemotaxis and motility: non-immune phenomenon with species specificity. Infect. Immun. 9:   27–33.

Wilkinson, P.C. (1980) Leukocyte locomotion and chemotaxis: effects of bacteria and viruses. Rev. Infect. Dis. 2:   293–317.

Woodin, A.M. (1970) Staphylococcal leukocidin In: S. J. Ajl, S. Kadis and T.C. Montie (Eds.),   Microbial Toxins Volume 3, Acad. Press. New York and London   pp 327–354.

Fehrenbach et al. (Eds.), Bacterial Protein Toxins, Zbl. Bakt. Suppl. 17
© Gustav Fischer, Stuttgart, New York, 1988

Vero Toxins (Shiga-Like Toxins) Produced by Escherichia Coli 0157:H7—Some Properties and Mode of Action

Y. Takeda, T. Yutsudo, H. Kurazono, M. Noda, T. Hirayama, C. Sasakawa, M. Yoshikawa, T. Takao[1], Y. Shimonishi[1]. K. Igarashi[2] and Y. Endo[3]

[1]The Institute of Medical Science, The University of Tokyo, Minato-ku, Tokyo 108
[2]Institute for Protein Research, Osaka University, Suita, Osaka 565
[3]Research Institute for Chemobiodynamics, Chiba University, Chiba 280
[4]Department of Biochemistry, Yamanashi Medical College, Yamanashi 409–38, Japan

ABSTRACT

It was found that the B subunit of VT1 has the same primary and disulfide bond structure as that of Shiga toxin and that the primary structure of the A subunit of VT1 and Shiga toxin is identical. Furthermore, nucleotide sequence of the gene encoding VT1 was determined.

VT2 was purified to its homogeneity. The purified VT2 showed a similar cytotoxicity to Vero cells to that of Shiga toxin. Lethal activity of VT2 is also similar to that of Shiga toxin. However, physico-chemical properties of VT2 were significantly different from those of Shiga toxin. Also VT2 and Shiga toxin were found to be immunologically unrelated.

Like Shiga toxin, VT1 and VT2 inhibited protein synthesis in rabbit reticulocyte lysates. These toxins inactivated 60S ribosomal subunits and inhibited EF-1 dependent aminoacyl-tRNA binding to ribosomes. Further study showed that VT2 and Shiga toxin released a fragment with 400-nucleotides from 28S ribosomal RNA of 60S ribosomal subunits after aniline treatment, which indicates RNA N-glycosidase activity of the toxins. The release of the fragment was parallel to the inhibition of protein synthesis and of EF-1 dependent aminoacyl-tRNA binding to ribosomes. Analysis of nucleotide sequence of the fragment indicated that an adenosine residue at position 4324 (A-4324) was absent in the 28S rRNA treated with the toxins. From these results, it was concluded that VT2 and Shiga toxin (and most probably VT1) show RNA N-glycosidase activity and cleave one N-glycoside bond at A-4324, thus preventing EF-1 dependent aminoacyl-tRNA binding to ribosomes and consequently inhibiting protein synthesis.

INTRODUCTION

Since the production of a cytotoxin to Vero cells by classical
enteropathogenic strains of Escherichia coli was first reported by
Konowalchuk and co-workers (1977), several investigators have
isolated a similar toxin from various serotypes, especially
O157:H7, of E. coli (Scotland and co-workers, 1980; O'Brien and
co-workers, 1982; Johnson and co-workers, 1983). O'Brien and co-
workers (1982) was the first to report that the cytotoxin to Vero
cells produced by some E. coli strains could be neutralized by
antibody against Shiga toxin produced by Shigella dysenteriae 1
and proposed to name this toxin as Shiga-like toxin. Recently,
Scotland and co-workers (1985) and Strockbine and co-workers
(1986) reported two immunologically distinct cytotoxins to Vero
cells from E. coli. One of these toxins is immunologically
identical to Shiga toxin, while the other is not (Scotland and co-
workers, 1985; Strockbine and co-workers, 1986; Noda and co-
worker, 1985; Yustudo and co-workers, 1987). Scotland and co-
workers (1985) named these toxins VT1 and VT2, respectively, while
Strockbine and co-workers (1986) named them Shiga-like toxin I and
Shiga-like toxin II respectively.

In this paper we report on the structural identity of VT1 and
Shiga toxin, on purification and some properties of VT2, and on
mode of action of VT1, VT2 and Shiga toxin.

STRUCTURAL IDENTITY OF VT1 AND SHIGA TOXIN

VT1 was purified from a strain of E. coli O157:H7 82-2035
(provided by Dr. H. Lior) isolated from a patient with hemorrhagic
colitis using the procedure described earlier (Noda and co-worker,
1987). The physico-chemical, biological and immunological properties of the purified VT1 were demonstrated to be identical to
that of Shiga toxin (Noda and co-workers, 1987). To compare the
structure of VT1 and Shiga toxin, the A and B subunits of VT1 and
Shiga toxin were isolated by HPLC on a reversed-phase $5C_{18}$ column,
and the isolated subunits were analyzed by Edman degradation of
their intact subunits and their tryptic or Achromobacter protease
I digests and by fast atom bombardment (FAB) mass spectrometry of
the digests (Takao and co-workers, 1987). It was shown that
primary structure of the B subunit of Shiga toxin was identical to
that reported by Seidah and co-workers (1986) and to that deduced
from the nucleotide sequence of the gene encoding the B subunit of
VT1 reported by Jackson and co-workers (1987). It also indicated
that the B subunit of VT1 has the same primary and disulfide bond
structure as that of Shiga toxin. The tryptic digests of the A
subunits of VT1 and Shiga toxin were analyzed directly by FAB mass
spectrometry. As shown in Fig. 1, the spectra of both A subunits
were quite identical indicating that the primary structure of the
A subunit of VT1 and Shiga toxin is identical. The fractions (TP-
3 and TP-3B) observed at m/z=3393.5 and 1709.6 in Fig. 1 did not
correlate with any sequences deduced from the nucleotide sequence
reported by Jackson and co-workers (1987). These fractions were
isolated from the tryptic digest and analyzed by Edman degradation.
As shown in Fig. 2, it was found that the amino acid residue at
position 45 is Thr instead of Ser as reported by Jackson and co-
workers (1987). This finding was compatible with the fact that

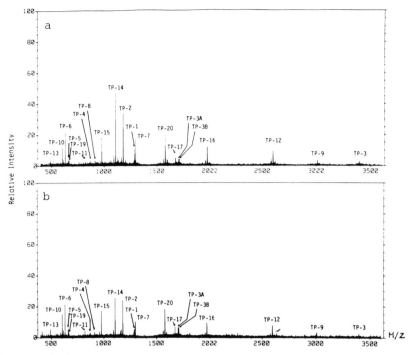

Fig. 1. Positive FAB mass spectra of the tryptic digests of the A
subunits of Shiga toxin and VT1. (a) Shiga toxin; (b) VT1.

the mass values of these sequences were 14 atomic mass units
larger than those deduced from the nucleotide sequence (Jackson
and co-workers, 1987). On Edman degradation, the A subunit of
Shiga toxin gave two main amino acid residues at each degradation
step up to about residue 25 from the N-terminus, suggesting that
the A subunit of Shiga toxin is composed of two peptide chains.
The FAB mass analysis of the tryptic digest of Shiga toxin showed
that the A subunit was nicked between Ala^{253} and ser^{254}: the A_1
fragment starting from the N-terminus ends at Ser^{247} and the A_2
fragment from Ser^{254} to the C-terminus, linked by a disulfide bond.

To analyze the nucleotide sequence of the gene encoding VT1, VT1-
converting phages were induced with UV from E. coli 0157:H7 strain
83-1386 and E. coli C600 was lysogenized with the VT1-converting
phage. EcoRI-fragments of the phage DNA from the lysogenized E.
coli C600 were ligated with EcoRI-digested pBR325 TC and it was
transformed into E. coli MC1061. Transformants with VT1 production commonly contained a 5.1Kb EcoRI-fragment. The restriction map of the EcoRI-fragment was prepared and it was found that
a 2.1Kb BamHI-BglII fragment coded VT1 production (Kurazono and
co-workers, 1987). The analysis of the nucleotide sequence of the
2.1Kb BamHI-BglII fragment showed that the sequence was identical

to that reported by Jackson and co-workers (1987) except one base
at position 364, which was T in our result instead of A as
reported by Jackson and co-workers (1987). This finding was
compatible with the fact that amino acid at position 45 from the
N-terminus of the A subunit was Thr.

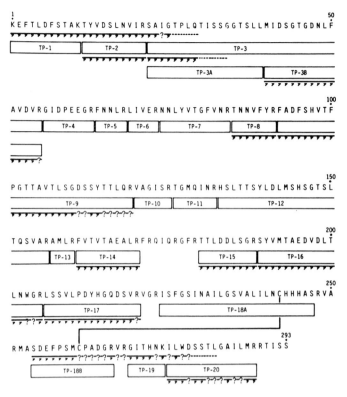

Fig. 2. Amino acid sequence of the A subunit of Shiga toxin. Arrows (⇁) indicate the amino acid residues identified by Edman degradation of the tryptic digests and boxes denote the sequences confirmed by FAB mass analysis.

PURIFICATION AND SOME PROPERTIES OF VT2

Although VT1 has been purified to its homogeneity (O'Brien and LaVeck, 1983; Noda and co-workers, 1987), little information is available on the purification and characterization of VT2. Thus, we attempted to purify and characterize VT2 from E. coli O157:H7. E. coli O157:H7, strain J-2 that was isolated from a patient with hemorrhagic colitis in Tokyo (Saku and co-workers, 1986), was cultured in a modified syncase medium at 37 C for 48 hours with vigorous shaking. Solid ammonium sulfate (561 g/1000 ml) was added at 4 C to the culture supernatant obtained by centrifugation of the cell culture at 13,000 x g for 20 minutes. The resulting precipitate was dissolved in about 1/15 volume of the original supernatant in 0.05M Tris-HCl buffer (pH 8.6) and dialyzed over-night against the same buffer. After removing the insoluble material by centrifugation, the sample was subjected to sequential chromatographies on DEAE-cellulose column, chromatofocusing column (twice) and TSK-gel G-2000 SW column for HPLC (twice) as described (Yutsudo and co-workers, 1987). In a typical purification procedure starting with 12 liters of culture supernatant, about 440 ug of the purified VT2 was obtained in a yield of about 22%. On

polyacrylamide gel disc electrophoresis, the purified VT2 gave a
single band staining for protein as shown in Fig. 3. The mobility
of VT2 was found to be quite different from that of VT1 and Shiga
toxin (Fig. 3), suggesting their molecular difference. On
polyacrylamide gel isoelectrofocusing, VT2, showed pI value of
4.1, while the pI value of VT1 and shiga toxin has been reported
to be 7.0 (Noda and co-workers, 1987). The amino acid composition
of VT2 showed significant difference from that of VT1 and Shiga
toxin. When the purified VT2 was subjected to SDS-polyacrylamide
slab gel electrophoresis, two bands staining for protein corresponding to the A and B subunits were observed. However, the two
subunits of VT2, especially the B subunit, migrated slower than
those of VT1 and Shiga toxin. The molecular weights of the A and
B subunits were estimated to be aobut 35,000 and 10,700,
respectively.

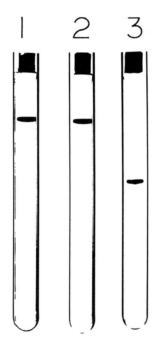

Fig. 3. Polyacrylamide disc gel electrophoresis of Shiga toxin,
VT1 and VT2. (1) Shiga toxin, (2) VT1, (3) VT2.

The purified VT2 showed similar cytotoxic activity as exhibited by
VT1 and Shiga toxin to Vero cells and killed about 50% of the Vero
cells in a well of a microtiter plate at 1 pg. The activity was
lost on heating the toxin at 80 C for 10 minutes, but not at 60 C
for 10 minutes. VT2 also showed lethal toxicity to mice when
injected intraperitoneally; the LD_{50} being 1 ng per mouse.

Figure 4 shows the result of Ouchterlony double gel diffusion test
of VT2 and Shiga toxin. It was found that anti-VT2 gave a precipitin line against VT2, but not against Shiga toxin, while anti-
Shiga toxin gave a precipitin line against Shiga toxin, but not
against VT2.

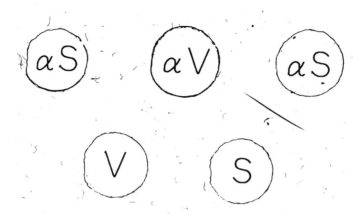

Fig. 4. Ouchterlony double gel diffusion test of Shiga toxin and VT2. S, Shiga toxin; V, VT2; S, anti-Shiga toxin; V, anti-VT2.

MODE OF ACTION OF VT1, VT2 AND SHIGA TOXIN

Shiga toxin inhibits protein synthesis (Brown and co-workers, 1986) and since VT2 and VT1 have similar biological activities as Shiga toxin we studied whether VT2 and VT1 show a similar mode of action as that of Shiga toxin. As shown in Fig. 5, VT2 inhibited polyU-dependent polyphenylalanine synthesis in the rabbit reticulocytes cell-free system, but not in the E. coli system. Slight inhibition of polyphenylalanine synthesis was observed in the wheat germ system. Globin synthesis in the rabbit reticulocyte system was also inhibited by VT2 (Fig. 5B) (Ogasawara and co-workers 1987). Almost the same results were obtained with VT and Shiga toxin (Igarashi and co-workers, 1987). The inhibition of protein syntheis by VT2 and VT1 was found to be due to inactivation of 60S rebosomal subunits of rabbit reticulocyte (Igarashi and co-workers, 1987; Ogasawara and co-workers, 1987). Furthermore, it was found that EF-1 dependent binding of phenylalanyl-tRNA to ribosomes was inhibited by VT2 (Ogasawara and co-workers, 1987). similar results were obtained with VT1 and Shiga toxin (Igarashi and co-workers, 1987).

Recently, it has been demonstrated some toxic lectins, such as ricin, abrin and modeccin inactivate 60S ribosomal subunits by hydrolyzing a single N-glycoside bond in the adenosine residue at position 4324 (A-4324) in 28S rRNA (Endo and co-corkers, 1987; Endo and Tsurugi, 1987). It was found, as in the case of ricin, when 28S rRNA obtained from VT1-, VT2-, and Shiga toxin-treated ribosomes was treated with aniline, the size of the 28S rRNA decreased with the concomitant appearance of a fragment of about 400 nucleotide in size. The phosphodiesterase bond of base-lacking residue is selectively cleaved by treatment with aniline at acidic pH (Peattie, 1979) and since exactly the same results have been observed with ricin and related lectins, it was concluded that they have RNA N-glycosidase activity (Endo and co-workers, 1987; Endo and Tsurugi, 1987). Thus, we conclude that VT2, VT1 and Shiga toxin also have a RNA N-glycosidase activity.

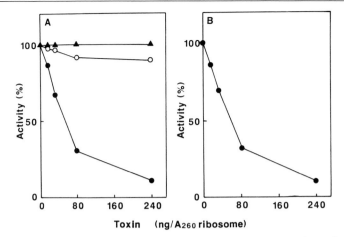

Fig. 5. Effect of VT2 on protein synthesis. (A) Polyplhenylalanine synthesis in cell-free system of E. coli (▲), wheat germ (o), and rabbit reticulocyte (o). (B) Globin synthesis in rabbit reticulocyte lysate.

To further support the notion that VT2 and Shiga toxin have an RNA N-glycosidase activity, determination of the nucleotide sequence of a fragment that migrated slightly slower than that of the untreated ribosomes on gel electrophoresis was carried out. This fragment was identified as a fragment of 3'terminus of 28S rRNA consisting of 553 nucleotides and it was found that the fragment is cleaved at the position of A-4324. Moreover, thin layer chromatography of the ethanol soluble fraction of the solution used for the toxin treatment of the ribosomes showed that VT2 and Shiga toxin released 0.87 and 0.81 mole of adenine per mole of the ribosomes, respectively.

REFERENCES

Brown, J. E., T. G. Obrig, M. A. Ussery, and T. P. Moran (1986). Shiga toxin from Shigella dysenteriae 1 inhibits protein synthesis in reticulocyte lysates by inactivation of aminoacyl-tRNA binding. Microb. Pathog., 1, 325-334.
Endo, Y., K. Mitsui, M. Motizuki, and K. Tsurugi (1987). The mechanism of action of ricin and related toxic lectins on eukaryotic ribosomes. The site and the characteristics of the modification in 28S ribosomal RNA caused by the toxins. J. Biol. Chem., 262, 5908-5912.
Endo, Y., and K. Tsurugi (1987). RNA N-glycosidase activity of ricin A-chain. Mechanism of action of the toxic lectin ricin on eukaryotic ribosomes. J. Biol. Chem., 262, 8128-8130.
Endo, Y., K. Tsurugi, T. Yutsudo, Y. Takeda, T. Ogasawara, and K. Igarashi (1987). The site of action of a Vero toxin (VT2) from Escherichia coli 0157:H7 and of Shiga toxin on eukaryotic ribosomes: RNA N-glycosidase activity of the toxins. submitted.
Igarashi, K., T. Ogasawara, K. Ito, T. Yutsudo, and Y. Takeda (1987). Inhibition of elongation factor 1-dependent aminoacyl-tRNA binding to ribosomes by Shiga-like toxin I (VT1) from Escherichia coli 0157:H7 and by Shiga toxin. FEMS Microb. Lett., in press.

Jackson, M. P., J. W. Newland, R. K. Holmes, and A. D. O'Brien (1987). Nucleotide sequence analysis of the structural genes for Shiga-like toxin I encoded by bacteriophage 933J from Escherichia coli. Microb. Pathog., 2, 147-153.

Johnson, W. M., H. Lior, and G. S. Bezanson (1983). Cytotoxic Escherichia coli O157:H7 associated with haemorrhagic colitis in Canada. Lancet, i, 76.

Konowalchuk, J., J. I. Speirs, and S. Staviric (1977). Vero response to a cytotoxin of Escherichia coli. Infect. Immun., 18, 775-779.

Kurazono, H., C. Sasakawa, M. Yoshikawa, and Y. Takeda (1987). Cloning of a Vero toxin (VT1, Shiga-like toxinI) gene from a VT1-converting phage isolated from Escherichia coli O157:H7. FEMS Microb. Lett., in press.

Noda, M., T. Yutsudo, N. Nakabayashi, T. Hirayama, and Y. Takeda (1987). Purification and some properties of Shiga-like toxin from Escherichia coli O157:H7 that is immunologically identical to Shiga toxin. Microb. Pathog., 2, 339-349.

O'Brien, A. D., and G. D. LaVeck (1983). Purification and characterization of a Shigella dysenteriae 1-like toxin produced by Escherichia coli. Infect. Immun., 40, 675-683.

O'Brien A. D., G. D. LaVeck, M. R. Thompson, and S. B. Formal (1982). Production of Shigella dysenteriae type 1-like cytotoxin by Escherichia coli. J. Infect. Dis., 146, 763-769.

Ogasawara, T., K. Ito, K. Igarashi, T. Yutsudo, N. Nakabayashi, and Y. Takeda (1987). Inhibition of protein synthesis by a Vero toxin (VT2 or Shiga-like toxin II) produced by Escherichia coli O157:H7 at the level of elongation factor 1-dependent aminoacyl-tRNA binding to ribosomes. submitted.

Peattie, D. A. (1979). Direct chemical method for sequencing RNA. Proc. Natl. Acad. Sci. USA, 76, 1760-1764.

Saku, K., K. Hikosaka, and M. Kashiwa (1986). Isolation of Escherichia coli O157:H7 and O157:H⁻ from patients with diarrhea (in Japanese). J. Jap. Assoc. Infect. Dis., 60, 640.

Scotland, S. M., N. P. Day, and B. Rowe (1980). Production of a cytotoxin affecting Vero cells by strains Escherichia coli belonging to traditional enteropathogenic serogroups. FEMS Microbiol. Lett., 7, 15-17.

Scotland, S. M., H. R. Smith, and B. Rowe (1985). Two distinct toxins active on Vero cells from Escherichia coli O157. Lancet, ii, 885-886.

Seidah N. G., A. Donohue-Rolfe, C. Lazure, F. Auclair, G. T. Keusch, and M. Chretien (1986). Complete amino acid sequence of Shigella toxin B-chain. J. Biol. Chem., 261, 13928-13931.

Strockbine, N. A., L. R. M. Marques, J. W. Newland, H. W. Smith, R. K. Holmes, and A. D. O'Brien (1986). Two toxin-converting phages from Escherichia coli O157:H7 strain 933 encode antigenically distinct toxins with similar biological activities. Infect. Immun., 53, 135-140.

Takao, T., T. Tanabe, H. Yeong-Man, T. Yutsudo, Y. Takeda, and Y. Shimonishi (1987). Primary structure of Shiga toxin of Shigella dysenteriae 1 and Shiga-like toxin I (VT1) of Escherichia coli O157:H7. submitted.

Yutsudo, T., Nakabayashi, T. Hirayama, and Y. Takeda (1987). Purification and some properties of a Vero toxin from Escherichia coli O157:H7 that is immunologically unrelated to Shiga toxin. Microb. Pathog., 3, 21-30.

Fehrenbach et al. (Eds.), Bacterial Protein Toxins, Zbl. Bakt. Suppl. 17
© Gustav Fischer, Stuttgart, New York, 1988

ADP-Ribosylation of Actin by Botulinum C2 Toxin

K. Aktories[1], M. Bärmann[2], K. H. Reuner[1], J. Vandekerckhove and B. Schering[1]

[1]Buchheim-Institut für Pharmakologie, [2]Institut für Pharmakologie und Toxikologie,
 Frankfurter Str. 107, D-6300 Gießen
[3]Laboratorium voor Genetika, Ledeganckstraat 35, B-9000 Gent

Keywords: Botulinum C2 toxin, ADP-ribosylation, actin, acceptor amino
acid.

Several microbial toxins such as diphtheria-, cholera- and pertussis
toxins interfere with eukaryotic cell functions by ADP-ribosylation
of regulatory proteins. Whereas diphtheria toxin modifies elongation
factor II, thereby inhibiting protein biosynthesis, pertussis- and
cholera-toxin affect GTP-binding proteins, which are involved in the
regulation of transmembrane signal transduction. Botulinum C2 toxin,
which is produced by certain strains of Clostridium botulinum Type C
and D, is another member of the family of ADP-ribosylating toxins. In
contrast to botulinum neurotoxins A to G, botulinum C2 toxin is unique
in function and structure. Botulinum C2 toxin is not neurotoxic but
increases intestinal secretion, vascular permeability and causes hypo-
tensive effects. Botulinum C2 toxin consists of two components C2I
and II with molecular weights of about 50 and 100 kDa, which are
neither linked by covalent nor non-covalent bonds. Thus, C2 toxin is
a real binary toxin: To elicit the toxic effects both components have
to act together. Whereas component II is apparently involved in the
binding of the toxin to the cell membrane of the eukaryotic cell,
component I possesses ADP-ribosyltransferase activity.

Recently it has been shown that actin is the substrate of botulinum
C2 toxin (Aktories and others, 1986). The toxin ADP-ribosylated non-
muscle actin in intact cells and isolated actin. Substrate of the
toxin was monomeric G-actin but not polymerized F-actin. Phalloidin,
which induced the polymerization of actin, blocked the ADP-ribosylation by C2 toxin. Isoforms (ß and γ) of non-muscle actin were ADP-
ribosylated by C2 toxin. The K_m value for NAD was 1 to 5 µM. Maximal
incorporation was about 0.5 mol ADP-ribose per mol actin. Actin was
apparently mono-ADP-ribosylated by the toxin. Treatment of ^{32}P-ADP
ribosylated actin with neutral hydroxylamine (0.5 M) for 60 min released about 22 % of the bound radioactivity. Tryptic digest of ^{32}P-
ADP-ribosylated actin produced two labelled peptides: an insoluble
peptide contained actin residues 148 - 183 and a soluble peptide residue 174 - 183. Digestion of these two peptides with thermolysin

generated the same radioactive peptide with residues 175 - 177. Amino acid sequence analysis determined Arg-177 as the ADP-ribosylated acceptor amino acid. Although Arg-177 is identical both in non-muscle and skeletal muscle actin, the latter actin species was only a very poor substrate of botulinum C2 toxin. It is possible that the exchange of Leu-176 in ß/γ-actin for Met in skeletal muscle actin renders the latter less susceptible to ADP-ribosylation by botulinum C2 toxin. ADP-ribosylation of isolated actin inhibited its ability to polymerize which was shown by viscometry and electron microscopy. These data may indicate that Arg-177 is located in an area which is involved in actin-actin binding. This view is supported by the finding that F-actin was protected from ADP-ribosylation by C2 toxin.

Treatment of chick embryo cells with botulinum C2 toxin induced rounding up of the cells, an effect which correlated with the ATP-ribosylation of actin in a time and concentration-dependent manner. The microfilament network stained by fluorescein-labelled phalloidin was destroyed by botulinum C2 toxin. Toxin treatment of intact cells decreased the amount of actin associated with the cytoskeleton, which was determined as Triton X-100 insoluble actin. On the other hand treatment of chick embryo cells with botulinum C2 toxin increased DNase-inhibiting activity of cell lysates in a concentration dependent manner indicating an increase in G-actin. The following model is proposed for the action of botulinum C2 toxin in intact cells: Botulinum C2 toxin disturbs the dynamic equilibrium between G and F-actin by ADP-ribosylation of G-actin. As ADP-ribosylated actin is unable to polymerize, the modified actin is trapped in its monomer form and accumulates. In order to restore the original equilibrium F-actin depolymerizes and thereby loses its cellular function.

REFERENCES

Aktories, K., M.Bärmann, I.Ohishi, S.Tsuyama, K.H.Jakobs and E.Habermann (1986). Botulinum C2 toxin ADP-ribosylates actin. Nature, 322, 390-392.

Fehrenbach et al. (Eds.), Bacterial Protein Toxins, Zbl. Bakt. Suppl. 17
© Gustav Fischer, Stuttgart, New York, 1988

Aeromonas Hydrophila Beta-Hemolysin

S. Bloch and H. Monteil

Laboratoire de Toxinologie Bactérienne, Institut de Bactériologie, 3, rue Koeberle, F-67000
Strasbourg

ABSTRACT

From our epidemiological study about Aeromonas hydrophila intestinal infections, the beta-hemolysin production is better correlated with the diarrhoeal
phenomenon than the enterotoxin production. In order to confirm that the beta-
hemolysin is the main virulence factor involved in the intestinal symptoms, we
have first purified this toxin from a clinical strain. Therefore some characteristics of this protein have been determined, especially its molecular
weight, isoelectric point and inactivation by various agents.

KEYWORDS

Aeromonas hydrophila, beta-hemolysin, purification, characterization, virulence
factor.

We carried out an epidemiological study for which we searched for Aeromonas
hydrophila in 7577 stool specimens (Brauer and co-workers, 1985). The 67 Aeromonas hydrophila strains were tested for their hemolytic activity upon rabbit
red blood cells and for their enterotoxic activity in rabbit ligated ileal
loops. The results revealed a statistically significant correlation between the
production of beta-hemolysin and the presence of diarrhoea but no correlation
between the presence of enterotoxin and the clinical symptoms. In order to
study the cellular and molecular effects of the beta-hemolysin which seems to
be involved in the intestinal troubles, we first purified this protein and
determined some of its physicochemical properties.

The strain used for this work was isolated in our laboratory from stool of a
patient who complained of diarrhoea and abdominal pains. The bacteria were
cultivated in a minimal synthetic medium supplemented with 1 % yeast extract
for 8 hours at 30°C with good aeration (beta-hemolysin excretion begins at the
end of the exponential growth phase - after 4 hours of culture - and increases
during the stationary phase). The culture supernatant had a hemolytic activity
but did not present any enterotoxic activity. After concentration by ultra-

filtration, the beta-hemolysin purification was performed according to the method of Asao and co-workers (1984), i.e. by acid precipitation after addition of a RNA solution followed by an anion exchange chromatography with a FPLC apparatus. The purified hemolysin was eluted between 0.22 and 0.25 M NaCl.

The molecular weight of the protein subunit estimated by SDS-PAGE analysis is 50,800 whereas native-PAGE in a gradient gel exhibits a proteic band at 149,000. This result will be confirmed by sedimentation equilibrium experiments. In isoelectric focusing, the protein separates at least into 2 bands, the main component being at pH 5.12. The beta-hemolysin is a protein containing neither lipids nor nucleic acids nor glucides. It is inactivated by heat and by proteolytic enzymes such as trypsin, chymotrypsin and pronase. This toxin possesses hemolytic and cytotoxic activities which are neutralized by anti-hemolysin antibodies. With regard to the immunological tests, we have compared our beta-hemolysin isolated from an European strain with an other one from a Japanese strain (Asao and co-workers, 1984). Both hemolysins are neutralized by the homologous and heterologous antisera and give a single precipitin line against the two antisera in the agar gel double-diffusion tests. These two toxins seem to have a complete immunological identity.

Although the culture supernatant had no effect in the rabbit ileal loop, the purified hemolysin gave a positive reaction when injected at a dose of 30 µg. We assume that the enterotoxic site of the molecule is exposed during the purification procedure. The three activities (hemolytic, cytotoxic and enterotoxic) seem to be carried by the same molecule which would be the main virulence factor responsible for diarrhoea.

REFERENCES

Asao, T., Y.Kinoshita, S.Kozaki, T.Uemura, and G.Sakaguchi (1984). Purification and some properties of Aeromonas hydrophila hemolysin. Infect. Immun., 46, 122-127.

Brauer, C., J.M.Scheftel, B.Rihn, and H.Monteil (1985). Isolement de Aeromonas hydrophila dans les diarrhées. Caractérisation des souches entérotoxinogènes et relations cliniques. Ann. Biol. Clin., 43, 725-731.

Fehrenbach et al. (Eds.), Bacterial Protein Toxins, Zbl. Bakt. Suppl. 17
© Gustav Fischer, Stuttgart, New York, 1988

A Sensitive, Microplate Assay for Pertussis Toxin Using Rabbit Neutrophils

F. F. Craig and R. Parton

Department of Microbiology, University of Glasgow, Glasgow G12 8QQ, Scotland

ABSTRACT

Nitroblue tetrazolium reduction (NBTR) is an indication of neutrophil superoxide production. Pre-incubation with pertussis toxin (PT) inhibited NBTR by rabbit neutrophils in response to N-formyl-methionyl-leucyl-phenylalanine (fMLP) but not to phorbol myristate acetate (PMA). Using a microplate assay for NBTR with fMLP as the stimulus, we detected $\geq$ 0.8 ng of PT per well by visual analysis and $\geq$ 0.4 ng by automated spectrophotometry. Pre-treatment with B.pertussis endotoxin or filamentous haemagglutinin did not affect NBTR by neutrophils stimulated with fMLP or PMA. The microplate NBTR assay is a fast, simple, sensitive technique which compares favourably with other in vitro assays for PT.

KEYWORDS

Bordetella pertussis, chemotactic peptide, neutrophil, pertussis, superoxide

INTRODUCTION

Pertussis toxin (PT) is a major virulence factor of Bordetella pertussis. The toxin is an A-B type toxin which ADP-ribosylates a membrane protein of M_r 39–41,000 kD in target cells (Tamura and others, 1982). Recent studies (Becker and others, 1986) found that pre-treatment with PT prevents neutrophil responses induced by certain chemotactic factors such as N-formyl-methionyl-leucyl-phenylalanine (fMLP). Nitroblue tetrazolium (NBT) can be reduced by neutrophil products, mainly superoxide, to a blue formazan derivative (Baehner and others, 1976). We have developed a microplate assay for NBT reduction (NBTR) using rabbit peritoneal neutrophils and phorbol myristate acetate (PMA) or fMLP as the neutrophil stimulus. The effects of pre-incubation with PT or other components of B.pertussis on the neutrophil response to these stimuli are described.

MATERIALS AND METHODS

Purified PT and endotoxin were obtained from LIST Biological Laboratories Ltd. Purified filamentous haemagglutinin (FHA) was provided by Dr. L.A.E. Ashworth (CAMR, Porton Down, Salisbury, U.K.). Other reagents were purchased from Sigma. Rabbit peritoneal neutrophils were elicited by glycogen, as described by Lackie (1977). The NBTR microplate assay involved the addition of neutrophils (0.05 ml of $2x10^7$ cells/ml) to 0.05 ml of serial dilutions of the test samples in microplate wells and subsequent incubation of the plate for 60 min at 37°C in a humidified box. The stimulus (0.05 ml of either 10^{-7} M fMLP or 10^{-6} M PMA) was then added and the plate left for a further 30 min before addition of 0.05 ml of 2.3 mM NBT. After a further 60 min the plate was examined visually for the yellow to blue colour change which occurs upon NBTR and also assayed spectrophotometrically using a Titertek Multiskan MC photometer (mode 1: filter 6). Test samples were compared to a control which contained buffer and NBT.

RESULTS AND DISCUSSION

Pre-incubation of neutrophils for 60 min with PT inhibited NBTR when fMLP but not PMA was used as the stimulus (Table); this agrees with other studies showing that PT inhibits neutrophil responses to fMLP but not to PMA (Becker and others, 1986). Inhibition of the neutrophil response to fMLP by PT was observed visually at doses $\geq$ 0.8 ng/well and spectrophotometrically at doses $\geq$ 0.4 ng/well. This compares favourably with other in vitro assays for PT (Sekura and others, 1985). A characteristic of PT is that its activity is destroyed by heating (80°C for 30 min) and we found that inhibitory activity was indeed abolished by such treatment. Other purified B.pertussis components, FHA and endotoxin, had no effect on NBTR by neutrophils induced by either fMLP or PMA. Inhibition of NBTR by PT was still detected in a semi-purified preparation of FHA (PT:FHA of 1:380, as determined by ELISA). Thus, neutrophil NBTR is a sensitive assay for PT and should be useful for monitoring PT activity in acellular vaccine preparations, during toxoiding procedures and possibly for measuring anti-PT antibodies.

Sample	Effect[1] on neutrophil response to:	
	fMLP	PMA
PT (unheated)	Inhibition at $\geq$ 0.4 ng*	None (up to 100 ng)
PT (80°C for 30 min)	None (at 100 ng)	Not done
FHA	None (up to 200 ng)	None (up to 200 ng)
PT/FHA (1:380) mixture[2]	Inhibition at $\geq$ 48 ng*	Not done
B.pertussis endotoxin	None (up to 2500 ng)	None (up to 2500 ng)

[1]The mean of $\geq$ 8 observations. [2]Prepared in our laboratory.
*Significantly different from control, by Student t-test.

ACKNOWLEDGEMENT

This work was financed by grant No. 16031/1.5 from the Wellcome Trust.

REFERENCES

Baehner, R.L., Boxer, L.A. and Davis, J. (1976). The biochemical basis of nitroblue tetrazolium reduction in normal human and chronic granulomatous disease polymorphonuclear leukocytes. Blood, 48, 309-313.
Becker, E.L., Kermode, J.C., Naccache, P.H., Yassin, R., Munoz, J.J., Marsh, M.L., Huang, C.-K., and Sha'afi, R.I. (1986). Pertussis toxin as a probe of neutrophil activation. Fed.Proc., 45, 2151-2155.
Lackie, J.M. (1977). The aggregation of rabbit polymorphonuclear leukocytes (PMN's): effects of agents which affect the acute inflammatory response and correlation with secretory activity. Inflammation, 2, 1-15.
Sekura, R.D., Moss, J. and Vaughan, M. (1985). Pertussis Toxin. Academic Press Inc., London.
Tamura, M., Nogimori, K., Murai, S., Yajima, M. Ito, K., Katada, T. Ui, M. and Ishii, S. (1982). Subunit structure of islet-activating protein, pertussis toxin, in conformity with the A-B model. Biochem., 21, 5516-5522.

Fehrenbach et al. (Eds.), Bacterial Protein Toxins, Zbl. Bakt. Suppl. 17
© Gustav Fischer, Stuttgart, New York, 1988

Purification, Characterization and Toxicity of the Sulfhydryl-Activated Hemolysin (Listeriolysin O) from Listeria monocytogenes

C. Geoffroy[1], J.-L. Gaillard[2], E. Alouf[1] and P. Berche[2]

[1]Unité des Antigènes Bactériens (Centre National de la Recherche Scientifique, UA O 40557), Institut Pasteur, 28, rue du Dr. Roux, F-75724 Paris Cédex 15[1]
[2]Faculté de Médecine Necker-Enfants Malades, Laboratoire de Microbiologie, F-75730 Paris Cédex 15

ABSTRACT

We purified and characterized an extracellular hemolysin produced by *Listeria monocytogenes* . Hemolysin production was greatly enhanced by growing bacteria in resin (Chelex)-treated medium. This hemolysin was separated as a homogeneous protein of 60,000 daltons by using thiol-disulfide exchange affinity chromatography. This protein was a sulfhydryl-activated toxin, termed listeriolysin O, which shared the classical properties of other bacterial sulfhydryl-activated toxins : (i) inhibition by very low amounts of cholesterol ; (ii) activation by reducing agents and suppression of the lytic activity by oxidation ; (iii) antigenic cross-reactivity with streptolysin O. However, listeriolysin O differed remarkably from the other sulfhydryl-activated toxins in that the cytolytic activity was maximum at low pH (~ 5.5) and was undetectable at pH 7.0 towards erythrocytes from various animal species. This suggests that the lytic activity of the toxin in host tissues might be better expressed in the acidic microenvironment, including macrophage phagosomes where bacteria presumably survive. Listeriolysin O was lethal to mice ($LD_{50} \sim 0.8$ µg) and induced a rapid inflammatory reaction when injected intradermally. These results favor the view that listeriolysin O might play a major role during intracellular replication of *Listeria monocytogenes* , ultimately promoting death of infected macrophages.

INTRODUCTION

The role of a hemolytic factor as a promoting factor of intracellular growth of *Listeria monocytogenes* has been suspected for many years, but previous attempts failed to isolate it in a sufficient homogeneous form and these results remained controversial. This work unambiguously demonstrated that this hemolytic factor belongs to the group of the SH-activated exotoxin.

RESULTS

Purification and characterization of the SH-activated hemolysin

Bacteria from strain EGD (Trudeau Institute) were grown for 18 h at 37°C in Chelex-treated medium (1) which allowed a remarkably greater hemolysin production. The hemolytic titer was about 1500 HU/ml in the chelated medium (10^9 bacteria/ml), as compared to 64 HU/ml in BHI (10^{10} bacteria/ml). Culture supernatant (27 liters) was concentrated to 650 ml by ultrafiltration. The concentrate was applied to thiopropyl-Sepharose 6 B columns, and the bound toxin was then eluted, concentrated to 16 ml and applied on Sephacryl-S-200 column. The pooled effluents that contained the peak of hemolytic activity were sequentially passed through Biogel P-100 and Fractogel HW-50 columns and the eluate was concentrated to 8 ml. This fraction exhibited a specific activity of *ca* 1,000,000 HU/mg and appeared as a single polypeptide chain of 60,000 visualized as one sharp band by SDS-PAGE after staining with Coomasie brilliant blue or silver nitrate. This protein displayed the usual properties of the SH-activated cytolysins. The hemolytic activity of the toxin was inhibited by cholesterol and was antigenically related to streptolysin O (SLO), since the pure toxin gave a single immunoprecipitate line by gel diffusion versus horse anti-SLO. The hemolytic activity of the purified hemolysin from *L. monocytogenes* as a function of pH was compared with SLO, perfringolysin O, pneumolysin and alveolysin. The activity of listerial hemolysin had the lowest optimum pH (pH 5.5) as compared to those of pneumolysin (pH 6.0), perfringolysin and alveolysin (pH 6.5) and SLO (pH 7.0). In contrast to the other four hemolysins, the listerial hemolysin exhibited a narrow pH range of activity and hemolysis was not observed at pH 7.0. The hemolytic activity was fully restored by lowering the pH from 7.0 to 5.5. The LD_{50} was estimated at about 0.8 µg per mouse (i.v.). The hemolysin lost all its lethal potential when treated with 1 mM of N-ethylmaleimide (3 h at 37°C), with cholesterol (0.2 wt/wt ; 30 min at 37°C) or with heating (1 h at 60°C).

It is concluded that the extracellular hemolytic factor secreted by *L. monocytogenes* is a SH-activated exotoxin, termed LISTERIOLYSIN O. This exotoxin is secreted by all strains of *L. monocytogenes* , as demonstrated by immunoblotting using a rabbit anti-listeriolysin O (unpublished data). These results are in agreement with the hypothesis that listeriolysin O is a major factor promoting intracellular growth of *L. monocytogenes* (2-4).

REFERENCES

1. Geoffroy, C., J-L. Gaillard, J.E. Alouf, and P. Berche. (1987). Purification, characterization and toxicity of the sulfhydryl-activated hemolysin listeriolysin O from *Listeria monocytogenes* Infect. Immun. 55, (in press).

2. Gaillard, J-L., P. Berche, and P. Sansonetti. (1986). Transposon mutagenesis as a tool to study the role of hemolysin in the virulence of *Listeria monocytogenes* . Infect. Immun. 52 : 50-55.

3. Berche, P., J.L. Gaillard, P. Sansonetti, C. Geoffroy, and J.E. Alouf. (1987). Towards a better understanding of the molecular mechanisms of intracellular growth of *Listeria monocytogenes* . Ann. Inst. Pasteur/Microbiol. 138 : 242-246.

4. Gaillard, J.L., P. Berche, J. Mounier, S. Richard, and P. Sansonetti. (1987). Penetration of *Listeria monocytogenes* into the host : a crucial step of the infectious process. Ann. Inst. Pasteur/Microbiol. 138 : 259-264.

Fehrenbach et al. (Eds.), Bacterial Protein Toxins, Zbl. Bakt. Suppl. 17
© Gustav Fischer, Stuttgart, New York, 1988

Inhibitory Effects of Streptolysin S on Selected Steps of in Vitro Translation System

W. Hryniewicz[1], S. Tyski[1], T. Twardowski[2]

[1]Department of Bacteriology, National Institute of Hygiene, P-00-791 Warsaw, Chocimska 24
[2]Institute of Bioorganic Chemistry, Polish Academy of Sciences, P-61-704 Poznan, Noskowskiego 12/14

INTRODUCTION

Streptolysin S (SLS), a cytolytic toxin is produced by most of Streptococcus pyogenes strains. It is composed of nonspecific carrier molecule (RNA, RNA-core, serum albumin, nonionic detergents, lipoteichoic acid, etc.). SLS can exert wide range of biological activity, even when used in subcytotoxic concentrations it may modify some cell functions (1-3).

Most of hitherto presented data on SLS biological action were concerned with different isolated cells and cell lines (1).

In this study an attempt was made to assess SLS activity on molecular level. An effect of SLS on protein synthesis at the translation level in cell free system was studied.

MATERIALS AND METHODS

RNA-core SLS was prepared from S. pyogenes C203S strain and purified as previously described and expressed in haemolytic units (HU) (4).
RNA-core (Sigma) was purified by the same procedure as SLS. This preparation contained 100% of RNA.
Haemolytic activity of SLS was measured by haemolytic test as described previously (4).
Ribosomes were isolated as described by Pulikowska (5), aminoacyl-tRNA-synthetases were isolated as described by Joachimiak (6), elongation binding factor 1 was purified according to the protocol published by Rafalski (8). The conditions for the binding assay were described in details elsewhere (5) and polymerisation of Phe on ribosomes programmed with poly-U was given by Twardowski and Legocki (9).

RESULTS AND DISCUSSION

It was shown in this study that SLS at the concentration of 0.3µg (90 HU) was a strong inhibitor of two out of three tested steps of translation. Namely, it had an inhibitory effect on binding of AA-tRNA to ribosomal A-site and on elongation of polypeptide chain (polymerisation) (Table 1). This latter step was the most sensitive to SLS action, being already influenced at the concentration of 0.03µg (9 HU).

RNA-core used as a control had no inhibitory effect when used at the same concentrations. To the contrary both SLS and RNA-core had no influence on the enzymatic process of tRNA aminoacylation despite of concentration used.

Table 1. PERCENTAGE OF INHIBITION OF SELECTED STEPS OF TRANSLATION.

Translation step	Streptolysin S[*]		RNA-core	
	0.03µg (9.0 HU)	0.3µg (90 HU)	0.03µg	0.3µg
Elongation of polypeptide chain	52 %	92 %	0 %	10 %
Binding of AA-tRNA to ribosomes	0 %	65 %	0 %	0 %
Aminoacylation of tRNA	0 %	10 %	0 %	15 %

[*] µg of protein determined by UV measurement.

The sigmoidal shape of the time curve (data unshown) suggests a complicated mechanism of inhibition i.e. binding and release between the components of the assay. This interesting biological activity of SLS first described in this study showing toxin-induced inhibition of some steps of translation process may lead to better understanding of SLS-mediated cytolysis and thus mechanism of action.

ACKNOWLEDGMENTS

This project was supported by the Polish Academy of Science within grant o4.12.1. We would like to thanks Ms. K. Ludwiczak for excellent technical assistance.

REFERENCES

1. Jeljaszewicz, J., Szmigielski, S. and Hryniewicz, W. (1978) In "Bacterial toxins and cell membranes." (Eds. J. Jeljaszewicz and T. Wadström) p. 185-227. Academic Press, London.
2. Hryniewicz, W., Pryjma, J. (1984) In "Bacterial Protein Toxins" (Eds. J.E. Alouf, F.J. Fehrenbach, J.H. Freer and J. Jeljaszewicz) p. 297-307, Academic Press, London.
3. Hryniewicz, W., Roszkowski, W., Rykiel, B., Kanclerski, K. and Jeljaszewicz, J. (1986), Zbl. Bakt. Hyg. I Abt. Orig. 261, 454-460.
4. Hryniewicz, W., Gray, E.D., Tagg, J., Wannamaker, L.W., Laible, N. and Kanclerski, K. (1979). Zbl. Bakt. Hyg. I Abt. Org. A 242, 327-338.
5. Palikowska, J., Barciszewska, M., Barciszewski, J., Joachimiak, A., Rafalski, A., Twardowski, T. (1979), Biochem. Biophys. Res. Comm. 1011-1017.
6. Joachimiak, A., Zwierzynski, T., Barciszewska, M., Rafalski, A., Twardowski, T., Barciszewski, J. (1986) Inter. J. Biol. Macromol., 3, 121-128.
7. Palikowska, J., Twardowski, T, (1982), Acta Biochim. Pol., 29, 245-258.
8. Rafalski, A., Barciszewski, J., Gulewicz, K., Twardowski, T., Keith, G. (1977) Acta Biochim. Pol. 24, 301-318.
9. Twardowski, T., Legocki, A. (1984) Biochim. Biophys. Acta.

Fehrenbach et al. (Eds.), Bacterial Protein Toxins, Zbl. Bakt. Suppl. 17
© Gustav Fischer, Stuttgart, New York, 1988

Erythrogenic Toxin Type A and Toxoid: Chemical Characterization and Biological Activities

H. Knöll[1], D. Gerlach[1], S. E. Holm[2], B. Wagner[1] and W. Köhler[1]

[1]Zentralinstitut für Mikrobiologie und experimentelle Therapie, Beutenbergstr. 11,
DDR-6900 Jena.
[2]University Umea, Department of Clinical Bacteriology, S-Umea

ABSTRACT

Erythrogenic toxin type A was purified to homogeneity from
Streptococcus pyogenes strain NY-5. Detoxification was performed
by formalin treatment for 20 days. The PI of the toxoid was found
to be 4.5 (PI of ET A: 5.2) and therefore it was clearly to
distinguish from native ET A.
During the detoxification process the toxin lost its mitogenicity
and pyrogenicity but maintained antigenicity. The binding of ET A
and toxoid on human peripheral blood lymphocytes was demonstrated
electron microscopically by direct labelling with ET A and toxoid
gold conjugate. The binding could be inhibited by antibody to
ET A. The antigenicity of toxoid was proved in a rabbit tissue
cage model; the antitoxic immunity protected against the pathogenicity of ET A.

KEYWORDS

Erythrogenic toxin type A, detoxification by formaldehyde treatment, mitogenicity, pyrogenicity, rabbit tissue cage model.

Erythrogenic toxins (syn. Dick toxin, scarlet fever toxin,
streptococcal pyrogenic exotoxin, streptococcal exotoxin) are
extracellular proteins which are produced by group A streptococci. Three serologically distinct toxin types (A, B and C)
have been identified and characterized.
The most detailed informations are available about the erythrogenic toxin type A (ET A); it has a molecular weight of about
26 kD and an isoelectric point of 5.2.
ET A produced and secreted by a heterologous host (S.sanguis)
carrying the cloned gene for ET A, was found to have properties
identical to ET A produced by S.pyogenes strain NY-5 (Gerlach
and co-workers, 1987).
The erythrogenic toxins display a variety of biological activities in vitro and in vivo, among others they are pyrogenic and

mitogenic for T lymphocytes. They are held to be responsible for scarlet fever rash. Soon after the discovery of erythrogenic toxin by Dick, G.F. and Dick, G.H. (1924) attempts were made to prevent scarlet fever by active immunization with a toxoid. The aim of the present study was to use a highly purified erythrogenic toxin type A for preparation of toxoid and to study the humoral and cell-mediated reactions after immunization with these antigens.

The process of detoxification of ET A was followed over a period of 20 days of exposure to formaldehyde. In isoelectric focusing a change of PI from 5.2 to 4.5 starting 15' after exposure to formaldehyde was accompanied by a loss of mitogenic activity.

TABLE 1 Biological Activities of ET A and Toxoid

activity	ET A	toxoid
antigenicity	+	+
direct binding to lymphocytes	+	+
skin reactivity	+	⊖
mitogenicity	+	⊖
pyrogenicity	+	⊖

The effectivity of toxoid immunization was proved in a rabbit tissue cage model (Knöll and co-workers, 1982, 1985). Immunization of rabbits with ET A or toxoid protected the animals in a challenge infection with an ET A producing streptococcal strain against the pyrogenic and enhancement activity of ET A.

REFERENCES

Dick, G.F., and Dick, G.H. (1924). A skin test for susceptibility to scarlet fever. J.Amer.Med.Ass., 88, 265-266.

Gerlach, D., Köhler, W., Knöll, H., Moravek, L., Weeks, C.R., and Ferretti, J.J. (1987). Purification and characterization of Streptococcus pyogenes erythrogenic toxin type A produced by a cloned gene in Streptococcus sanguis. Zbl.Bakt.Hyg.Orig.A, in press.

Knöll, H., Holm, S.E., Gerlach, D., and Köhler, W. (1982). Tissue cages for study of experimental infection in rabbits. I. Production of erythrogenic toxins in vivo. Immunobiol., 162, 128-140.

Knöll, H., Holm, S.E., Gerlach, D., Kühnemund, O., and Köhler, W. (1985). Tissue cages for study of experimental streptococcal infection in rabbits. II. Humoral and cell-mediated immune response to erythrogenic toxins. Immunobiol., 169, 116-127.

Fehrenbach et al. (Eds.), Bacterial Protein Toxins, Zbl. Bakt. Suppl. 17
© Gustav Fischer, Stuttgart, New York, 1988

Streptococcal Outbreaks and Erythrogenic Toxin Type A

W. Köhler, D. Gerlach and H. Knöll

Zentralinstitut für Mikrobiologie und experimentelle Therapie, Beutenbergstr. 11,
DDR-6900 Jena

ABSTRACT

Streptococcus pyogenes strains were examined by ELISA and double
immunodiffusion tests for their ability to produce erythrogenic
toxin type A. Reference strains, isolated from scarlet fever
cases at the beginning of this century, produce large amounts of
ET A (up to 16,000 µg/l). Recent epidemic strains are weak toxin
producers (type 3 epidemic in 1972/73 mean value 68 µg/l; type 1
epidemic 1982/83 mean value 8 µg/l). Because ET A must be considered as a pathogenicity factor the decrease in toxin production may be one reason for the present mild form of scarlet
fever.

KEYWORDS

Erythrogenic toxin A, synthesis of ET A, scarlet fever, scarlet
fever outbreaks, group A streptococci.

Reference strains of Streptococcus pyogenes as well as strains
from recent epidemics and from sporadic cases of scarlet fever
were examined for their ability to produce erythrogenic toxin
type A (ET A) by an ELISA and double immunodiffusion (Ouchterlony)
test using an anti-ET A antibody purified by affinity chromatography. Of the reference strains (most of them isolated before
1945) 16/51 produced more or less ET A. Toxin synthesis is
strain-specific but not type-specific (f.i. type 12 strain NY-5
(Dochez) is a strong ET A producer, strain K56 (Kjems)
synthesizes no toxin). Well-known toxin producers like strains
NY-5, 594 or "Smith" produce up to 16,000 µg/l under optimal
culture conditions. Type 3 strains isolated from scarlet fever
patients during the outbreak 1972/73 (incidence 47.3/100 000)
seem to belong to one clone as evidenced by the uniform SDS-PAGE
pattern. They were found to produce 5-200 µg/l (mean 68 µg/l)
ET A only. After appearance of type 3 strains in 1980, causing
sporadic cases of scarlet fever, they were found to produce only

low amounts of ET A or not at all (0-138 μg/l, mean 30 μg/l). Strains of type 1, causing the epidemic in 1982/83 (incidence: 34/100 000) synthesized only low amounts of ET A being detectable only by ELISA but not by Ouchterlony tests (range 0.75-10 μg/l), mean about 8 μg/l). Only a few strains of S.pyogenes isolated 1984 or later synthesized ET A but they were found more often to produce ET B (proteinase precursor) even in batch cultures. These results were confirmed by Ferretti and co-workers using a specific probe consisting of 606 bases within the spA gene. The ELISA and the DNA-hybridization techniques gave the same results.

The difference of ET A production by scarlet fever strains from periods of high mortality (beginning of this century) and recent epidemic strains is of a quantitative nature. As a result of our experiments using the rabbit tissue cage infection model, ET A was found to be a pathogenicity factor. Immunization with a toxoid of ET A resulted in decline of fever reaction, and no deaths occured after infection.

The decline in mortality of scarlet fever seems to be caused among others by the evolution of strains producing only low amounts of ET A.

Fehrenbach et al. (Eds.), Bacterial Protein Toxins, Zbl. Bakt. Suppl. 17
© Gustav Fischer, Stuttgart, New York, 1988

Specificity of Human Immunological Response to Pneumolysin

Krzysztof Kanclerski[1,2], and Roland Möllby[1]

[1]National Bacteriological Laboratory, S-105 21 Stockholm
[2]National Institute of Hygiene, Chocimska Street 24, P-00-791 Warsaw

INTRODUCTION

In an earlier study (1) we have shown that pneumolysin can be used as an
antigen in an ELISA for serological diagnosis of pneumococcal pneumonia with
a sensitivity of 80% for bacteremic patients.

MATERIALS AND METHODS

Pneumolysin.
The pneumolysin was produced and purified as described previously (2).
Streptolysin O
The standard crude preparation of streptolysin O was obtained form the
Serological Departement of the National Bacteriological Laboratory.
Enzyme Linked Immunosorbent Assay.
The assay was described in detail previously (1). Briefly, cobalt irradiated
polystyrene microplates (Dynatech M 129 B, Plochigen, West Germany) were
coated with antigen overnight at room temperature (22°C). The optimal coating
dose was determined to 2.5 µg/ml by antigen titration. Patient sera diluted
10^{-3}, or more if necessary, were added to two wells and the plates were
incubated for 1 h at room temperature. Specific alkaline phosphatase
conjugated antiserum (Orion, Diagnostica, Finland) was added and incubation
was done overnight at room temperature. Volumes of 100 µl were used in each
step and all washings were done three times with isotonic phosphate buffered
saline supplemented with 0.05% Tween 20. The ELISA titer was defined as the
absorption at 405 nm multiplied by the serum dilution factor.
Neutralization test.
The standard method (3) adapted for microtiter plates was used.
Sera.
Antibodies to pneumolysin were studied in serum samples from the following
groups of patients:
- 184 healthy individuals 0 to 80 years of age.
- 35 patients with high anti-streptolysin O titer.
- 40 patients with pneumococcal pneumonia.

RESULTS AND DISCUSSION

The distribution of antibody titers to pneumolysin depended on age, with low values in children under 7 years of age and adults older then 70 years. These groups are most prone to develop pneumococcal disease. The highest values were found in children 8 to 15 years old.

The antipneumolysin titers in acute serum samples drawn within five days after onset of respiratory symptoms from the patients with pneumococcal pneumonia were significantly lower than in healthy age-matched controls. Titers above 200 were found in only 9/37 (24%) of these patients while in the control 26/47 (55%).

Sera from patients with pneumococcal pneumonia demonstrating high titers in the pneumolysin ELISA were analysed for antistreptolysin 0 titers. No correlation (r=-0.112) was found between antibody titers measured by the two assays. In sera from patients with high antistreptolysin 0 titers the same lack of correlation to antipneumolysin titers was found (r=-0.313).

Antibody titers to pneumolysin in sera with high antistreptolysin 0 titers were also compared to a healthy age-matched control group. No difference in titer distribution between these two groups was found.

CONCLUSIONS

Antibodies to pneumolysin and to streptolysin did not crossreact in the clinical sera studied. Thus, the use of the pneumolysin-ELISA for clinical diagnostic purposes will not be disturbed by crossreactions with antibodies against streptolysin.

REFERENCES
1. Kalin, M., L. Kanclerski, M. Granström, R. Möllby (1987). Diagnosis of pneumococcal pneumonia by measurement of antibodies to pneumococcal hemolysin (pneumolysin) with ELISA. J.Clin. Microbiol., 25.
2. Kanclerski, K. and R. Möllby (1987) Production and purification of Streptococcus pneumoniae hemolysin (pneumolysin). J. Clin. Microbiol., 25.
3. Rantz, L.A., Randall, E. (1945) A modification of the technique for determination of the antistreptolysin titer. Proc. Soc.. Exp. Biol. Med., 59.

Fehrenbach et al. (Eds.), Bacterial Protein Toxins, Zbl. Bakt. Suppl. 17
© Gustav Fischer, Stuttgart, New York, 1988

Another Verotoxin-Oedema Disease Principle

M. A. Linggood and J. M. Thompson

Unilever Research, Colworth House, Sharnbrook, Beds MK44 1LQ, U.K.

ABSTRACT

Strains of Escherichia coli isolated from documented cases of disease in
pigs and belonging to a wide range of pathogenic serotypes were tested for
their ability to produce a heat labile verotoxin (VT). The strains
isolated from oedema disease all produced VT, indicating that the cytotoxin
detected by the vero cell assay was identical to oedema disease principle.
Strains belonging to the serotypes associated with enterotoxic diarrhoea
were VT^-. Not all the strains belonging to the recognised oedema disease
serotypes (0141:K85,0139:K82 and 0138:K81) produced VT, but the VT^- strains
were not associated with outbreaks of clinical disease.
Keywords: Escherichia coli, verotoxin, oedema disease, pig.

INTRODUCTION

Oedema disease attacks thriving pigs about one week after weaning, the
major feature being progressive incoordination leading to partial or
complete paralysis and death. The E.coli strains associated with the
disease are confined to the intestinal tract and so it has been assumed
that they produce a neurotoxin, oedema disease principle, which is absorbed
and gives rise to the pathological signs. Many srains belonging to
serotypes associated with post-weaning disease in pigs (oedema disease or
diarrhoea) produce a factor cytopathic for vero cells so it is possible
that oedema disease principle is also a verotoxin (VT).

In order to clarify the role of VT in the virulence of E.coli for pigs we
examined a large number of strains isolated from healthy and diseased
animals in order to determine whether there was any real correlation
between the observed clinical symptoms of oedema disease or diarrhoea and
the presence of a VT^+ strain.

MATERIALS AND METHODS

Most of the strains tested were isolated during the period 1978-1985 from
pig farms in the UK. They were serotyped and their toxin pattern (VT,LT
and ST) determined. VT was assayed by the vero cell method of Konowalchuk,
Speirs and Stavric (1977) before and after heat treatement at 70°C for 30
mins. LT was assayed by ELISA and ST by the suckling mouse test.

RESULTS AND DISCUSSION

The porcine verotoxin was not neutralised by antisera to shiga toxin or to either of two verotoxins produced by human strains of E.coli.   The human verotoxins were inactivated by heat treatment at 80°C but were stable at 70°C.   The verotoxins produced by all the porcine strains were inactivated by heat treatment at 70°C.

Strains associated with neonatal diarrhoea in piglets were generally VT^- but 67% of the strains associated with post-weaning disease in pigs (serotypes 0141:K85,0139:K82 and 0138:K81) were found to be VT^+.   Previous studies had revealed this general association of VT with serotype (Dobrescu, 1983; Smith, Green and Parsell, 1983) but we found that an analysis of the strains based on the clinical signs in the infected pigs, rather than simply on serotype, provided much stronger evidence for the role of verotoxin in virulence (Linggood & Thompson, 1987).   Verotoxin producing E.coli strains were isolated from all cases of oedema disease but when the same serotypes were isolated from healthy pigs, or pigs suffering from post-weaning diarrhoea, they were usually VT^-.

0141:K85 strains showed three different toxin patterns: (i) $VT^+ST^-LT^-$ types isolated from pigs with oedema disease (ii) $VT^-ST^+LT^-$ types isolated from pigs with diarrhoea and (iii) $VT^-ST^-LT^-$ types found as part of the mixed faecal flora of healthy animals.   No 0139:K82 strains produced LT or ST or were associated with cases of diarrhoea but VT producing strains were isolated from animals with oedema disease. VT^- 0139 strains were not associated with clinical oedema disease even when the strains were present in almost pure culture in faecal swabs.

Our major observation was that verotoxicity in porcine E.coli was associated with the ability to cause oedema disease.   Not all of the strains belonging to the implicated serotypes were VT^+ but the VT^- strains were not associated with clinical outbreaks of the disease. Therefore for accurate identification of a potential oedema disease pathogen a toxin assay is necessary in addition to serological typing.

REFERENCES

DOBRESCU, L. (1983). New biological effect of edema disease principle and its use as an in vitro assay for this toxin. Amer.J.Vet.Res.,44, 31-44

KONOWALCHUK,J., J.I.SPEIRS and S.STAVRIC (1977). Vero response to a cytotoxin of E.coli. Inf.Imm.,18. 775-779.

LINGGOOD,M.A. and J.M.THOMPSON, (1987). Verotoxin production among porcine strains of E.coli and its association with oedema disease. J.Med.Microbiol., in press.

SMITH.H.W., P.GREEN and Z.PARSELL (1983). Vero cell toxins in E.coli and related bacteria: transfer by phage and conjugation and toxic action in laboratory animals, chickens and pigs. J.Gen.Microbiol.,129,3121-3137.

Fehrenbach et al. (Eds.), Bacterial Protein Toxins, Zbl. Bakt. Suppl. 17
© Gustav Fischer, Stuttgart, New York, 1988

Comparison of Toxins from Clostridium sordellii and Clostridium difficile

M. R. Popoff

Service des Anaérobies, Institut Pasteur, 25 rue du Dr Roux, F-75724 Paris Cédex 15

ABSTRACT

Clostridium sordellii toxins has been compared to C. difficile
toxins. Some similarities exist between C. sordellii lethal toxin
and C. difficile cytotoxin, and C. sordellii haemorrhagic toxin
and C. difficile enterotoxin respectively.

KEYWORDS
Clostridium sordellii,Clostridium difficile,toxins.

INTRODUCTION
Clostridium difficile has been recognized as the aetiological
agent of pseudomembranous colitis and some post antibiotic colitis
in man. C. sordellii is an agent of gas gangrene, and induces also
enteritis, haemorrhagic enteritis and enterotoxaemia in animals.
C. difficile produces 2 toxins: an enterotoxin or toxin A and a
cytotoxin or toxin B. C. sordellii synthetizes also 2 major
toxins:the lethal toxin (LT) and the haemorrhagic toxin(HT).

RESULTS AND DISCUSSION
The biochemical characteristics and the biological activities of
these toxins are summarized in table 1.
C. sordellii LT and HT are related to C. difficile cytotoxin and
enterotoxin respectively. Furthermore, antigenic similarities
exist between C. sordellii and C. difficile cytotoxin. Antibodies
against LT neutralize biological activities of LT and C. difficile
cytotoxin but not those of C. sordellii HT or C. difficile
enterotoxin. However, the neutralization titer of anti LT
antiserum was 40 fold higher with LT than with C. difficile
cytotoxin. These data suggest that partial immunological identity
exist between C. sordellii LT and C. difficle cytotoxin. On the
other hand, several differences exist between C. sordellii LT and
C. difficile cytotoxin.Indeed, C. sordellii LT causes rounding up
of the culture cells (Vero, MRC5), but does not produce
actinomorphic alterations like C. difficile cytotoxin. LT is not
inhibited by proteolytic enzymes and is activable by DTT .
Moreover, unlike C. difficile enterotoxin, C. sordellii HT is
produced during sporulation and is not cytotoxic for culture
cells.

The molecular mechanism of C. sordellii LT remains unknown. LT does not induce an early inhibition of protein synthesis in Vero cells by (measuring incorporation of (^{14}C)-leucine).However, a slight decrease of ^{14}C-leucine incorporation was observed when morphological alterations of cells were evident (about 4-5 h after inoculation of 3 10^{-8}mM of LT for 10^5 cells). In addition, no ADP-ribosyl transferase activity was found associated with LT, using (^{32}P)-NAD and Xenopus oocytes microinjected with toxin,and LT does not induce change in the basal activity of adenylate cyclase from rat brain synaptosomes.

Table 1: Properties of C. sordellii and C. difficile toxins.

Biochemical and biological properties	C. sordellii LT	C. sordellii HT	C. difficile (1) Cytotoxin	C. difficile (1) Enterotoxin
Molecular Weight of native molecule (10^3 kDa)	250	440	150-440	440-550
Isoelectric point	4.5	?	5.2-5.7	4.1-4.7
NaCl concentration for elution from DEAE Trisacryl ion exchange	0.12-0.18M	0.06-0.12M	0.1-0.25M	0-0.1M
Cytotoxicity (CU/mg of protein)	6.1 10^4	0	2 10^{11}	1 10^5
Lethality for mouse (LD100/mg protein)	3.4 10^5	0	2 10^4	2 10^4
Increased vascular permeability (skin test)	6.4 10^5 U/mg prot	dermo-necrosis	Yes	Yes
Intestinal haemorrhage	No	Yes	No	Yes
Inactivation of activity inactivation by heat	10min at 60°C		6min at 56°C	
interval pH of stability	5-8.5		4-10	5-9
inactivation by trypsin	No		Yes	Yes
" " by oxydized-glutathion at	7mM		No	No
" " by N-bromo-succinimide at	0.01mM		0.01mM	0.01mM
" " by N-chloro-succinimide at	0.01mM		-	-
" " by chloramine T	0.05mM		-	-
" " by sulfhydryl reagents	No		No	No
activation by DTT	2-4 times		No	No

(1) according to Lyerly and others,1986;Pothoulakis and others,1986;Thelestam and Florin,1984.

REFERENCES

Lyerly,D.M.,M.D.Roberts,C.J.Phelps and T.D.Wilkins (1986) Purification and properties of toxins A and B of Clostridium difficile.FEMS Microbiol. Let. 33,31-35.

Popoff M.R.(1987).Purification and characterization of Clostridium sordellii lethal toxin and cross-reactivity with Clostridium difficile cytotoxin.Infec.Immun. 55,35-43.

Pothoulakis C.,L.M.Barone,R.Ely,B.Faris,M.E.Clark,C.Franzblau and J.T.Lamont (1986).Purification and properties of Clostridium difficile cytotoxin .J.Biol.Chem.261,1316-1321.

Thelestam M. and I. Florin (1984).Cytopathogenic action of Clostridium difficile toxins.J.Toxicol.Rev.3,139-180.

Fehrenbach et al. (Eds.), Bacterial Protein Toxins, Zbl. Bakt. Suppl. 17
© Gustav Fischer, Stuttgart, New York, 1988

Production of Vero Cytotoxins by Strains of Escherichia coli Isolated from Human Infections and Correlation with Hybridisation with Gene Probes for VT1 and VT2

S. M. Scotland, H. R. Smith, G. A. Willshaw, H. Chart and B. Rowe

Division of Enteric Pathogens, Central Public Health Laboratory, 61 Colindale Avenue, London NW9 5HT, U.K.

ABSTRACT

78 strains of Escherichia coli that hybridised with specific gene probes for Vero cytotoxins VT1 and VT2 were isolated in the British Isles from cases of haemorrhagic colitis, haemolytic uraemic syndrome and diarrhoea in infants. Probe tests correlated well with tests for VT in filtered culture supernatants. There were three classes of E.coli producing either VT1, or VT2, or VT1 and VT2 and we suggest that both Vero cytotoxins are important in human disease.

KEYWORDS

Escherichia coli, Vero cytotoxin, DNA hybridisation, haemorrhagic colitis, haemolytic uraemic syndrome.

Certain strains of Escherichia coli (VTEC) produce a heat-labile cytotoxin, termed Vero cytotoxin (VT), active on Vero cells (Konowalchuk, Speirs and Stavric, 1977). Immunologically distinct VTs have been recognised, and VT1 and VT2 have been described in strains of E.coli 0157 (Scotland, Smith and Rowe, 1985). VT1 is immunologically related to Shiga toxin whereas VT2 is not. Phages encoding VT have been isolated and gene probes for VT1 and VT2 have been developed from them (Willshaw and others, 1987).

VTEC have been isolated from patients with haemorrhagic colitis (HC) and haemolytic uraemic syndrome (HUS) in North America and Japan and we have recently reported their isolation from these diseases in the United Kingdom (Scotland and others, 1987; Smith and others, 1987). VT probes have been used to examine these strains and also strains of classic enteropathogenic serogroups (EPEC) from outbreaks and sporadic cases of diarrhoea in infants. Filtered culture supernatants were tested on monolayers of Vero cells for VT. The toxin titre was the highest dilution giving a cytotoxic effect after 4 days at 37°C. Serum neutralisation tests were performed as described previously (Scotland, Smith and Rowe 1985). Hybridisation was by the method of Willshaw and others (1985). Two DNA probes for VT1 were developed from sequences cloned from a phage from strain H19 (E.coli 026.H11). They were a HincII fragment of 0.75kb and a HindIII–BgIII fragment of 0.65kb and probably cover most of the sequences encoding VT1. The probe for VT2 sequences was a 0.85kb AvaI–PstI fragment obtained from a phage from strain E32511 (E.coli 0157.H⁻). The VT1 and VT2 probe sequences did not cross hybridise under stringent conditions.

30 patients with HC and 15 patients with HUS yielded strains of E.coli 0157. 40 of these strains were flagellar type H7 and 5 were non-motile (H-). 44 of the 45 strains hybridised with the VT2 probe and 18 of these also hybridised with the VT1 probes. A single strain hybridised with only the VT1 probes. All produced VT at titres greater than 1250. Neutralisation experiments with 10 strains confirmed the production of either VT1 or VT2 or both toxins in agreement with the hybridisation tests.

Three other patients with HC and 4 with HUS yielded strains of E.coli which were not 0157 but which hybridised with the probes. The strains from HC were: 091.H- (VT1 and VT2), 0?H8 (VT2) and 0?H25 (VT1). The strains from HUS were: 026.H11 (VT1), 0153.H25 (VT1 and VT2), 0163.H19 (VT2) with 0 rough.H51 (VT2) and 0104.H2 (VT2) with 0?H25 (VT1). Two of the HUS patients yielded two different strains. The two 0?H25 strains hybridised with the HincII VT1 probe but not the HindIII-BgIII probe; they did not produce VT in cell tests and probably had incomplete VT sequences. The other 7 strains produced VT at titres ranging from 50 to 156250.

The epidemic strains from each of 12 well-documented outbreaks of infantile diarrhoea were studied and they did not produce VT or hybridise with the DNA probes. An earlier study of strains belonging to 11 different EPEC serogroups showed that a few strains of serogroups 026 and 0128 produced VT (Scotland, Day and Rowe, 1980). VTEC of these serogroups were examined for hybridisation. All strains of serogroup 026 hybridised with the VT1 probes only whereas, with one exception, the 0128 strains hybridised with both VT1 and VT2. The 026 and 0128 strains produced VT at titres greater than 250.

There is good correlation between VT production detected using filtered culture supernatants in Vero cell tests and the possession of VT genes as indicated by hybridisation with specific DNA probes. VTEC produced either VT1 or VT2 or both toxins and our results indicate that both Vero cytotoxins may be virulence factors in human disease.

REFERENCES

Konowalchuk, J., Speirs, J.I. and Stavric, S. (1977). Vero response to a cytotoxin of Escherichia coli. Infect. Immun., 18, 775-779.

Scotland, S.M., Day, N.P. and Rowe, B. (1980). Production of a cytotoxin affecting Vero cells by strains of Escherichia coli belonging to traditional enteropathogenic serogroups. FEMS Microbiol. Lett. 7, 15-17.

Scotland, S.M., Rowe, B., Smith, H.R., Willshaw, G.A. and Gross, R.J. (1987). Vero cytotoxin-producing strains of Escherichia coli from children with haemolytic uraemic syndrome and their detection by specific DNA probes. J. med. Microbiol. Accepted for publication.

Scotland, S.M., Smith, H.R. and Rowe, B. (1985). Two distinct toxins active on Vero cells from Escherichia coli 0157. Lancet, ii, 885-886.

Smith, H.R., Rowe, B., Gross, R.J., Fry, N.K. and Scotland, S.M. (1987). Haemorrhagic colitis and Vero cytotoxin-producing Escherichia coli in England and Wales. Lancet, i, 1062-1065.

Willshaw, G.A., Smith, H.R., Scotland, S.M., Field, A.M. and Rowe, B. (1987).Heterogeneity of Escherichia coli phages encoding Vero cytotoxins: comparison of cloned sequences determining VT1 and VT2 and development of specific gene probes. J. gen. Microbiol. 133, 1309-1317.

Willshaw, G.A., Smith, H.R., Scotland, S.M. and Rowe, B. (1985). Cloning of genes determining the production of Vero cytotoxin by Escherichia coli. J. gen. Microbiol. 131, 3047-3053.

Fehrenbach et al. (Eds.), Bacterial Protein Toxins, Zbl. Bakt. Suppl. 17
© Gustav Fischer, Stuttgart, New York, 1988

Induction of Murine Cytolytic T-Lymphocytes by Pseudomonas Aeruginosa Exotoxin A

T. Zehavi-Willner

Israel Institute for Biological Research, P. O. B. 19, Ness-Ziona 70450, Israel

KEYWORDS

Pseudomonas exotoxin A, cytolytic T-lymphocytes (CTL), splenocytes, mitogenesis.

Pseudomonas exotoxin A (PA) is considered the most toxic substance produced by this organism, and as such, may have a significant role in its pathogenicity. PA, being an highly potent protein synthesis inhibitor, acts as a cytolytic agent on a whole range of mammalian cells including cells of the immune system (Holt, 1985). The data presented in this communication demonstrates that PA is a weak T cell mitogen for murine splenocytes. Maximal stimulation of ^{3}H-thymidine incorporation is obtained with 10-100ng toxin per ml of culture, following a 4 day induction (Fig. 1). The indicated optimal toxin concentrations for mitogenic induction, are slightly inhibitory to protein biosynthesis in freshly prepared and 24 h cultured splenocytes. Protein biosynthesis in toxin treated splenocytes cultured over 24 h, followed the general pattern of ^{3}H-thymidine incorporation, namely protein synthesis was markedly enhanced (Fig.1.).

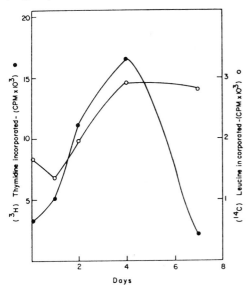

Fig. 1. The effect of PA on ^{3}H-thymidine and ^{14}C-leucine incorporation into cultured murine splenocytes. Spleen cells (2 x 10^6/ml) were incubated at 37°C in the presence of 100ng PA for various times. At the time indicated, the cultured splenocytes were isolated on Ficoll paque, resuspended in fresh medium and their incorporating activity of ^{3}H-thymidine and ^{14}C-leucine (1µCi per well) was tested separately. Closed circles-splenocytes cultured with PA. Open circles – control splenocytes.

PA was also shown to be a polyclonal activator of cytolytic T lymphocytes (CTL) effective against Concanavaline A treated target cells (Fig. 2). The effective PA dose for CTL induction was as for mitogenic stimulation, only with a prolonged priming time (7 days).

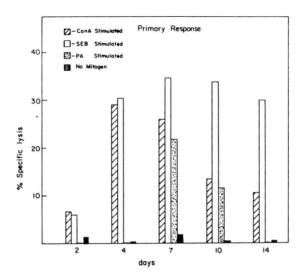

Fig. 2.: Kinetics of PA as compared to ConA and SEB induced cytolytic cell response. Splenocytes isolated from BALB/C mice were incubated alone, with 100 ng/ml PA, 2μg/ml ConA, or with 1 μg/ml SEB and were tested daily for cytolytic activity against ConA treated ^{51}Cr-EL-4. Effector target ratio was 10:1.

In summary, the results presented in this study, indicate that PA at low concentrations is mitogenic to cells of the immune system. Furthermore, PA induces CTL activity, a phenomenon which also may be triggered by the mitogenic properties of the toxin. Finally, it is feasable that the exposure of animals to sublethal doses of PA, enhances cytolytic activity in vivo.

1. Holt, P.S. and M.L. Misfeldt (1985). Induction of an immune response in athymic nude mice to thymus-dependent antigens by Ps. aeruginosa exotoxin A. Cellular Immunol. 95, 265-275.

Applied Toxinology

Fehrenbach et al. (Eds.), Bacterial Protein Toxins, Zbl. Bakt. Suppl. 17
© Gustav Fischer, Stuttgart, New York, 1988

Interleukin-2 Receptor Targeted Toxicity: Genetic Construction and Properties of a Diphtheria Toxin-Related Interleukin-2 Fusion Protein

D. P. Williams[1][2], P. Bacha[3], C. Waters[3], W. Bishai[4], K. Parker[3], T. B. Strom[5], and J. R. Murphy[1]

[1]Evans Department of Clinical Research and Department of Medicine, The University, Hospital, Boston, MA 02118, U.S.A.
[2]Department of Microbiology, Boston University School of Medicine, Boston, MA 02118, U.S.A.
[3]Seragen Inc., Hopkinton, MA 01748, U.S.A.
[4]Department of Microbiology and Molecular Genetics, Harvard Medical School, Boston, MA 02115, U.S.A.
[5]Charles A. Dana Research Institute, Harvard Thorndike Laboratory of the Beth Israel Hospital, Harvard Medical School, Boston, MA 02215, U.S.A.

ABSTRACT

The diphtheria toxin receptor binding domain has been genetically replaced with a cDNA encoding the T-cell growth factor interleukin-2 (IL-2). The toxin-related / IL-2 fusion gene encodes, in mature form, a 68,086 dalton protein that retains immunologic determinants intrinsic to both its diphtheria toxin and IL-2 components. The chimeric IL-2-toxin has been purified from periplasmic extracts of recombinant Escherichia coli and is shown to selectively inhibit protein synthesis in IL-2 receptor bearing T-cells in vitro. The action of IL-2-toxin is shown to be mediated through the IL-2 receptor, to require an acidification step in the entry process, and to catalyse the ADP-ribosylation of elongation factor 2 in target cells.

KEYWORDS

Fusion gene, chimeric toxin, diphtheria toxin, interleukin-2, recombinant DNA, protein engineering

INTRODUCTION

The expression of interleukin-2 (IL-2) and the induction of the interleukin-2 receptor (IL-2R) on the surface of activated normal T-cells constitute critical events in the generation of an immune response (Smith, 1984). Upon stimulation with either antigen or mitogen in the presence of interleukin-1 (IL-1), IL-2R are expressed de novo (Cotner et al., 1983; Williams et al., 1984). The IL-2R has been shown to fall into "high" and "low" affinity classes (Robb et al. 1984;

Lowenthal et al. 1985). Recent work has shown that the "high" affinity receptor is composed of a 55,000 and 70,000 dalton glycoprotein heterodimer (Robb et al., 1987; Kuo et al., 1986). Each subunit has been shown to bind IL-2 and constitute a "low" affinity receptor; however, only the "high" affinity receptor appears to mediate the internalization of IL-2 (Fugii et al., 1986; Weissman et al., 1986). In the presence of the "high" affinity receptor and IL-2 there is clonal expansion and continued viability of activated T-cells. Since the high affinity IL-2R appears to be limited in distribution to activated T-cells, some recently activated B-cells, and macrophages, a potent cytotoxic agent directed toward this receptor may have therapeutic application for a variety of autoimmune disorders, and acute allograft rejection.

In the case of retroviral HTLV-I associated adult T-cell leukemia (ATL), there is evidence suggesting the viral tat gene product functions as a transactivator and induces the expression of "high" affinity IL-2R genes (Haseltine et al., 1984). In this instance, IL-2R are found in increased number on the T-cell surface. As a result, a cytoxic agent directed against the IL-2R on ATL cells may also have therapeutic application. Indeed, treatment of ATL patients with a monoclonal antibody, anti-Tac, directed against the IL-2R has resulted in a moderate rate of remission (Waldmann, 1986), even though murine antibodies poorly fix human complement. Moreover, monoclonal antibody bound to the Tac antigen (55,000 dalton glycoprotein) is not internalized by the cell (Weissman et al., 1986), and therefore this subunit of the IL-2R should not be effective in delivering the toxophore of an immunotoxin to Tac antigen positive cells.

Using protein engineering and recombinant DNA methodologies, Murphy et al. (1986) have recently shown that the diphtheria toxin receptor binding domain could be functionally replaced with peptide hormone sequences. In this study, a synthetic gene encoding α-melanocyte stimulating hormone (α-MSH) was genetically fused to the 3'-end of the diphtheria toxin structural gene. The fusion protein expressed by this chimeric gene was composed, in mature form, of amino acids Gly1 to Ala485 of diphtheria toxin fused to Ser1 through Val13 of α-MSH. The chimeric protein was found to be selectively cytotoxic for α-MSH receptor bearing human malignant melanocytes; whereas, cells devoid of this receptor were found to be resistant to its action. We have used a similar strategy to genetically construct a fusion gene encoding amino acids 1 through 485 of diphtheria toxin linked to Pro2 through Thr133 of IL-2. The mature form of the diphtheria toxin-related / IL-2 fusion protein, IL-2-toxin, has a deduced molecular weight of 68,086. In the present report, we show that IL-2-toxin retains immunologic determinants of both of its components. Further, we show that IL-2-toxin is specifically directed to the IL-2R on HTLV-I infected transformed T-cells, and that the subsequent inhibition of protein synthesis is due to the ADP-ribosylation of target cell elongation factor 2.

MATERIALS AND METHODS

Bacterial strains, plasmids, and eukaryotic cell lines. The bacterial strains, plasmids, and eukaryotic cell lines used in this study are listed in Table 1.

Nucleic acids. Plasmid DNAs were prepared by the alkaline lysis method and purified by cesium chloride / ethidium bromide centrifugation as described by Maniatis et al. (1982). Plasmid DNA was digested with restriction endonucleases as recommended by the manufacturer (New England Biolabs, Beverly, MA). Restriction fragments were analysed by electrophoresis on horizontal 1.0% agarose gels in TBE buffer (89 mM boric acid, 89 mM Trisma base [Sigma Chemical

CO., St. Louis, MO], 2.5 mM disodium ethylenediaminetetraacetic acid [EDTA]). DNA fragments were cloned into plasmid vectors according to standard methods (Maniatis et al., 1982). DNA sequencing was performed by the dideoxy chain termination method essentially as described by Sanger et al. (1977). Portions of the chimeric IL-2-toxin gene were recloned into the M13mp18 and/or M13mp19 vectors, and sequencing reactions were initiated with the universal primer.

TABLE 1 Prokaryotic and eukaryotic cell lines.

Prokaryotic strains.	source or reference
Escherichia coli SY327	(Isberg et al., 1982)
Escherichia coli SY327(pABC508)	(Bishai et al., 1987a)
Escherichia coli SY327(pABI508)	(Williams et al., 1987)
Escherichia coli JM101(M13mp18)	New England Biolabs, Beverly, MA
Escherichia coli JM101(M13mp19)	New England Biolabs, Beverly, MA

Eukaryotic cell lines.	
C91/PL	Robert Schwartz
C8215	John Williams
CTLL-2	(Gillis et al., 1977)
CEM-3	ATCC, TIB-195
Karpas	Robert Schwartz
U937	ATCC, CRL-1593

Protein purification. E. coli SY327(pABI508) was grown in 10 liter volumes of Luria broth (10 g Tryptone [Difco], 10 g NaCl, and 5 g yeast extract per liter) at 30°C for 15-18 hours. Bacteria were harvested by centrifugation, washed, and resuspended in TES buffer (50 mM Tris-HCl, pH8.3, 1 mM EDTA, 20% sucrose) at 4°C. Periplasmic extracts were prepared as previously described (Leong et al., 1983). Bacteria were treated with lysozyme (100 µg/ml) for 20 min, and the spheroplasts were sedimented by centrifugation. The crude periplasmic extract was then treated with ammonium sulfate which was added to 65% saturation. Following centrifugation the pellet was resuspended in 10 mM Tris-HCl, pH 8.3, and applied to an anti-IL-2 immuno-affinity column (Celltech, Berkshire, U.K.). Following extensive washing, IL-2-toxin was eluted from the column with 4 M guanidine hydrochloride in 100 mM Tris-HCl, pH 9.0. Chimeric toxin preparation were exhaustively dialysed and stored at -76°C until used.

Cytoxicity assays. Eukaryotic cells were seeded in 96 well plates at 2 x 10^5 cells/ml in Dulbecco's Modified Eagle Medium (DMEM) supplemented with 10% fetal bovine serum, 2 mM glutamine, 1% non-essential amino acids, and penicillin and Streptomycin to 50 IU and 50 µg/ml, respectively. Diphtheria toxin or IL-2-toxin was added and the plates were incubated at 37°C under 5% CO_2. Following incubation, the medium was removed and replaced with fresh leucine free medium (Spectamine, GIBCO) containing 2% fetal bovine serum and labeled for 2 hr with 0.5 µCi [14C]-leucine (>280 mCi/mmol; New England Nuclear, Boston, MA). Cells were collected on Whatman GF/A filters. Filters were then washed with 5% trichloroacetic acid, phosphate buffered saline, and then were dried and counted in Econofluor (New England Nuclear). Experiments were performed in quadruplicate. Dose response curves compare the incorporation of [14C]-leucine by an untreated control culture to that incorporated by culture exposed to either of the toxins.

Immunoblot analysis. Periplasmic extracts of recombinant E. coli SY327 (pABI508), or purified preparations of diphtheria toxin and IL-2-toxin were electrophoresed in 12.5% polyacrylamide gels containing 0.1% sodium dodecyl sulfate (SDS) essentially as described by Laemmli (1970). Proteins were transferred to nitrocellulose paper as described by Towbin et al. (1979), and immunoblot analysis was performed as described by Robb et al. (1982), except for the incubation buffer which contained 0.15 M NaCl. Antisera to diphtheria toxin was obtained from Connaught Laboratories (Toronto, Canada), and rabbit anti-rIL-2 was obtained from Genzyme (Boston, MA).

Determination of elongation factor 2 levels available for ADP-ribosylation. The level of elongation factor 2 (EF2) that was available for ADP-ribosylation was determined essentially as described by Moynihan and Pappenheimer (1981). Cells were seeded in 24 well plates at a density of 5×10^5/well in 1 ml of medium. Diphtheria toxin, or IL-2-toxin was added to each well in 100 µl medium. Following 24 hr incubation, the cell suspension was transferred to micro-centrifuge tubes and centrifuged for 4 min. The cell pellets were lysed and assayed for the level of EF2 available for ADP-ribosylation by the addition of purified diphtheria toxin fragment A to 2 µg/ml and [32P]-NAD to 1 - 2 Ci/ml. Assays were performed in triplicate.

RESULTS

The chimeric diphtheria toxin-related / IL-2 fusion gene was assembled from plasmid pABC508 and a modified cDNA encoding IL-2. Plasmid pABC508 encodes the diphtheria tox promoter and the tox structural gene from fMet-25 to Ala485 (Bishai et al., 1987). The region of the tox gene that encodes Ala485 is also defined by a unique Sph1 restriction endonuclease site. Cleavage of the tox gene at the Sph1 site and cleavage of vector sequences at a HindIII site results in the deletion of the C-terminal 50 amino acids of diphtheria toxin. Murphy et al. (1986) have recently demonstrated that this region of diphtheria toxin is required for the formation of the toxin's receptor binding domain.

Williams et al. (1987) have modified the 5'-end of the cDNA encoding IL-2 by the insertion of an oligonucleotide linker that introduces a unique Sph1 restriction site such that Pro2 of mature IL-2 could be fused in correct translational reading frame to Ala485 of the tox gene. This genetic construct should then encode a 70,546 molecular weight precursor form of a diphtheria toxin-related / IL-2 fusion protein, IL-2-toxin. In this instance, the C-terminal 50 amino acids of diphtheria toxin will be replaced by 132 amino acids of IL-2. In mature form, IL-2-toxin should be a single chain protein of 617 amino acids with a deduced molecular weight of 68,086. Following ligation and transformation, Williams et al. (1987) isolated several clones of E. coli that were found to carry recombinant plasmids with the restriction endonuclease digestion patterns predicted for the toxin-related / growth factor fusion gene. One of these strains was selected and the recombinant plasmid was designated pABI508 in accordance with the nomenclature proposed by Bishai et al. (1987). In order to insure that the correct translational reading frame was maintained through the fusion junction, the DNA sequence of this region was determined. As seen in Fig. 1, Ala485 of the diphtheria tox gene is fused in correct translational reading frame to Pro2 of IL-2, and the fusion junction is also characterized by an Sph1 restriction site.

Diphtheria tox gene products that are expressed from the tox promoter and contain the tox signal sequence have been shown to be constitutively produced and exported to the periplasmic compartment of recombinant E. coli (Leong et al., 1983; Tweten and Collier, 1983; Bishai et al., 1987b). Following growth and extraction of E. coli(pABI508), we have analyzed crude periplasmic extracts by SDS polyacrylamide gel electrophoresis and immunoblot with anti-diphtheria toxin serum and monoclonal antibody to recombinant IL-2. As shown in Fig. 2, anti-toxin serum was found to react with polypeptides of M_r 68,000, 56,000,

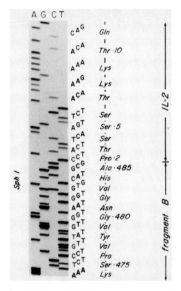

Fig. 1: DNA and deduced amino acid acid sequence of the junction region between the diphtheria tox gene and the cDNA encoding IL-2.

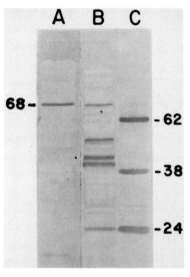

Fig.2: Immunoblot analysis of peri-extracts of E. coli(pABI508). Lane A, anti-rIL-2; Lane B, anti-toxin; Lane C, diphtheria toxin standard probed with anti-toxin

43,000, 41,000, and 24,000 molecular weight. In contrast, anti-IL-2 was found to react with only the M_r 68,000 species. The detection of a 68,000 molecular weight polypeptide that contains immunologic determinants of both diphtheria toxin and IL-2 is in excellent agreement with the deduced molecular weight and antigenic properties expected for the chimeric toxin. It is of interest to note that many of the degradation products of IL-2-toxin have apparent molecular weights that are identical to that of the degradation products of α-MSH-toxin and are likely to be the result of the action of E. coli endopeptidase(s) (Swamy and Goldberg, 1982; Murphy et al., 1986).

Williams et al. (1987) have partially purified IL-2-toxin from crude periplasmic extracts of E. coli(pABI508) by immuno-affinity chromatography using immobilized monoclonal antibody to recombinant IL-2 (Fig. 3). Following elution with 4 M guanidine hydrochloride in 100 mM Tris-HCl, pH 8.3, IL-2-toxin was exhaustively dialysed and tested for biologic activity against a variety of eukaryotic cell lines. As seen in Table 2, there is a direct correlation between the sensitivity of a given cell line to IL-2-toxin mediated inhibition of protein synthesis and the presence of "high" affinity IL-2R on the cell surface.

In order to demonstrate that the cytotoxic effect of IL-2-toxin on IL-2R bearing cells was mediated through the IL-2R, Bacha et al. (1987) have examined the effect of several competitive inhibitors. As can be seen in Table 3, both excess free recombinant IL-2 and a monoclonal antibody, 33B.3, directed against the Tac antigen of the IL-2R were effective in blocking the cytoxic action of IL-2-toxin in vitro. In contrast, the addition of transferrin or a monoclonal antibody, 4F2, that is directed toward an early activation antigen on the T-cell surface had no effect on the action of IL-2-toxin.

TABLE 2 Comparison of the Sensitivity of Various IL-2R$^+$ and IL-2R$^-$ Eukaryotic Cell Lines to IL-2-toxin [adapted from Williams et al., 1987].

cell line	source	IL-2R	IL-2-toxin sensitivity
C91/PL	human, T-cell	+	+
CTLL-2	murine, T-cell	+	+
C8215	human, T-cell	+	+
CEM-3	human, T-cell	−	−
Karpas	human, T-cell	−	−
U937	human, myeloid leukemia	−	−

+, IC50 <1 x 10^{-9}M;   −, IC50 >5 x 10^{-8}M

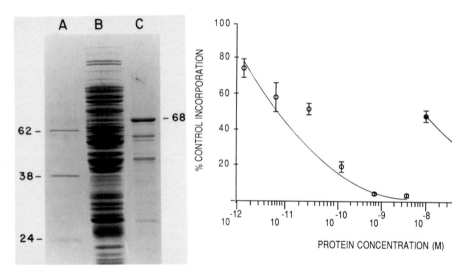

Fig. 3: SDS-polyacrylamide gel analysis of partially purified IL-2-toxin. Lane A, molecular weight standards; Lane B, periplasmic extracts of E. coli(pABI508); Lance C, immuno-affinity purified IL-2-toxin.

Fig. 4: Dose response analysis of IL-2-toxin (○) and diphtheria toxin (●) on the IL-2R$^+$ human C91/Pl T-cell line.

Following binding to specific receptors on the surface of sensitive cells, diphtheria toxin has been shown to be concentrated in coated pits and to be internalized by receptor mediated endocytosis (Moya et al., 1985). It is widely known that lysozomatrophic agents that prevent acidification of the endosome block the entry of diphtheria toxin fragment A into the cytosol (Kim and Groman, 1965; Sandvig et al., 1985). In experiments to further characterize the mechanism of IL-2-toxin entry into IL-2R$^+$ T cells, Bacha et al. (1987) has found that the addition of chloroquine to 6 x 10^{-6}M to C91/PL cells in culture completely blocks the action of IL-2-toxin (Table 3). These results demonstrate that IL-2-toxin, like diphtheria toxin, must pass through an acidic vesicle in order to deliver its ADP- ribosyl transferase to the cytosol.

TABLE 3 Incorporation of [14C]-leucine by Human C91/PL IL-2R[+] T-cells
Following a 24 Hour Exposure to IL-2-toxin in the Presence or Absence
of Various Additions [adapted from Bacha et al., 1987].

IL-2-toxin concentration	additions	% control incorporation
-	-	100
4×10^{-9}M	-	14
"	IL-2 (10^{-7}M)	111
"	33B.3 (10^{-7}M)	72
"	transferrin (10^{-7}M)	17
"	4F2 (10^{-7}M)	15
-	chloroquine (6 x10^{-6}M)	85
1×10^{-9}M	-	38
"	chloroquine (6 x 10^{-6}M)	90

Bacha et al. (1987) have further characterized the sensitivity of human T-cell
lines to both IL-2-toxin and diphtheria toxin by dose response analysis. As
shown in Fig. 4, in C91/PL cells the IC_{50} for IL-2-toxin and diphtheria toxin
were found to be 1×10^{-11}M and 1×10^{-8}M, respectively. Similar results have
been obtained for a variety of human "high" affinity IL-2R[+] T-cell lines (Bacha,
unpublished observations). In striking contrast, human T-cells that are devoid
of the "high" affinity IL-2R are resistant to the action of IL-2-toxin (Fig. 5).

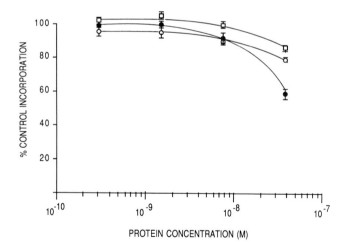

Figure 5: Dose response analysis of IL-2-toxin
on a variety IL-2R[-] cell lines. (□), CEM-3;
(○), Karpas; (●), U937.

Finally, in order to demonstrate that the IL-2-toxin mediated inhibition of
protein synthesis in T-cells was not due to stearic hindrance imposed by
blocking the IL-2R, we have measured the levels of elongation factor 2 (EF2) in

TABLE 4 Murine CTLL-2 and Human C91/PL Elongation Factor 2 that is Available for ADP-ribosylation Following 24 Hour Exposure to Either IL-2-toxin or Diphtheria Toxin [adapted from Bacha et al., 1987].

cell line	toxin and concentration	% control level of EF2 available for ADP-ribosylation
CTLL-2	diphtheria (10^{-7}M)	98
	IL-2-toxin (10^{-8}M)	8
C91/PL	diphtheria (10^{-6}M)	<5
	IL-2-toxin (10^{-8}M)	<5

C91/PL and CTLL-2 cells that was available for ADP-ribosylation following exposure to IL-2-toxin. As shown in Table 4, murine CTLL-2 cells which are resistant to diphtheria toxin have reduced levels of EF2 available for ADP-ribosylation only after exposure to IL-2-toxin. In the case of human C91/PL cells which are sensitive to both IL-2-toxin and diphtheria toxin, reduced levels of EF2 available for ADP-ribosylation were found after exposure to either toxin.

DISCUSSION

We have used protein engineering and recombinant DNA methodologies for the genetic assembly of a fusion gene in which the diphtheria toxin receptor binding domain has been replaced with the lymphocytotrophic factor IL-2. The resulting chimeric IL-2-toxin has been cloned in E. coli K-12 and is constitutively expressed from the diphtheria tox promoter and exported to the periplasmic compartment. The mature form of the fusion protein is composed of diphtheria toxin sequences from Gly1 to Ala485 which is linked to Pro2 through Thr133 of IL-2 by a peptide bond. Williams et al. (1987) have demonstrated that IL-2-toxin selectively inhibits protein synthesis in IL-2R$^+$ HTLV-I transformed human T-cell lines, as well as the IL-2 dependent murine CTLL-2 cell line. In both instances, the action of IL-2-toxin may be blocked with agents that bind to the IL-2R; whereas, agents that bind to other receptors or antigens on the T-cell surface fail to inhibit the action of IL-2-toxin.

Bacha et al. (1987) have shown that IL-2-toxin appears to be internalized by receptor mediated endocytosis into vesicles which become acidified. Since chloroquine blocks IL-2-toxin mediated inhibition of protein synthesis, we conclude that IL-2-toxin must pass through an acidic vesicle in order to deliver its ADP-ribosyl transferase across the endosomal membrane. In addition, Bacha et al. (1987) have demonstrated that both murine and human IL-2R$^+$ T-cells that have been exposed to IL-2-toxin have reduced levels of EF2 available for ADP-ribosylation. These results demonstrate that the inhibition of protein synthesis in IL-2R$^+$ target T-cells the result of the classic diphtheria toxin fragment A catalysed reaction.

It is of particular interest to note that the diphtheria toxin-related IL-2-toxin is active against the murine CTLL-2 T-cell line. It is widely known that cell lines derived from diphtheria toxin resistant species (e.g., mouse and rat) are resistant to the action of diphtheria toxin. Since the EF2 derived from these cell lines is sensitive to ADP-ribosylation in vitro, it was not known whether the intact cell resistance to diphtheria toxin was due to a non-functional toxin receptor, a defect in the internalization process, or alternatively to a defect in a putative processing event that may be involved in the intoxication process. The sensitivity of CTLL-2 cells to IL-2-toxin clearly demonstrates that the binding of a diphtheria toxin-related fusion protein to a functional receptor (IL-2R) results in the internalization of IL-2-toxin, and the subsequent delivery of its fragment A to the cytosol. These results would suggest that if the diphtheria toxin receptor were present on the surface of murine cells, it is non-functional. If the receptor is present, then one would predict that either it fails to internalize bound toxin, or fails to bind diphtheria toxin. Alternatively, the diphtheria toxin receptor may simply not be present on the surface of mouse or rat cells.

ACKNOWLEDGMENTS

This work was supported in part by Public Health Service grants AI21628 (J.R.M.) and AI22882 (T.B.S.) from the National Institute of Allergy and Infectious Diseases, and CA41746 (J.R.M.) from the National Cancer Institute (J.R.M.). We thank Dr. Robert Schwartz, Tufts Medical School, Boston, MA, and Dr. John Williams, Harvard Medical School, Boston, MA for providing eukaryotic cell lines. In addition, we thank Dr. Donna Akiyoshi for assistance in DNA sequencing and Dr. Frank Genbauffe for many helpful discussions.

REFERENCES

Bacha, P., C.Waters, J.Williams, J.R.Murphy, and T.B. Strom (1987). Interleukin 2 receptor targeted cytotoxicity. II. Selective action of a diphtheria toxin-related interleukin-2 fusion protein. J.Exp.Med., (submitted for publication).

Bishai, W.R., A.Miyanohara, and J.R.Murphy (1987). Cloning and expression in Escherichia coli of three fragments of diphtheria toxin truncated within fragment B. J.Bacteriol., 169, 1554-1563.

Bishai, W.R., R.Rappuoli, and J.R.Murphy (1987b). High level expression of a proteolytically sensitive diphtheria toxin fragment in Escherichia coli. J.Bacteriol., (Submitted for publication).

Cotner, T., J.M.Williams, L.Christenson, T.Reddish, H.J.Shapiro, T.B.Strom, and J.Strominger (1983). Simultaneous flow cytometric analysis of human T-cell activation antigen expression and DNA content. J.Exp.Med., 157, 461-472.

Fugii, M., K.Sugamura, K.Sano, M.Naki, K.Sagita, and Y.Hinuma (1986). High-affinity receptor-mediated internalization and degradation of interleukin-2 in human T-cells. J.Exp.Med., 163, 550-562.

Gillis, S., and K.A.Smith (1977). Long-term culture of cytotoxic T-lymphocytes. Nature (London) 268, 154-156.

Haseltine, W.A., J.Sodroski, R.Patarca, D.Briggs, D.Perkins, F.Wong-Stall (1984). Structure of 3' terminal region of type II human T lymphotrophic virus: Evidence for a new coding region. Science 225, 419-421.

Isberg, R.R., A.L.Lazaar, and M.Syvanen (1982). Regulation of Tn5 by the right repeat proteins: control at the level of the transposition reaction? Cell, 30, 883-892.

Kim, K., and N.B.Groman (1965). In vitro inhibition of diphtheria toxin action by ammonium salts and amines. J.Bacteriol., 90, 1557-1562.

Kuo, L.-M., C.M.Rusk, and R.J.Robb (1986). Structure function relationships for the IL-2 receptor system. 2. Localization of an IL-2 binding site on high and low affinity receptors. J.Immunol., 137, 1544-1551.

Laemmli, U.K. (1970). Cleavage of structural proteins during the assembly of the head of bacteriophage T4. Nature (London), 227, 680-685.

Leong, D., K.D.Coleman, and J.R.Murphy (1983). Cloned diphtheria toxin fragment A is expressed from the tox promoter and exported to the periplasm by the SecA apparatus of Escherichia coli K12. J.Biol.Chem., 258, 15016-15020.

Lowenthal,.J.W., R.H.Zubler, M.Nabholz, and H.R.MacDonald (1985). Similarities between interleukin-2 receptor number and affinity on activated lymphocyte-T and lymphocyte-B. Nature (London), 325, 669-672.

Maniatis, T., E.F.Fritsch, and J.Sambrook (1982). Molecular cloning: a laboratory manual. Cold Spring Harbor Laboratory, Cold Spring Harbor, New York

Moya, M., A.Dautry-Varsat, B.Goud, D.Louvard, and P.Boquet (1985). Inhibition of coated pit formation in Hep2 cells blocks the cytotoxicity of diphtheria toxin but not that of ricin. J.Cell Biol., 101, 548-559.

Moynihan, M., and A.M.Pappenheimer, Jr. (1981). Kinetics of adenosine diphos-phorribosylation of elongation factor 2 in cells exposed to diphtheria toxin. Infect.Immun., 32, 575-582.

Murphy, J.R., W.Bishai, M.Borowski, A.Miyanohara, J.Boyd, and S.Nagle (1986). Genetic construction, expression, and melanoma-selective cytotoxicity of a diphtheria toxin-related -melanocyte stimulating hormone fusion protein. Proc.Natl.Acad.Sci.USA, 83, 8258-8262.

Robb, M., J.C.Nichols, S.K.Whoriskey, and J.R.Murphy (1982). Isolation of hybridoma cell lines and characterization of monoclonal antibodies against cholera toxin and its subunits. Infect.Immun., 38, 267-272.

Robb, R.J., W.C.Greene, and C.M.Rusk (1984). Low and high affinity receptors for interleukin-2: implications for the level of Tac antigen. J.Exp.Med., 160, 1126-1146.

Robb, R.J., C.M.Rusk, J.Yodoi, and W.C.Greene (1987). Interleukin-2 binding molecule distinct from the Tac protein: analysis of its role in formation of high-affinity receptors. Proc.Nalt.Acad.Sci.USA, 84, 2002-2006.

Sandvig, K., T.I.Tonnessen, O.Sand, and S.Olsnes (1986). Requirement of a transmembrane pH gradient for the entry of diphtheria toxin into cells at low pH. J.Biol.Chem., 261, 11639-11644.

Sanger, F., S.Nicklen, and A.R.Coulson (1977). DNA sequencing with chain terminating inhibitors. Proc.Natl.Acad.Sci.USA, 74, 5463-5467.

Swamy, K.H.S., and A.L.Goldberg (1982). Subcellular distribution of various proteases in Escherichia coli. J.Bacteriol., 149, 1027-1033.

Smith, K.A. (1984). Interleukin-2. Annu.Rev.Immunol., 2, 319-333.

Towbin, H., T.Staehelin, and J.Gordon (1979). Electrophoretic transfer of proteins from polyacrylamide gels to nitrocellulose sheets: procedure and applications. Nature (London), 76, 4350-4354.

Tweten, R.K., and R.J.Collier (1983). Molecular cloning and expression of gene fragments from corynebacteriophage encoding enzymatically active peptides of diphtheria toxin. J.Bacteriol., 156, 680-685.

Waldmann, T.A. (1986). The interleukin-2 receptor on malignant cells: a target for diagnosis and therapy. Cell.Immun., 99, 53-60.

Weissman, A.M., J.B.Harford, P.B.Svetlik, W.L.Leonard, J.M.Depper, T.A.Waldmann, and W.C.Greene (1986). Only high affinity receptor for interleukin-2 mediate internalization of ligand. Proc.Natl.Acad.Sci.USA, 83, 1463-1466.

Williams, D.P., K.Parker, W.Bishai, M.Borowski, F.Genbauffe, T.B.Strom, and J.R.Murphy (1987). Interleukin-2 receptor targeted cytotoxicity: I. Genetic construction, expression, and purification of a diphtheria toxin-related interleukin-2 fusion protein. J.Exp.Med., (submitted for publication).

Williams, J.M., R.Loertscher, T.Cotner, M.Reddish, H.J.Shapiro, C.B.Carpenter, J.Strominger, and T.B.Strom (1984). Dual parametric flow cytometric analysis of DNA content, activation antigen, and T-cell subset proliferation in the human lymphocyte reaction. J.Immunol., 132, 2330-2337.

Fehrenbach et al. (Eds.), Bacterial Protein Toxins, Zbl. Bakt. Suppl. 17
© Gustav Fischer, Stuttgart, New York, 1988

Antibody-DT Conjugates in the Study of Surface Antigen Properties and DT Cytotoxic Mechanism[1]

M. Colombatti[1], L. Dell'Arciprete[1], L. Greenfield[2], R. J. Youle[3], R. Rappuoli[4], G. Tridente[1]

[1]Ist. di Scienze Immunol., Univ. of Verona Italy
[2]Cetus Corporation, San Francisco, U.S.A.
[3]Natl. Inst. of Health, Bethesda, U.S.A.
[4]Centro di Ricerche Sclavo, Siena, Italy

ABSTRACT

Antibody-toxin conjugates (Immunotoxins) made with ricin and diphtheria toxin (DT) and with monoclonal antibodies (mAb) against different T-cell antigens (Ag), CD5 (T101) and CD3 (UCHT1, OKT3) were studied. UCHT1-DT and OKT3-DT immunotoxins (IT) were 10-100 fold more toxic for Jurkat T leukemia cells than native DT. The kinetics of UCHT1-DT were 6-30 times faster than other IT. We suggest that the T3 antigen may have a role in facilitating the transport of DT to the cytosol. We have also investigated the role of discrete domains of DT B chain in cytosol entry and cytotoxicity by linking UCHT1 mAb to DT, DT A chain or to a genetically engineered form of DT (MspSA) lacking the C-terminal 17 Kd end of the B subunit. Addition of increasing lenghts of DT B to the IT increased toxicity considerably. A mutant of DT (CRM 1001) with a cys→tyr substitution in the 17 Kd C-terminus of DT B was 1,000-10,000 fold less toxic for Jurkat and Vero cells. The OKT3-CRM 1001 IT was 1,000 fold less toxic than OKT3-DT for Jurkat target cells. Entry of CRM-1001 via an alternate receptor did not seem to overcome its translocation block.

KEYWORDS

Diphtheria toxin, cell surface antigens, antibody-toxin conjugates, penetration mechanisms.

INTRODUCTION

Antibodies to cell surface Ag have been chemically coupled to DT, ricin or their subunits to synthesize cell type-specific cytotoxic reagents (for a review see Youle and Colombatti,1986a). Ricin and DT are 60-65 Kd proteins with two functionally distinct subunits : the A chain inhibits enzymatically the protein synthesis of the target cell and the B chain binds cell surface receptors and facilitates

[1]Our work has been supported in part by PFCCN, CNR, Rome (Italy)

the passage of the A subunit to the cytosol (Pappenheimer, 1977).
Ricin IT are rendered cell-specific by adding lactose to the culture media (Youle, Murray and Neville, 1979). We describe in this paper a very potent intact DT IT directed against sensitive human cells. This IT, synthesized with mAb to the human lymphocyte Ag T3 linked to DT (UCHT1-DT) showed exceptional properties: we concluded that the differentiation Ag T3 has a role in facilitating DT penetration and toxicity.

DT B chain facilitates the entry of DT A chain to the cytosol and its presence in intact DT IT renders them more toxic although less specific. The 17 Kd C-terminal region of DT B contains the cell surface binding domain (Eisenberg and others, 1984). Three other hydrophobic domains are found within the N-terminal region of DT B chain. These hydrophobic regions facilitate DT entry by membrane insertion at low pH (Sandvig and Olsnes, 1981). The role of discrete DT B subdomains in cell entry as distingueshed from cell binding has been investigated by comparing the cytotoxic activity of anti T3 mAb (UCHT1, OKT3) linked to DT, DT A chain, MspSA (a genetically engineered DT lacking the C-terminal 17 Kd region) or the DT mutant CRM-1001.

MATERIALS AND METHODS

Reagents

Ricin was purified according to Nicolson, Blaustein and Etzler (1974). DT was purchased from List Biologicals and from Calbiochem. DT A chain was purified according to Chang and Collier (1977) and Sandvig and Olsnes (1981). UCHT1 (IgG$_1$) was a gift from Unilever, T101 (IgG$_{2a}$) was provided by Hybritech and OKT3 (IgG$_{2a}$) was purified from ascites obtained by injecting hybridoma cells intra peritoneally into BALB/c mice. MspSA is a recombinant derivative of DT synthesized in E.coli and consisting of aminoacids 1 through 382 of the native DT sequence (Youle and others, 1986b). After purification MspSA was obtained as a >95% pure protein of 45 Kd according to SDS-PAGE. CRM-1001 obtained >95% pure from culture filtrates of the appropriate strain of C.diphtheriae after phenyl-sepharose chromatography, has a cys→tyr subsitution at position 471 of DT B chain. Toxin-mAb conjugates cross-linked with SPDP or MBS (Pierce) were separated from unreacted toxins or antibodies by gel filtration on HPLC.

Protein Synthesis Assay

Protein synthesis was assayed essentially as described (Youle and Neville, 1982), by evaluating incorporation of ^{14}C- leucine in treated or control cells. Ricin IT were assayed in the presence of 100 mM lactose to block non target cell binding of ricin.

RESULTS

Toxicity of UCHT1-DT for Human Cells and Kinetics of Target Cell Killing

The toxicity of anti T3 IT was assayed against a human T3$^+$ leukemia cell line (Jurkat). As shown in Table 1 UCHT1-DT had the fastest kinetics killing 90% of target cells within 2 hrs. At 4x10^{-9} M UCHT1-DT was not toxic for T3$^-$ target cells (not shown). All other IT examined killed cells with a 6 to 30 fold slower kinetics at similar concentrations. UCHT1-ricin killed 1 log of target cells in 20 hrs. We investigated the cytotoxicity via another T cell associated surface

TABLE 1 Comparison of IT Kinetics

Immunotoxin	Concentration (M)	Target Cell	$t_{10}(hr)^a$	Reference
UCHT1-DT	4×10^{-9}	Jurkat	2	our work
UCHT1-ricin	2×10^{-9}	Jurkat	20	our work
T101-ricin	4×10^{-9}	Jurkat	20	our work
T101-DT	2×10^{-9}	Jurkat	20	our work
T101-RTA[b]	2×10^{-8}	CEM	60	Casellas,1984
Transferrin-RTA	10^{-7}	K562	20	Raso, 1984
Thy1.1-ricin	10^{-9}	AKR-SL2	12	Youle, 1982
α-murine IgG-RTA	10^{-7}	Murine B cells	60	Miyazaki, 1980

[a] t_{10} is the time required for 90% inhibition of protein synthesis.

[b] RTA, ricin A chain.

antigens (CD5) recognized by the mAb T101. T101 IT had 10-30 fold slower kinetics than UCHT1-DT. T101 mAb has more binding sites on Jurkat cells than UCHT1 mAb and has a higher affinity (not shown). Therefore, mAb subclass, number of binding sites or affinity cannot explain the differences between UCHT1-DT and the other IT.

Role of DT B Chain Domains in IT Toxicity and Penetration

We have compared the cytotoxic activity of UCHT1 and OKT3 anti T3 mAb linked to DT, to two size-derivatives of DT and to a mutant form of DT with an aminoacid substitution in the 17 Kd C-terminus of DT B chain. As shown in Table 2, UCHT1-DTA, UCHT1-MspSA and UCHT1-DT had increasing toxicity for Jurkat target cells. The DT IT was therefore about 100-fold more toxic than the MspSA IT and about 10,000-fold more toxic than the DTA IT. DT was about 30 fold less toxic than UCHT1-DT and OKT3-DT, and CRM-1001 was 10-fold less toxic than OKT3-CRM 1001. The same difference in toxicity observed between DT and CRM-1001 (about 800-fold) was also observed between OKT3-DT and OKT3-CRM 1001 (about 1400-fold).

The specificity of the IT was demonstrated by blocking cytotoxicity with excess nonconjugated mAb or by the reduced cytotoxic effect for non target cells. Control experiments ruled out differences in ADP-ribosylation activity of DT A chain, binding activity of the IT or cross-linking methods as the cause of cytotoxicity differences (not shown), so we conclude that the large differences in toxicity were due to the different DT B chain domains.

TABLE 2 Role of DT B Chain Domains in Anti T3 IT Activity

Immunotoxin	IC_{50}[a]	Specificity Factor[b]
UCHT1-DT	3×10^{-12}	100
UCHT1-MspSA	3×10^{-10}	>10
UCHT1-DTA	2×10^{-8}	not det.
OKT3-DT	5×10^{-12}	100
OKT3-CRM 1001	7×10^{-9}	>100
DT	8×10^{-11}	—
CRM 1001	7×10^{-8}	—

[a] The IC_{50} is the molar concentration of the IT required to inhibit the protein synthesis of target cells to 50% of control values in a 24 hr assay.

[b] The specificity factor represents the difference between the IC_{50} of the IT on untarget cells and the IC_{50} of the IT for target cells.

DISCUSSION

We have studied the properties of an anti T3 DT conjugate and compared its cyto-toxic activity with that of other IT. We found that the cytotoxic kinetics via the T3 antigen is extremely rapid. UCHT1-DT killed target cells 6-30 times faster than any other IT examined. The 17 Kd C-terminus of DT B chain binds cell surface receptors; DT is successively internalized by receptor-mediated endocytosis and passage through an acidic compartment. At low pH the hydrophobic domains of DT B are exposed and then the toxin crosses the membrane.

UCHT1-DT has a faster kinetics than DT (not shown), T101-DT or UCHT1-ricin. Therefore, the activity that facilitates DT entry does not facilitate ricin entry; moreover, rapid penetration of DT is linked to the T3 Ag but not the T101 Ag. The T3 Ag has several peculiar properties that may explain the fast entry rate of UCHT1-DT : 1) rapid and efficient modulation upon Ab binding (Rinnooy and others, 1983); 2) function in lymphocyte activation coupled to an increase in intracellular Ca^{++} levels. Modulated and internalized T3 may compartmentalize in a low pH environment which facilitates DT entry but not ricin entry, which is instead degraded in the lysosomes (Casellas and others, 1984).

We have also studied the role of DT B chain in cell penetration as distinguished from cell binding by adding a new binding moiety to various size derivatives of DT and to one DT mutant, CRM-1001 which appears to be defective in transmembrane translocation. UCHT1 mAb linked to DT A chain had low toxicity, but addition of the 21 Kd N-terminus of DT B (as in UCHT1-MspSA) with its three hydrofobic domains, augmented the IT efficacy about 100 fold. Addition of the 17 Kd C-terminal

domains of DT B by linking intact DT to UCHT1 mAb increased toxicity 100-200 fold more. The additional hydrophobic domain of the DT B C-terminus might be responsible for the high cytotoxic efficacy of UCHT1-DT. Linkage of CRM-1001 to an anti T3 mAb and penetration via an alternate receptor did not increase its entry rate. The cys→tyr substitution in the 17 Kd C-terminus could have affected DT penetration a)by altering the 17 Kd C-terminal domain conformation or b)its hydrophobic interactions or c) by eliminating a residue directly involved in cell entry. Immunotoxins are widely used for in vitro cell depletion and have great potential for in vitro cancer therapy (Youle and Colombatti, 1987).
Intact toxins IT are very potent, but may have too much nontarget cell toxicity for in vivo use. Identification of different functional activities within different toxin B chain subdomains may be helpful in designing IT with high cytotoxicity and low nonspecific side effects.

REFERENCES

Casellas,P., B.J. Bourrie, and F.K. Jansen (1984). Kinetics of cytotoxicity induced by immunotoxins. Enhancement by lysosomotropic amines and carboxilic ionophores. J. Biol.Chem., 259, 9359-9364.

Chang,D.W.,and R.J.Collier (1977). The mechanism of ADP-ribosylation of elongation factor 2 catalyzed by fragment A from diphtheria toxin. Biochem.Biophys. Acta, 483, 248-257.

Eisenberg,D., E.Schwarz, M.Komaromy, and R.Wall (1984). Analysis of surface protein sequence with the hydrophobic moment plot. J.Mol.Biol., 179, 125-132.

Nicolson,G.L., J.Blaustein, and M.E.Etzler (1974). Characterization of two plant lectins from Ricinus communis and their quantitative interaction with a murine lymphoma. Biochemistry, 13, 196-202.

Pappenheimer,A.M. Jr (1977). Diphtheria toxin. Annu.Rev.Biochem., 46, 69-94.

Rinnooy Kan,E.A., C.Y.Wang, L.C. Wang, and R.L.Evans (1983). Noncovalently bonded subunits of 22 and 28 Kd are rapidly internalized by T cells reacted with anti-Leu-4 antibody. J.Immunol., 131, 536-538.

Sandvig,K., and S.Olsnes (1981). Rapid entry of nicked Diphtheria toxin into cells at low pH. Characterization of the entry process and effects of low pH on the toxin molecule. J.Biol.Chem., 256, 9068-9076.

Youle,R.J., G.J.Murray, and D.M.Jr Neville (1979). Ricin linked to monophosphopentamannose binds to fibroblast lysosomal hydrolase receptors resulting in a cell-type specific toxin. Proc.Natl.Acad.Sci. USA, 75, 5559-5562.

Youle,R.J., and D.M.Jr Neville (1982). Kinetics of protein synthesis inactivation by ricin-anti Thy 1.1 monoclonal antibody hybrids. J.Biol.Chem., 257, 1598-1601.

Youle,R.J., and M.Colombatti (1986a).Immunotoxins: monoclonal antibodies linked to toxic proteins for bone marrow transplantation and cancer therapy. In: J.Roth (Ed.), Monoclonal antibodies for the diagnosis and therapy of cancer, Futura Publishing Co., New York, pp. 173-213.

Youle,R.J., F.M.Uckun, D.A.Vallera, and M.Colombatti (1986b). Immunotoxins show rapid entry of diphtheria toxin but not ricin via the T3 antigen. J.Immunol., 136, 93-98.

Fehrenbach et al. (Eds.), Bacterial Protein Toxins, Zbl. Bakt. Suppl. 17
© Gustav Fischer, Stuttgart, New York, 1988

Novel Approaches to Vaccine Production

N. F. Fairweather, V. A. Lyness, D. Maskell and G. Dougan

Bacterial Genetics Group, Department of Molecular Biology, Wellcome Research Laboratories, Beckenham, Kent, BR3 3BS, England

ABSTRACT

The cloning of the gene for tetanus toxin and expression of non-toxic fragments in E.coli is described. Mice immunised with these protein fragments survived challenge with tetanus toxin, demonstrating that it is possible to construct tetanus vaccine in E.coli. The use of live attenuated Salmonella strains as a carrier for a new generation of tetanus vaccines is discussed. The virulence factors of B.pertussis are described briefly, in the context of the composition of possible acellular pertussis vaccines.

KEYWORDS

Vaccine, tetanus, pertussis, live oral vaccine, recombinant DNA, Salmonella.

INTRODUCTION

Many pathogenic bacteria produce one or more protein toxins, some of which are presumed to be of importance in the pathogenesis of the disease process. Several bacterial toxins have been studied as possible protective antigens after inactivation by, for example, formaldehyde. However for many bacterial infections, the protective effect of vaccines based on one isolated toxin is poor, reinforcing the idea that for most bacterial infections there are several important virulence factors.

This article will concentrate on two bacterial vaccines, pertussis and tetanus. Both Bordetella pertussis, the causative agent of whooping cough and C.tetani, which is responsible for tetanus, produce protein toxins. However while tetanus toxin is solely responsible for the clinical symptoms of tetanus, pertussis toxin is only one of many virulence factors produced by B.pertussis which appear to contribute to the disease caused by the organism.

PERTUSSIS VACCINE

Over the past few years, there has been much research into the development of an acellular vaccine against whooping cough. This is due largely to the low acceptance of the current whole cell vaccine, which is composed of heat killed B.pertussis cells. Ideally an acellular vaccine will be composed of only those cellular components which are essential for providing long term protective immunity against B.pertussis infection. Much of the research into a new vaccine has concentrated on genetic cloning and characterisation of those components which are thought to contribute to the virulence of the organism (Weiss and co-workers, 1983). Hopefully such work will lead to the analysis of the structure and function of many of these factors, increasing our knowledge of their role in virulence. In addition, cloning will allow the production of large amounts of these proteins, possibly in a heterologous host, eg E.coli. These components may then be tested as vaccine constituents of acellular vaccines.

Much of the work so far has concentrated on pertussis toxin (see Rappouli and co-workers, this volume), and a great deal of knowledge concerning the regulation and sub-unit structure of this toxin has been obtained (Locht and Keith, 1986; Nicosia and co-workers,1986). One acellular vaccine composed of pertussis toxin and filamentous haemagglutinin has been used in Japan for several years now, (for a review, see Manclark and Cowell, 1984) and clinical trials currently underway in Sweden should give an indication of the efficacy of these vaccines.

There are however many virulence factors of B.pertussis which could be considered as components of an acellular vaccine including pertussis toxin, filamentous haemagglutinin, dermonecrotic toxin, tracheal cytotoxin, agglutinogens, lipopolysaccharide, adenylate cylase and outer membrane proteins (for a review see Weiss and Hewlett, 1896). The genes for several of these have been cloned (eg. Nicosia and co-workers, 1986; Locht and Keith, 1986; Brownlie and co-workers 1986; Brown and Parker, 1987) and we can expect to see detailed structures for many of these B.pertussis antigens in the next few years. We can also expect to have several different candidate acellular vaccines based on one or more of these antigens, and hopefully clinical trials will be arranged to determine which antigens are most suitable for an effective and safe acellular vaccine against whooping cough.

TETANUS VACCINE

Tetanus is one of the most effective toxoid based vaccines used today. The clinical symptoms of tetanus are caused solely by tetanus toxin which is produced by C.tetani. Immunisation with tetanus toxoid induces anti-toxin antibodies which completely neutralise the effects of this toxin, and completely prevent the symptoms of the disease.

Tetanus toxin is produced intracellularly by C.tetani as a single polypeptide of molecular weight 150,000. Upon cell lysis, the toxin is cleaved into the 50,000 light chain disulphide bonded to the 100,00 dalton heavy chain (Matsuda and Yoneda, 1975). The toxin may be cleaved by papain to yield a 50,000 dalton carboxy terminal fragment C (Helting and Zwisler, 1977). See Fig. 1.

The current tetanus vaccines have changed little over the past twenty years, largly because the vaccines offer complete protection to those individuals receiving a full vaccination course. The vaccine consists of whole toxin which has been formaldehyde treated. The production of this vaccine has been reviewed (Bizzini, 1974). Fragments of the toxin have been used as experimental vaccines (Helting and Nau, 1984) showing that the entire toxin is not necessary for generation of protective antibodies.

Recombinant DNA tetanus vaccines

In order to investigate the requirement for various portions of the tetanus molecule for immunisation, we are studying the toxin at the molecular level. We have described previously the cloning of part of the tetanus gene coding for fragment C (Fairweather and co-workers, 1986), and have recently completed the cloning and DNA sequencing of the entire toxin gene (Fairweather and Lyness,1986). We cloned the gene from total C.tetani DNA as a series of overlapping fragments in E.coli plasmid vectors. The orientation of the fragments and a restriction map is presented in Fig. 1. Only one open reading frame was found, giving a protein of the expected size of 150,000 daltons.

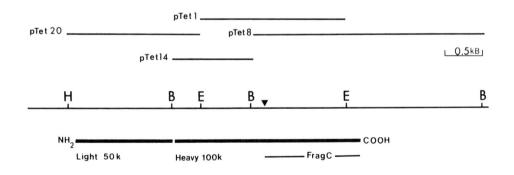

Fig. 1: Structure of tetanus toxin and the fragments of the gene cloned in E.coli. The restriction map is presented below the fragments cloned. E, EcoRI; B, BamHI; H, HindIII. The position of the protein fragments is shown in the bottom line.

The DNA sequence is identical to that deduced for the tetanus gene from a different strain of C.tetani by Eisel and co-workers (1986). The similarity is not surprising as both our strain, CN3911, and that used by Eisel and co-workers are vaccine production strains and most probably originate from the strain isolated by Meuller and Miller (1954) as a high toxin producer.

The availability of the entire DNA sequence allowed us to design several expression constructs in E.coli where defined portions of the toxin molecule were expressed (Fairweather and co-workers 1986). In this article we will describe the properties of one plasmid (pTet18) which expresses a 63,000 protein comprising 121 amino acids of fragment B and the entire 451 amino acids of fragment C (see Fig. 1). We chose initially to concentrate on clones expressing fragment C because it is completely non-toxic and will induce protective antibodies in animals (Helting and Zwisler, 1977). The synthesis of pTet18 protein is under the control of the tac promoter and is induced by the addition of IPTG. The E.coli produced pTet18 protein was found to be insoluble and this provided us with a simple way of partially purifying this protein by differential centrifugation. pTet18 protein was analysed by SDS polyacrylamide gel electrophoresis and Western blotting and was shown to cross react with anti-fragment C antibodies, verifying that the protein is a fragment of tetanus toxin (data not shown).

TABLE 1 Immunisation of Mice Against Tetanus with E.coli Derived Fragments

Protein	Amount (ug) [a]	Adjuvant	ABT_{50} [b]	Survivors [c]
pTet18	100	Yes	734	10/10
"	10	Yes	368	10/10
"	1	Yes	232	10/10
"	0.1	Yes	79	1/10
Fragment C	10	Yes	2137	10/10
"	1	Yes	304	10/10
"	0.1	Yes	48	2/10
"	0.01	Yes	40	0/10
pTet18	100	No	ND [d]	10/10
"	10	No	ND	10/10
"	1	No	ND	10/10
"				

(a) Mice were given 1 shot of vaccine with or without CFA.
(b) Titre of anti-tetanus toxoid antibodies.
(c) Mice were challenged with 10 LD_{50} tetanus toxin.
(d) ND not determined.

As fragment C is protective in animals, it was of interest to determine whether the pTet18 protein could also induce protective antibodies. Mice were immunised with various amounts of pTet18 protein, either with or without complete Freunds adjuvant (CFA). Table 1 shows the results of these experiments. Mice given one shot of various amounts of either pTet18 (from E.coli) or fragment C (from C.tetani) in CFA developed dose-dependant titres of anti-tetanus toxoid antibodies. The mice were challenged with 10 LD_{50} tetanus toxin, and survivors were recorded after 4 days. Amounts of 1ug or more pTet18 gave complete protection, whereas 0.1 ug gave only partial protection. The requirement for an adjuvant was investigated by immunising mice with 1, 10 or 100 ug pTet18 protein without adjuvant. All these doses gave complete protection from toxin challenge, indicating that an adjuvant is not necessary with pTet18 to obtain protection.

LIVE ATTENUATED SALMONELLA STRAINS AS CARRIERS OF ANTIGENS

These experiments show that it is possible to prepare tetanus vaccine in E.coli. So far the possibility of this being used as a vaccine is slight, particularly as the existing vaccine is so effective. However in the Third World tetanus is still considered a major problem, with over one million cases every year. This is largely due to the difficulty of vaccinating people in these countries, and the fact that three doses of tetanus vaccine are required for effective prevention of tetanus. How then can a recombinant tetanus vaccine help in this regard? One way is to investigate the use of an alternative delivery system of the antigen that does not rely on injection, such as oral immunisation.

One promising oral immunisation system is based upon attenuated Salmonella strains. Various live attenuated Salmonella vaccines have been proposed. S.typhi galE mutants (Germanier & Furer, 1975) have been successfully used in field trials (Wahdan and co-workers, 1982; Levine and co-workers, 1987a) and auxotrophic mutants of S.typhi have also recently been tested in human volunteers (Levine and co-workers, 1987b). These S.typhi mutants were developed after extensive work using mouse-virulent salmonellae, such as S.typhimurium, in mouse models of typhoid (Germanier,1970, 1972; Hoiseth & Stocker, 1981).

Several defined mutations in biochemical pathways have been introduced into S.typhimurium strains, and the growth of such strains in vivo has been extensively studied (for a review, see Dougan, Hormaeche and Maskell, 1987). Attenuated S.typhimurium strains have also been used to deliver foreign antigens to the immune system. Many bacterial antigens have been cloned and expressed to a high level in E.coli. Several clones expressing antigens have been introduced into S.typhimurium strains attenuated via deletion mutations in the aromatic amino acid biosynthesis pathway, and the immune response to these antigens has been measured in mice immunised both orally and intravenously with the recombinant S.typhimurium strains. For example, an S.typhimurium aroA strain (SL3261 (Hoiseth & Stocker, 1981)) carrying the gene for the B subunit of E.coli heat-labile toxin (LT-B) induced anti LT-B antibodies in both the serum and the gut if given orally to mice (Maskell and co-workers, 1987; Clements and co-workers, 1986).

So far the use of attenuated Salmonella strains as carriers of foreign antigens has been confined to experimental animals. However, attenuated S.typhi strains are showing considerable promise as vaccines against typhoid and we can look forward to the development of human Salmonella strains carrying foreign antigens as vaccines against heterologous diseases. One example of such a vaccine might be a live oral tetanus vaccine, although perhaps it is too early to speculate in this fashion. Such vaccines may have benefits compared to conventional vaccines, for example better stability and perhaps the requirement for fewer doses to achieve complete immunisation.

REFERENCES

Bizzini, B. (1984). Tetanus. In: R. Germanier (Ed.), Bacterial Vaccines. Academic Press. pp. 37-67.

Brown, D.R. and C.D. Parker (1987). Cloning of the filamentous haemagglutinin of Bordetella pertussis and its expression in Escherichia coli. Infect.Immun., 55, 154-161.

Brownlie, R.M., J.G. Coote and R. Parton (1986). Complementation of mutations in Escherichia coli and Bordetella pertussis by B.pertussis DNA cloned in a broad-host range cosmid. J.Gen.Microbiol., 132, 3221-3229.

Clements, J.D., F.L. Lyon, K.L. Lowe, A.L. Farrand and G. El-Morshidy (1986). Oral immunisation of mice with attenuated Salmonella enteritidis containing a recombinant plasmid which encodes for production of the B subunit of heat-labile Escherichia coli enterotoxin. Infect.Immun., 53, 685-692.

Dougan, G., C.E. Hormaeche and D.J. Maskell (1987). Live oral Salmonella vaccines: potential use of attenuated strains as carriers of heterologous antigens to the immune system. Parasite Immunology, 9, 151-160.

Eisel, U., W. Jarausch, K. Goretzki, A. Henschen, J. Engels, U. Weller, M. Kendel, E. Haberman and H. Niemann (1986). Tetanus toxin: primary structure, expression in E.coli and homology with botulinum toxins. EMBO J., 10, 2495-2502.

Fairweather, N.F., V.A. Lyness, D.J. Pickard, G. Allen and R.O. Thomson (1986). Cloning, nucleotide sequencing and expression of tetanus toxin fragment C in E.coli. J.Bacteriol., 165, 21-27.

Fairweather, N.F. and V.A. Lyness (1986). The complete nucleotide sequence of tetanus toxin. Nucleic Acid Res., 14, 7909-7912.

Germanier, R. (1970). Immunity in experimental salmonellosis I. Protection induced by rough mutants of Salmonella typhimurium. Infect.Immun., 2, 309-315.

Germanier, R. (1972). Immunity in experimental Salmonellosis III. Comparative immunisation with viable and heat-inactivated cells of Salmonella typhimurium. Infect.Immun., 5, 792-797.

Germanier, R. and E. Furer (1975). Isolation and characterisation of galE mutant Ty21a of Salmonella typhi: a candidate for a live oral typhoid vaccine. J.Infect.Dis., 131, 553-558.

Helting, T.B. and O. Zwisler (1977). Structure of tetanus toxin. J.Biol.Chem., 252, 187-193.

Helting, T.B. and H.H. Nau (1984). Analysis of the immune response to papain digestion products of tetanus toxin. Acta.Pathol.Microbiol., Sect. C., 92, 59-63.

Hoiseth, S. and B.A.D. Stocker (1981). Aromatic dependent Salmonella typhimurium are non-virulent and effective as live vaccines. Nature, 291, 238-239.

Levine, M.M., R.E. Black, C. Ferreccio, M.L. Clements, C. Lanata, J. Rooney, R. Germanier and Chilean Typhoid Committee (1987a). Field trials of efficacy of attenuated Salmonella typhi oral vaccine strain Ty21a. In: J. Robbins (Ed.), in press. Proceedings of International Symposium on Bacterial Vaccines.

Levine, M.M., D. Herrington, J.R. Murphy, J.G. Morris, G. Losonsky, B. Tall, A.A. Linberg, S. Svenson, S. Bagar, M.F. Edwards and B. Stocker (1987b). Safety, infectivity, immunogenicity and in vivo stability of two attenuated auxotrophic mutants of Salmonella typhi, 541Ty and 543Ty, as live oral vaccine candidates. J.Clin.Invest., 79, 888-902.

Locht, C. and J.M. Keith (1986). Pertussis toxin gene: nucleotide sequence and genetic organisation. Science, 232, 1258-1264.

Manclark, C.R. and J.L. Cowell (1984). Pertussis. In: R. Germanier (Ed.), Bacterial Vaccines. Academic Press, pp. 69-106.

Maskell, D.J., K.J. Sweeney, D. O'Callaghan, C.E. Hormaeche, F.Y Liew and G. Dougan (1987). Salmonella typhimurium aroA mutants as carriers of the Escherichia coli heat-labile enterotoxin B subunit to the murine secretory and systemic immune systems. Microbial Pathogenesis, 2, 211-221.

Nicosia, A., M. Pergini, C. Franzini, M.C. Casagli, M.G. Borri, G. Antoni, M. Almani, P. Neri, G. Ratti and R. Rappouli (1986). Cloning and sequencing of the pertussis toxin genes: operon structure and gene duplication. Proc.Natl.Acad.Sci., 83, 4631-4635.

Wahdan, M.H., C. Serie, Y Cerisier, S. Sallam and R. Germanier (1982). A controlled field trial of live Salmonella typhi strain Ty21a oral vaccine against typhoid: three year results. J.Infect.Dis., 145, 292-295.

Weiss, A.A., E.L. Hewlett, G.A. Myers and S. Falkow (1983). Tn-5 induced mutations affecting virulence factors of Bordetella pertussis. Infect.Immun., 42, 33-41.

Weiss, A.A. and E.L. Hewlett (1986). Virulence factors of Bordetella pertussis. Ann.Rev.Microbiol., 40, 661-686.

Fehrenbach et al. (Eds.), Bacterial Protein Toxins, Zbl. Bakt. Suppl. 17
© Gustav Fischer, Stuttgart, New York, 1988

Pertussis Toxin as a Tool to Investigate Growth Factor Signalling Pathways in Fibroblasts

K. Seuwen, J.-C. Chambard, G. L'Allemain, I. Magnaldo, S. Paris and J. Pouysségur

Centre de Biochimie, Parc Valrose, F-06034 Nice Cédex

ABSTRACT

Human α-thrombin, Epidermal growth factor (EGF) and fibroblast growth factor (FGF) are mitogens for CCL39 fibroblasts. Whereas thrombin activates a phosphoinositide specific Phospholipase C in these cells, EGF and FGF have no effect on this signalling pathway. Pretreatment of cells with pertussis toxin selectively inhibits thrombin- induced activation of phospholipase C and mitogenesis in quiescent cultures of CCL39 cells, presumably by ADP-ribosylation of a G protein coupling the thrombin receptor to the phospholipase C, whereas the toxin has no effect on EGF/FGF- induced mitogenesis. We conclude that activation of the phospholipase C by thrombin is essential for thrombin- induced mitogenesis and requires a G protein sensitive to pertussis toxin. The mitogenic signals produced by EGF and FGF are not generated by activation of the phospholipase C. Transfection of CCL39 cells with the activated Ha-ras oncogene renders the cells tumorigenic but does not lead to persistent activation nor to abrogation of the pertussis toxin sensitivity of the phospholipase C signalling pathway. Therefore, the GTP binding protein encoded by the Harvey ras oncogene can not replace the G protein mediating thrombin action.

KEYWORDS

Growth factors, phospholipase C, pertussis toxin, ras oncogene

INTRODUCTION

Mammalian cells require the presence of specific peptide molecules in the culture medium to be maintained and grown in vitro. These "growth factors" play a crucial role in processes like development and differentiation, immune response, wound repair and neoplasia.
Much of our current knowledge concerning growth factors and control of cell proliferation has been accumulated using established (immortal) cell lines of rodent fibroblasts, that could be isolated and maintained in culture with relative ease.
These cells can be grown in media supplemented with calf serum and become reversibly

arrested in the G_0/G_1 phase of the cell cycle when the serum factors are withdrawn. If growth factors are added again, a new round of DNA synthesis and cell proliferation can be reinitiated. Much research is aimed to understand the sequence of events leading from growth factor addition to commitment to cell division.

Research on growth factors has advanced considerably with the purification of certain mitogens to de facto homogeneity. Today, some growth factors can even be produced pure and in considerable quantities using recombinant DNA technology. This allows us to study the effects of defined molecules and their synergistic interaction on cell proliferation and biochemical signalling pathways inside cells.

Since many years it is known that the turnover of membrane polyphosphoinositides plays an important role in signal generation in a variety of biological systems responding to external stimuli (Michell, 1975).

Upon binding to appropriate receptors, stimulatory molecules activate a phosphatidyl-inositoldiphosphate (PIP_2) specific phospholipase C (PLC), wich cleaves PIP_2 yielding diacylglycerol, an activator of protein kinase C, and inositoltrisphosphate, which causes release of calcium from intracellular stores (reviewed by Berridge and Irvine, 1984; Nishizuka, 1984; Majerus and co-workers, 1986).

In quiescent fibroblasts, activation of this biochemical pathway correlates very well with the mitogenic stimulation by a variety of growth factors (Rozengurt, 1986).

It has been proposed that the activation of the PLC is mediated by a GTP binding protein (Cockroft and Gomperts, 1985), in analogy to the well characterized adenylate cyclase system (Gilman, 1984).

In agreement with this notion it was subsequently found that stimulation of the PLC in several cell systems (Ohta, Okajima and Ui, 1985; Volpi and co-workers, 1985) is sensitive to the toxin secreted by Bordetella Pertussis, named "islet activating protein" or pertussis toxin (PT), which was allready known to inactvate the inhibitory G protein (G_i) of the adenylate cyclase system (Ui, 1986).

Normal fibroblasts in vitro can become tumorigenic and partially independent of growth factors, if they (over-) express different oncogenes (Bishop, 1987).

One type of oncogenes severely deregulating cell proliferation is designated the *ras* gene family. The *ras* genes encode closely related proteins of 21 kd molecular weight, termed p21*ras*. Nontransforming versions of p21*ras* exist in every normal cell, but several different point mutations can activate the proteins to become tumorigenic (Levinson, 1986).

The *ras* proteins are GTP binding proteins showing considerable sequence homology to other known G proteins. Activated forms of p21*ras* seem to be characterized by a decreased intrinsic GTPase activity or by a modified GTP/GDP exchange rate (Walter, Clark and Levinson, 1986).

It has been speculated that *ras* proteins might couple growth factor receptors to the PLC system in fibroblasts and that mutated forms of p21*ras* might transform cells by persistently activating the PLC signalling pathway (Fleischmann, Chahwala and Cantley, 1986; Wakelam and co-workers, 1986).

Using CCL39 hamster fibroblasts as a model system to study growth factor signalling, we have recently shown that thrombin, a potent mitogen for CCL39 cells, activates the phospholipase C (L'Allemain and co-workers, 1986). This activation seems to be mediated by a G protein, as the PLC can be activated by GTP in vitro (Magnaldo and co-workers, 1987) and by the AlF_4^- complex in vivo (Paris and Pouysségur, 1987).

In the following we present evidence demonstrating that the activation of the PLC is not an obligatory event in mitogenic stimulation, as growth factors exist that do not activate this enzyme (EGF, FGF). We show that thrombin- induced activation of PLC as well as its mitogenicity is strongly inhibited by pertussis toxin, whereas EGF/FGF induced mitogenicity is not. Finally we demonstrate that transformation of CCL39 fibroblasts by the activated Ha-*ras* oncogene is not accompanied by persistent activation of the PLC.

METHODS

Cell Culture

The Chinese hamster fibroblast cell line CCL39 (American Type Culture Collection) was cultivated in Dulbecco's modification of Eagle's medium (DME) containing 5% fetal calf serum (FCS).
Quiescent cells were obtained by incubating confluent monolayers for 24h in serum- free medium.

Measurement of DNA synthesis reinitiation

Quiescent cultures were stimulated with growth factors in medium containing [^{3}H]-thymidine (3 uM, 1 uCi/ml). After 24h, radioactivity incorporated into trichloracetic acid precipitable material was counted.
When pertussis toxin was used, it was added to the cells 4h before the growth factors.

Measurement of PLC activity

PLC activity was determined as described by Paris and Pouysségur (1987). Briefly, cells were rendered quiescent in serum free medium containing [^{3}H]- Inositol (2 uCi/ml). This medium was aspirated and replaced by fresh Hepes buffered DME containing 20 mM LiCl. Li$^+$ inhibits the dephosphorylation of inositolmonophosphate, which accumulates. After 10 minutes, the cells were stimulated with growth factors at 37°C. The reaction was stopped by aspiration of the medium and addition of perchloric acid (10% w/v). The acid extracts containing inositol and inositolphosphates were neutralized with KOH and loaded onto anion exchange columns. Radioactivity incorporated into the different inositolphosphate fractions eluted with an ammoniumformate gradient was counted.
When pertussis toxin was used, it was added to the cultures 4h before the beginning of the experiment into the medium used to prelabel the cells.

RESULTS

Mitogenic activity of different defined growth factors in CCL39 cells is not strictly correlated with activation of phospholipase C

Upon removal of growth factors from growing cultures of CCL39 fibroblasts, >99% of the cells become arrested in the G_0/G_1 phase of the cell cycle within 24 h. Defined growth factors can be used to reinitiate DNA synthesis and cell proliferation in these quiescent cultures. Potent growth factors for CCL39 cells are human α-thrombin, epidermal growth factor (EGF) and fibroblast growth factor (FGF). Insulin like growth factor 1 (IGF1), that can be replaced by high concentrations of Insulin, is not mitogenic but potentiates the activity of the other growth factors cited.
Other growth factors active for example in 3T3 fibroblasts (Rozengurt, 1986) are only weakly (platelet derived growth factor) or not at all mitogenic (bombesin, bradykinin, vasopressin) in CCL39 cells.
Figure 1A shows the mitogenic potencies of thrombin, EGF, FGF and insulin in CCL39 cells administered either alone or in combination compared to the effect of 10% FCS.
Thrombin is the most potent mitogen, a similar effect can be achieved only with a combination of EGF, FGF and Insulin.
As is demonstrated in Fig. 1B, thrombin- and serum- induced mitogenesis is paralelled by a

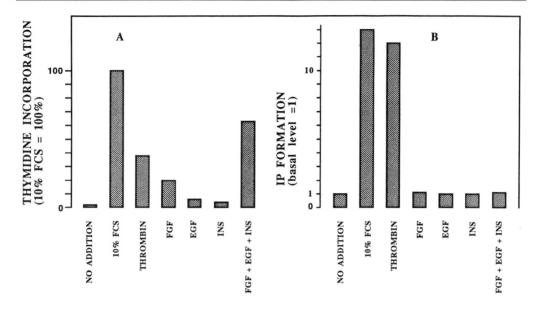

<u>Fig. 1:</u> Effect of different growth factors on reinitiation of DNA synthesis (A) and activation of phospholipase C (B) in quiescent CCL39 cells.

Reinitiation of DNA synthesis and activation of PLC was measured as described in the methods section. The growth factors were used in the following concentrations: Thrombin: 10 nM, FGF: 100 ng/ml, EGF: 50 ng/ml, Insulin: 5 ug/ml.
The data shown in (B) are the Inositolphosphates accumulated during 20 minutes in the presence of Lithium and growth factors, relative to the basal level measured in the absence of Lithium.

strong activation of PLC, whereas EGF and FGF, even in combination, do not stimulate this signalling pathway.
These results clearly prove that activation of PLC can not be considered as an obligatory event in mitogenesis.

<u>Pertussis toxin inhibits thrombin induced mitogenesis and activation of phospholipase C but not EGF and FGF induced mitogenesis</u>

Evidence for the role of a G protein in the activation of PLC in CCL39 cells includes stimulation of the enzyme by GTP in vitro (Magnaldo and co-workers, 1987) and by AlF_4^- and vanadate in vivo (Paris and Pouysségur, 1987).
As we show here in fig. 2, PLC activation is sensitive to pertussis toxin. Maximal inhibition (50% of thrombin stimulated activity and 70% of AlF_4^- stimulated activity) is observed at a toxin concentration of 10 ng/ml.
As we have shown above that only thrombin besides serum activates PLC in CCL39 cells but EGF and FGF do not, it was tempting to speculate that thrombin- induced mitogenesis was pertussis toxin sensitive but EGF/FGF- induced mitogenesis was not.

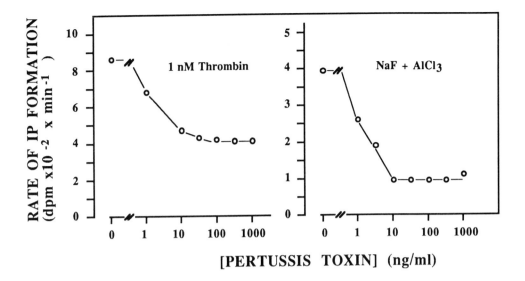

<u>Fig. 2:</u> Effect of pertussis toxin on thrombin- and AlF_4^-- induced activation of phospholipase C

Cells pretreated with different concentrations of the toxin were stimulated with 1 nM thrombin or 5 uM $AlCl_3$ + 10 mM NaF in the presence of Li^+. The initial rate of inositolphosphate formation was measured as the radioactivity accumulating per minute in the inositolphosphate fractions collected (see "methods"). Inositol-phosphate accumulation was linear for 2 minutes (thrombin) and for 10 minutes (AlF_4^-).

As is evident from the data plotted in Fig. 3A, this is indeed the case. Pertussis toxin inhibits >90% of thrombin- induced DNA synthesis, whereas FGF- induced mitogenesis is completely unaffected. As CCL39 cells respond only weakly to EGF (see Fig. 1A), we have tested the sensitivity of EGF- induced mitogenesis to pertussis toxin in secondary cultures of Chinese hamster lung fibroblasts, where EGF is much more mitogenic. Pertussis toxin does not inhibit EGF- induced reinitiation of DNA synthesis in these cells (data not shown).

This observation extends to cell growth in a defined medium supplemented with thrombin or EGF/FGF, respectively. CCL39 cell proliferation in the presence of thrombin is completely suppressed by pertussis toxin, whereas growth in the presence of EGF/FGF is unaffected (data not shown).

The inhibitory effects of pertussis toxin on CCL39 cells stimulated by thrombin correlate well with ADP- ribosylation of a 41 kd protein present in the cell membrane (Fig. 3B).

Whether inhibitory effects of pertussis toxin on cell proliferation can be observed seems to depend entirely on the type of growth factor used to stimulate cell growth.

We propose that pertussis toxin can efficiently distinguish between growth factors activating the PLC (thrombin, bombesin, bradykinin) and growth factors (EGF, FGF, PDGF) that have been reported to activate receptor tyrosine kinases (Heldin and Westermark, 1984).

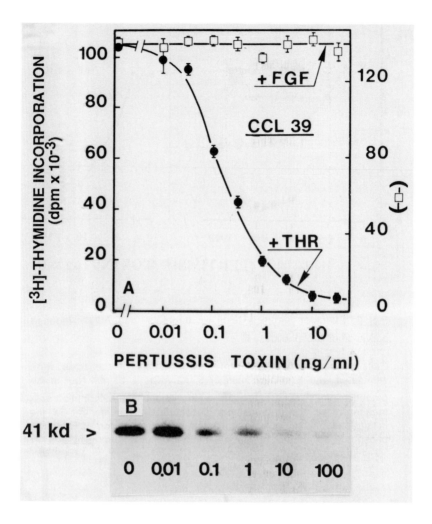

Fig. 3: Effect of pertussis toxin on thrombin- and FGF- induced reinitiation of DNA synthesis (A) and ADP- ribosylation of a 41 kd cellular protein (B)

A: Qiescent CCL39 cells pretreated with different concentrations of toxin were stimulated with thrombin (1 nM) or FGF (100 ng/ml) (see "methods"). Cell incorporated [^{3}H]-thymidine is plotted as a function of toxin concentration.

B: Total cell homogenates were prepared from cells pretreated with different concentrations of toxin and were incubated for 30 min at 37°C with 5 ug/ml of pertussis toxin and 10 uM [^{32}P]-NAD$^+$ (20 uCi/ml) under the conditions described by Ribeiro-Neto (1976). The homogenates were solubilized in 2% SDS and proteins were separated by electrophoresis in 15% SDS- polyacrylamide gels. Pretreatment of cells with pertussis toxin in vivo ADP- ribosylates the protein, which can not be ADP- ribosylated anymore in the following in vitro step.

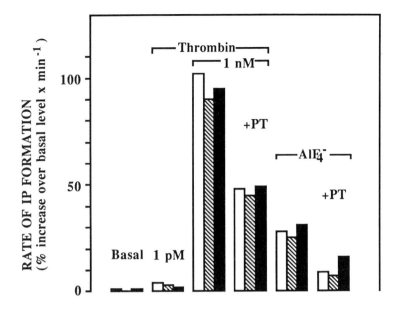

<u>Fig. 4:</u> Unstimulated and stimulated PLC activity in CCL39 cells and cells transfected with the normal and activated Ha-*ras* oncogene. Sensitivity to pertussis toxin.

Initial rates of Inositolphosphate formation were measured as described under "methods" and in the legend to fig. 2. The data were normalized to the basal inositolphosphate levels observed in each cell type to allow comparison of the rates determined.
Open bars: CCL39 cells; shaded bars: cells transfected with normal Ha-*ras*; filled bars: cells transfected with T24-Ha-*ras*.
Basal: Activity detected in the presence of Li$^+$ only.
PT: Cells pretreated with 20 ng/ml pertussis toxin.

<u>Activated forms of the Ha-*ras* oncogene do not transform cells by persistent activation of phospholipase C</u>

We have transfected CCL39 fibroblasts with plasmids carrying the normal and a mutated form (from T24 bladder carcinoma) of the Ha-*ras* oncogene (Spandidos and Wilkie, 1984).
All cell clones isolated after transfection with the activated oncogene were morphologically transformed, partially independent of growth factors, formed colonies in soft agar and induced tumors in nude mice whereas cells transfected with the normal version of the gene were not different from wild type cells (Seuwen, Lagarde and Pouysségur, submitted).
To see if expression of the oncogene modified PLC activity, we have measured the basal rate of phosphoinositide turnover and the activity stimulated by thrombin and AlF$_4^-$ as well as the sensitivity to pertussis toxin in the transfectants obtained. The *ras* proteins can not be ADP-ribosylated by pertussis toxin (Beckner, Hattori and Shih, 1985). If they were able to substitute for the G protein coupling the thrombin receptor to the PLC, this should render PLC activation less sensitive to pertussis toxin.

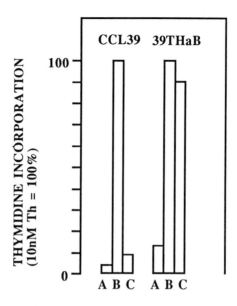

Fig. 5: Sensitivity of thrombin induced reinitiation of DNA synthesis in cells transfected with T24-Ha-*ras*.

Reinitiation of DNA synthesis was measured as described under "methods". 39THaB: cells transfected with T24-Ha-*ras*.
A: No growth factor added; B: 10 nM thrombin; C: 10 nM thrombin, cells pretreated with 20 ng/ml pertussis toxin.

The results of our experiments are summarized in Fig. 4. Both the cells transfected with normal Ha-*ras* as well as those transfected with T24-Ha-*ras* show no significant differences compared to wild type cells. There is no basal PLC activity detectable and activation of the system by thrombin and AlF_4^- is of the same order of magnitude.

Expression of p21*ras*, either normal or activated, does not abrogate the sensitivity of PLC activation to pertussis toxin.

We conclude that activated p21Ha-*ras* does not transform cells by persistent activation of PLC and that the oncogene protein can not replace the pertussis toxin sensitive G protein mediating the activation of PLC by thrombin.

However, as is shown in Fig. 5, cells transformed by T24 Ha-*ras* have lost the sensitivity of the thrombin induced mitogenic response to pertussis toxin. This indicates that these cells have become less dependent on the G protein sensitive to pertussis toxin. We are currently investigating whether this effect is specific for *ras* or if it can be observed in other transformed cells as well.

CONCLUSION

We have shown that growth factors mitogenic in CCL39 cells can be divided into a class activating PLC and another class acting via other signalling pathways, presumably by stimulating receptor tyrosine kinases. Pertussis toxin can be used to selectively block the PLC pathway. Therefore, the toxin might be a useful tool to help isolate mutant cells deficient in PLC activity and to study the relevance of this signalling pathway for growth factor relaxation and carcinogenesis. We have allready shown that deregulation of growth by the T24-Ha-*ras* oncogene does not involve persistent activation of this pathway.

REFERENCES

Beckner, S.K., Hattori, S., and Shih, T.Y. (1985). The ras oncogene product p21 is not a regulatory component of adenylate cyclase. Nature. 317, 71-72.

Berridge, M.J., and Irvine, R.F. (1984). Inositol trisphosphate, a novel second messenger in cellular signal transduction. Nature. 312, 315-321.

Bishop, J.M. (1987). The molecular genetics of cancer. Science. 235, 305-311.

Cockroft, S., and Gomperts, B.D. (1985). Role of guanine nucleotide binding protein in the activation of polyphosphoinositide phosphodiesterase. Nature. 314, 534-536.

Fleischman, L.F., Chahwala, S.B., and Cantley, L. (1986). Ras-transformed cells: Altered levels of phosphatidylinositol-4,5-bisphosphate and catabolites. Science. 231, 407-410.

Gilman, A.G. (1984). G proteins and dual control of adenylate cyclase. Cell. 36, 577-579.

Heldin, C.H., and Westermark, B. (1984). Growth factors: Mechanism of action and relation to oncogenes. Cell. 37, 9-20.

L'Allemain, G., Paris, S., Magnaldo, I., and Pouysségur, J. (1986). Thrombin- induced inositol phosphate formation in G0- arrested and cycling hamster lung fibroblasts: Evidence for a protein kinase C- mediated desensitization response. J. Cell. Physiol.. 129, 167-174.

Levinson, A.D. (1986). Normal and activated ras oncogenes and their encoded products. Trends in Gen.. p81-85.

Magnaldo, I., Talwar, H., Anderson, W.B., and Pouysségur, J. (1987). Evidence for a GTP-binding protein coupling thrombin receptor to PIP2-phospholipase C in membranes of hamster fibroblasts. FEBS Lett.. 210, 6-10.

Majerus, P.W., Connoly, T.M., Deckmyn, H., Ross, T.S., Bross, T.E., Ishii, H., Bansal, V.S., and Wilson, D.B. (1986). The metabolism of phosphoinositide derived messenger molecules. Science. 234, 1519-1526.

Michell, R.H. (1975). Inositol phospholipids and cell surface receptor function. Biochem. Biophys. Acta. 415, 81-147.

Nishizuka, Y. (1984). The role of protein kinase C in cell surface signal transduction and tumour promotion. Nature. 308, 693-698.

Ohta, H., Okajima, F., and Ui, M. (1985). Inhibition by islet-activating protein of a chemotactic peptide- induced early breakdown of inositol phospholipids and Ca++ mobilization in guinea pig neutrophils. J. Biol. Chem.. 260, 15771-15780.

Paris, S., and Pouysségur, J. (1987). Further evidence for a phospholipase C- coupled G protein in hamster fibroblasts. J. Biol. Chem.. 262, 1970-1976.

Ribeiro-Neto, F. (1976). Meth. Enzym.. 45, 566-573.

Rozengurt, E. (1986). Early signals in the mitogenic response. Science. 234, 161-166.

Spandidos, D.A., and Wilkie, N.M. (1984). Malignant transformation of early passage rodent cells by a single mutated human oncogene. Nature. 310, 469-475.

Ui, M. (1984). Islet- activating protein. Trends in Pharm. Sc.. p277-279.

Volpi M., Naccache, P.H., Molski, T.E.P., Shefcyk, J., Huang, C.-K., Marsh, M.L., Munoz, J., Becker, E.L., and Sha'afi, R.I. (1985). Pertussis toxin inhibits fMet-Leu-Phe- but not phorbol ester stimulated changes in rabbit neutrophils: role of G proteins in excitation response coupling. Proc. Natl. Acad. Sci. USA. 82, 2708-2712.

Wakelam, M.J.O., Davies, D.S., Houslay, M.D., McKay, I., Marshall, C.J., and Hall, A. (1986). Normal p21N-ras couples bombesin and other growth factor receptors to inositol phosphate production. Nature. 323, 173-176.

Walter, M., Clark, S.G., and Levinson, A.D. (1986). The oncogenic activation of human p21ras by a novel mechanism. Science. 233, 649-652.

Fehrenbach et al. (Eds.), Bacterial Protein Toxins, Zbl. Bakt. Suppl. 17
© Gustav Fischer, Stuttgart, New York, 1988

Molecular Organization and Applications of Bacillus thuringiensis Delta Endotoxins

H. Höfte, W. Chungjatupornchai, J. Van Rie, S. Jansens and M. Vaeck

Plant Genetic Systems N.V. Plateaustraat 22, B-9000 Gent

INTRODUCTION:

The gram positive bacterium Bacillus thuringiensis (B.t.) produces crystals during sporulation. These crystals are composed of proteins, called delta endotoxins and are specifically toxic against certain insect larvae. The delta endotoxins are protoxins which, upon solubilization in the insect midgut, are proteolytically degraded into toxic polypeptides. In susceptible insects, the activated toxins interact with the membrane of the midgut cells. These consequently swell and lyse, eventually provoking the death of the larvae. B.t. strains producing toxins active against Lepidoptera, Diptera and Coleoptera have been described (for a recent review see Whiteley and Schnepf, 1986). The variation in the insecticidal spectrum of different B.t. strains can be a result of different factors. The proteases and/or the pH in the larval midgut can differ, which can have an influence on the efficiency of both the solubilization and the activation of the delta endotoxins (Jacquet and coworkers, 1987). Different insects may have different specific receptors on the midgut epithelium. Components of the diet could interfere with the activity of the toxin. Also certain cellular defense mechanisms could play a role (Chiang and coworkers, 1987). Finally, the polypeptide composition of the crystals varies for the different B.t. strains.
The results described in this report, demonstrate that crystals generally are composed of different proteins. These proteins can show individual differences in their insecticidal spectrum. We also provide evidence that functionally different toxins are structurally related which suggests a similar mode of action.
In addition, as exemplified by our present data, biologically active B.t. toxins can be expressed not only in different procaryotic hosts, but also in eucaryotic cells (higher plants). This opens interesting perspectives for the development of new, effective and environmentally safe methods for the biocontrol of insects.

RESULTS AND DISCUSSION.

Insecticidal spectrum of different B.t. crystals.

1. Three different pathotypes: Lepidoptera, Diptera and Coleoptera-specific crystals.

Purified crystals of the three major pathotypes show a high and specific activity (Table 1).

B.t. strain	M.sexta (Lepidoptera) LC50 (ng/cm^2) 1st instar	A.aegypti (Diptera) LC50 (ng/ml) 3rd instar	L.decemlineata (Coleoptera) LD50 (ng/larva) 1st instar
berliner cry	7.5	-	-
Bt2	6	-	-
israelensis cry	-	9	-
Bt8	-	25	-
tenebrionis cry	-	-	13
Bt13	-	-	20

TABLE 1: Toxicity of Three types of B.t. Delta Endotoxins ("-"= not toxic).

2. Different specificities of Lepidoptera specific toxins.

Also within the pathotypes clear differences in insecticidal spectrum could be observed for different B.t. strains (Fig.1).

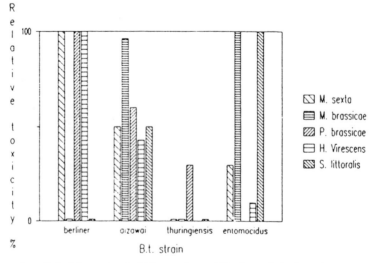

Fig. 1: Relative toxicities of purified, solubilized B.t. crystals. The percentages express the relative toxicities of the crystals of the different strains against each insect.

Polypeptide composition of the B.t. crystals.

1.Three types of Lepidoptera specific toxins.

In order to investigate a possible relationship between the protein composition of the crystals and the insecticidal spectrum, the crystals of a series of B.t. strains were analysed using a set of monoclonal antibodies (mab's) raised against purified crystal proteins. Based upon their immunological properties and the size of the protease resistant core fragment, three different classes of crystal proteins could be distinguished in the strains considered. These toxin classes could be correlated with a specific insecticidal spectrum (Table 2). The proteins of the three classes can exist in different combinations in the crystals of different B.t. strains. These combinations eventually determine the toxicity spectrum of the whole crystals.

Group	M.W. crystal protein (kDa)	M.W. tryptic-fragm. (kDa)	MAB's	example of strain	– LC50 – M. sexta (ng/cm^2)	M. brassicae (ng/cm^2)	LD50 P. brassicae (ng/larva)
I	130	60	1.7;4.8	B.t. berliner	6	> 1350	1.6
II	140	70-55	4F11;4G11	B.t. berliner	> 600	> 1300	2.8
III	130	63	1H12;4B10	B.t. aizawai	n.d.	45	n.d.

TABLE 2: Three Types of Lepidoptera Specific B.t Delta Endotoxins and the Toxicity Spectrum of the Solubilized Proteins (MAB's = monoclonal antibodies).

2.Structural comparison of toxins against Lepidoptera, Diptera and Coleoptera.

The protein compositions of crystals representing the three major pathotypes are shown in Fig. 2. B.t.berliner crystals contain a 130 kDa and a 140 kDa polypeptide. B.t.israelensis crystals contain at least three major proteins of 28 kDa, 65 kDa and 130 kDa respectively. The crystals of B.t.tenebrionis contain one major 66 kDa protein.

Three genes encoding delta endotoxins of the three major pathotypes, were cloned, sequenced and expressed in E.coli. The recombinant proteins were purified and their toxicity was determined (Fig. 2 and Table 1). Bt2, a 130 kDa crystal protein derived from B.t.berliner shows a toxicity against M.sexta comparable to that of intact B.t.berliner crystals (Höfte and co-workers, 1986). Bt8, a 130 kDa protein derived from B.t.israelensis shows a somewhat lower toxicity against A.aegypti larvae than the crystals (Chunjatupornchai and co-workers, in prep.). The crystals could have a higher toxicity as a result of synergistic effects between the different crystal components (Wu and Chang, 1985).

Bt13, cloned from B.t.tenebrionis, has a toxicity to L.decemlineata comparable to that of the intact crystals. In B.t. this protein is produced as a 72 kDa precursor which is proteolytically cleaved into a 66 kDa polypeptide, before the assembly of the crystal. This processing is apparently incomplete in the E.coli clone.

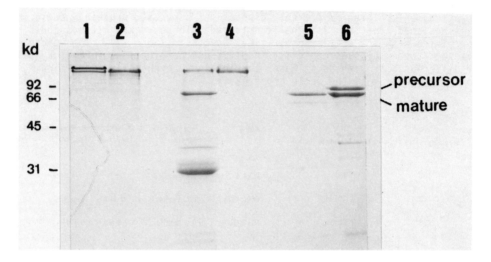

Fig. 2: SDS-PAGE (10%) of the crystals of the three major pathotypes and the recombinant proteins purified from the E.coli clones. 1: B.t.berliner crystals, 2: Bt2, 3: B.t.israelensis crystals, 4: Bt8, 5: B.t.tenebrionis crystals, 6: Bt13.

The structural comparison of the three cloned toxins revealed the following structural similarities.
    -Bt2, Bt8 and Bt13 are all protoxins. The active toxin is a proteolytic fragment of around 60 kDa.
    -This toxic fragment is localized in the N-terminal half of the protoxin. Bt13 can be considered as a protoxin without its C-terminus (Fig. 3).
    -Several sequence elements are conserved for all three toxins (Fig. 4).
    -The distribution of the hydrophobic and hydrophylic amino acids is remarkably conserved in the N-terminus of the three toxins.

Taken together, these results indicate that the three toxins can be considered as members of one family of proteins which probably have a similar mode of action. The significance of the conserved sequence elements for the toxic activity can now be investigated using site directed mutagenesis techniques combined with functional assays.

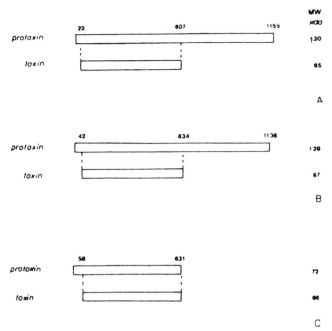

Fig. 3: Localisation and size of the active toxic fragment in the B.t. delta endotoxins of the three major pathotypes. A: Bt2 (Lepidoptera), B: Bt8 (Diptera), C: Bt13 (Coleoptera). The amino acid positions delineating the toxic fragments are indicated.

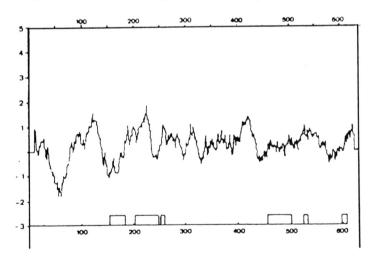

Fig. 4: Hydrophylicity plot (according to Kyte and Doolittle) of the first 620 amino acids of Bt2, containing the toxic fragment. The boxes represent the sequence elements that are conserved for Bt2, Bt8 and Bt13.

Expression of modified B.t. genes in transgenic plants.

Starting from bt2, modified toxin genes have been constructed: truncated genes encoding the active toxin and gene fusions containing 5'-fragments of bt2 fused to the neomycin phosphotransferase gene II (neo) of Tn5. This gene confers resistance against aminoglycoside antibiotics, such as Kanamycin (Km) and G418. The resulting fusionproteins were stable and as toxic as intact Bt2. They exhibited specific neomycin phosphotransferase II (NPTII) activity, comparable to that of the original NPTII enzyme (Vaeck and coworkers, in press). These bifunctional fusion proteins allow to select for plant transformants with a high expression of the B.t.-gene by selecting for resistance against high doses of Km or G418. Chimeric genes consisting of these modified toxin genes, flanked by the regulatory sequences of plant genes, have been transfered to tobacco plants, using Agrobacterium vectors. Transgenic plants were obtained expressing active toxins in their tissue. The expression levels were sufficiently high to substantially protect the plants from feeding damage caused by larvae of M.sexta. The insect resistance trait was stably inherited. These experiments exemplify the feasibility of expressing biologically active B.t.toxins in higher plants. Transfer of different B.t. genes into a variety of crop species may provide agriculture with a new and environmentally safe method to control destructive pests.

REFERENCES.

Chiang, A.S., D.F.Yen and W.K.Peng (1987) J.Inv.Path.47, 333-339.
Höfte,H., H.de Greve, J.Seurinck, S.Jansens, J.Mahillon, C.Ampe,
        J.Vandekerckhove, H.Vanderbruggen, M.van Montagu, M.Zabeau and
        M.Vaeck (1986) Eur.J.Biochem.161, 273-280.
Jacquet,F.,R.Hütter and P.Lüthy (1987) Appl.Environ.Microbiol.53,500-504.
Vaeck,M., A.Reynaerts, H.Höfte, S.Jansens, M.De Beuckeleer, C.Dean,
        M.Zabeau, M. Van Montagu and J. Leemans.
Whiteley,H.R. and Schnepf, H.E. (1986) Ann.Rev.Microbiol.40, 546-576.
Wu,A. and F.N.Chang (1985) FEBS 190, 232-236.

Fehrenbach et al. (Eds.), Bacterial Protein Toxins, Zbl. Bakt. Suppl. 17
© Gustav Fischer, Stuttgart, New York, 1988

New Simple Exact Method for Determination of Haemolytic Activity.

K. Kanclerski[1,2] and R. Möllby[1]

[1]National Bacteriological Laboratory, S-105 21 Stockholm
[2]National Institute of Hygiene, Chocimska Street 24, P-00-791 Warszawa

INTRODUCTION

The haemolytic activity is conventionally determined through serial dilution and the titer is expressed as the dilution of the toxin that results in 50% lysis of a standardized erythrocyte suspension. The test is usually performed in tubes and released haemoglobin is measured visually or in an ordinary spectrophotometer (1,2,5).

The aim of the study was to develop a simple and precise haemolytic test based on direct reading of the optical density of the unlysed erytrocytes in micro-titer plates by using a vertical spectrophotometer connected to a personal computer (4).

MATERIALS AND METHODS

Standardization of erythrocyte suspension.

Washed sheep erythrocytes in isotonic phosphate buffered saline, pH 7.4 (PBS) were resuspended as a 1% (v/v) suspension in PBS. One ml of this suspension was centrifuged, the supernatant was carefully removed and the erythrocytes were lysed by adding 2 ml of distilled water. The absorbance of liberated haemoglobin was red in a spectrophotometer in a 1 cm glass cuvette and, if necessary, adjusted to 1.0 by titration with distilled water. The erythrocyte suspension was then standardized by adding PBS, according to this titration.

Haemolysin preparation.

Five different preparations of highly purified haemolysin of Streptococcus pneumoniae (pneumolysin) with different haemolytic activities were used. The preparation and purification methods of the toxin were described in detail previously (3). The toxin was activated by incubation in PBS supplemented with 0.1% of bovine albumin and 10mM of dithiothreitol (PBS-D) for 30 min at room temperature. Serial 2^x times predilutions were made, where x was 0 to 2.2 at 0.1 intervals.

Haemolysis test in tubes.

Serial two-fold dilutions of each predilution were made in 1 ml of PBS-D with the help of an automatic pipette. The tips were changed after each step of dilution. To each tube 1 ml of standardized erythrocyte suspension was added and the tubes were incubated for 30 min at $37^{\circ}C$ in a water bath. After centri-fugation the absorbance of released haemoglobin was measured in a spectrophoto-meter at 542 nm in a 1 cm cuvette. The reference absorbance value for 50% lysis was obtained by lysing 0.5 ml of the erythrocyte suspension with 1.5 ml of undiluted toxin.

Haemolysis test in Microtiter plates.
Serial two-fold dilutions of each predilution in a microtiter plate were
prepared in a volume of 100 µl instead of 1 ml with the help of an 8-channel
automatic pipette. To each well, 100 µl of the standardized erythrocyte
suspension was added and the plates were incubated at 37°C for 30 min with
constant shaking. After incubation, settled erythrocytes were carefully
resuspended through sucking up and down with the 8-channel pipette and, if
necessary, air bubbles were removed through slight flaming. The density of the
remaining cells was measured in a vertical spectophotometer at 620 nM. The
reference value for 50% lysis was obtained by mixing 50 µl of RBC suspension
with 150 µl of diluting buffer.
Calculation of haemolytic titer.
A haemolytic unit (HU) was defined as the amount of active haemolysin present
in the dilution that resulted in lysis of 50% if the erythrocytes.
The titer in HU/ml was obtained as the inverted value of a fictive dilution
corresponding exactly to 50% lysis, and was calculated as follows:

$$\text{Titer (HU/ml)} = 2^{x}$$

$$x = n + \frac{A(50) - A(n)}{A(n+1) - A(n)}$$

where

HU	= haemolytic units
n	= the last dilution number that resulted in lysis of less then 50%
A(50)	= 50% lysis reference absorbance value
A(n)	= absorbance value of the dilution number n
A(n+1)	= absorbance value of the dilution number n+1

The activity of a haemolysin preparation was then obtained through
multiplication with the predilution factor.
Computer help
For the microplate test the absorbance values were automatically transferred
from the spectrophotometer to the computer and the titers were directly
calculated and printed out.

RESULTS AND DISCUSSION
The relation between the concentration and the absorbance of the erythrocytes
was not strictly linear but showed a slightly curved shape. However, when the
absorbance was plotted against $-\log_2$ of the haemolysin dilution, the curve was
found to be linear in a wide range for both tube and microtiter method. This
linearity suggested that only two points, representing the dilution before and
after 50% lysis, should be enough to calculate the exact titer by
interpolation.

In order to prove this hypothesis the activity of five different pneumolysin
preparations prediluted as described in materials and methods was determined.
The obtained titers were identical for both tube and microtiter method. The
standard variations obtained with the different predilutions for each
haemolysin preparation were found to be only 3-8%, i.e. a SE of 1.3-3.6%.
CONCLUSION
A simple and rapid method for determination of an exact haemolytic titer was
obtained. The method has a high precision and can easily be performed in
microplates in large numbers.

REFERENCES
1. Bernheimer, A.W. (1947). J. Gen. Microbiol., 30, 455-468.
2. Johnson, M.K. (1972). Infect. Immun., 6, 755-760.
3. Kanclerski, K. and R. Möllby (1987). J. Clin. Microbiol., 25.
4. Kanclerski, K. and R. Möllby (1987). Acta Microbiol. Scand. Sect B.
5. Paton, H.C., R.A. Lock, D.J. Hansman (1983). Infect. Immun., 40, 548-552.

Fehrenbach et al. (Eds.), Bacterial Protein Toxins, Zbl. Bakt. Suppl. 17
© Gustav Fischer, Stuttgart, New York, 1988

Radioimmunoassay of Delta Toxin from Bacillus thuringiensis

S. Tyski[1] and C.-Y. Lai[2]

[1]Department of Bacteriology, National Institute of Hygiene, P-00-791 Warsaw, Chocimska 24
[2]Department of Protein Biochemistry, Roche Research Center, Hoffmann-La Roche Inc.,
 Nutley, NJ 07110, U.S.A.

KEYWORDS:

Bacillus thuringiensis, delta toxin, radioimmunoassay.

INTRODUCTION

Bacillus thuringiensis - Gram positive, aerobic, sporeforming rods form a true microcrystal of protein within the cell at the time of sporulation. This crystal, described as delta endotoxin, is insecticidal for the larval stages of several economically important lepidoptera.

In this study faster, more effective radioimmunoassay (RIA) for delta toxin detection, instead of less sensitive and very laborious bioassay, was elaborated.

MATERIALS AND METHODS

Bacillus thuringiensis var. kurstaki HD-1 strain was used in this study. Delta toxin was extracted from spore-crystals mixture with alkaline-reducing buffer (1). Such obtained high molecular weight (100 - 130 kD) form of toxin was digested with proteolytic enzymes (trypsin, papain, chymotrypsin, insect juice).

Rabbit antisera were obtained by i.m. injection of either the holotoxin or purified 60 kD active fragment. Antibodies to low molecular weight form of delta toxin were used in RIA technique.
Immobilization antibodies to IGG-Sorb (The Enzyme Center Inc.) and RIA were performed, with minor modification according to the conditions described previously (2). Radiolabelled-iodinated delta toxin was prepared according to Markwell (3), using iodobeads (Pierce). Results of the assay were expressed as percentage of hot delta toxin amount displaced by cold toxin. Insecticidal activity was assayed by modified procedure of Dulmage et al. (4), where LD_{50} for one day old tobacco budworms were calculated after 3 days of feeding with delta toxin preparation.

Influence of high temperature ($60^{o}C$) of incubation on delta toxin activity was also investigated by bioassay as well as by RIA.

RESULTS AND DISCUSSION

Proteolysis study showed that no loss of activity of the insecticidal activity was observed when delta toxin was incubated either with trypsin or with crude insect juice for up to 22 hrs at room temperature. Chymotrypsin caused partial inactivation (about 10%) after 22 hrs of incubation. SDS-UREA-PAGE of the digests taken at different intervals revealed that major polypeptide with m.w. of 60 kD was produced by trypsin digestion of the native protein (5).
Double diffusion analysis in agar of the 60 kD active fragment with rabbit anti-serum raised against the native delta toxin, and vice versa showed completely fused immuno-precipitation lines. It indicates identical immunogenicity of the investigated proteins.

Attempt was made to replace very laborious bioassay by more sensitive, easy to use, RIA. LD_{50} for the pure 60 kD delta toxin was calculated as 350 ng/ml. This amount of toxin was able to displace hot toxin in 60%. Linear correlation of bioassay and RIA was observed in range of 100 - 190 ng of delta toxin.

It was shown, that twenty five minutes incubation at $60^{o}C$ caused about 30% loss of activity estimated by bioassay as well as by RIA. It was also found, that changes of protein molecular conformation were more evident when bioassay was performed, although RIA changes would be also observed.

Exact insecticidal activity of delta toxin can be estimated by bioassay only, since radioimmunoassay although very sensitive detects whole amount of toxin present without specifying its activity. It should be underline, that RIA is much faster, more effective and simpler method to perform than bioassay, and can be used for delta toxin detection.

REFERENCES
1. Lai, C.-Y., Tyski, S., Wu, S.-L. and Fujii, Y. (1985) Fed. Proc. 44, 1803.
2. Rush, R. A., Kindler, S. H., and Underfrend, S. (1975). Clin. Chem. 21, 148-150.
3. Markwell, M. A. K. (1982). Anal. Biochem. 125, 427-432.
4. Dulmage, H. T., Martinez, A. Y. and Pena, T. (1976). US Dept. Agric. Tech. Bull. 1528. 5.
5. Tyski, S., Fujii, Y. and Lai, C.-Y. (1986). Biochem. Biophys. Res. Commun. 141, 106-111.

Authors' Index

Subject Index

Systematic and Applied Microbiology

Formerly: Zentralblatt für Bakteriologie, Mikrobiologie und Hygiene
I. Abt. Originale, Series C

Executive Editor: Prof. Dr. O. Kandler, München

Systematic and Applied Microbiology (formerly – up to Vol. 3, 1982 – "Zentralblatt für Bakteriologie und Hygiene, I. Abt. Originale, Serie C") was started in 1980. Molecular approaches to the systematics and phylogeny of microorganisms and analyses of microbial populations of natural and man-made habitats – including fermented food – have been main subjects of this journal from its inception.

The majority of papers having found their way into this journal have dealt with the new description or emendations of bacterial taxa, and with the taxonomical and phylogentical implications of nucleic acid hybridization and sequence data. Because of the systematically and phylogentically important spin-off from the archaebacteria concept, the journal has published the papers presented at the two workshops on Archaebacteria (1981 and 1985) and at the "EMBO Workshop on Molecular Genetics of Archaebacteria" (1985) in Volumes 3 and 7, respectively, thus supplying the reader with the most comprehensive collection of current papers respective of this rapidly developing research area.

Aims and scope of the journal:

1. Systematics: e.g. new descriptions and revisions of taxa; methods for the determination of taxonomical and genealogical relationships.

2. Physiology and biochemistry: comparative studies of fine structure, metabolism, chemical composition, etc., particularly concerning the classification or phylogenetic assignment of the considered organisms, their way of life and role in the natural material budget and their importance for agriculture as well as for food processing and biotechnology.

3. Applied microbiology: all aspects of agricultural, industrial, food and sewage microbiology, inasmuch as the main emphasis concerns the role or characteristics of the microorganisms.

4. Ecology: all aspects of soil, water and air microbiology including the analysis of populations present in natural and man-made habitats, their role in the material cycle and the effect of human activity upon them.

1988. Volume 10
DM 310,– plus postage and handling,
Single issue DM 124,–

Three issues form one Volume. 1 Volume per Year. Contributions and Summaries in English language.

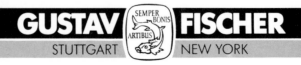

GUSTAV FISCHER

STUTTGART · NEW YORK